S·U·R·V·I·V·O·R·S

OF

CHILDHOOD CANCER

Assessment and Management

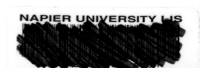

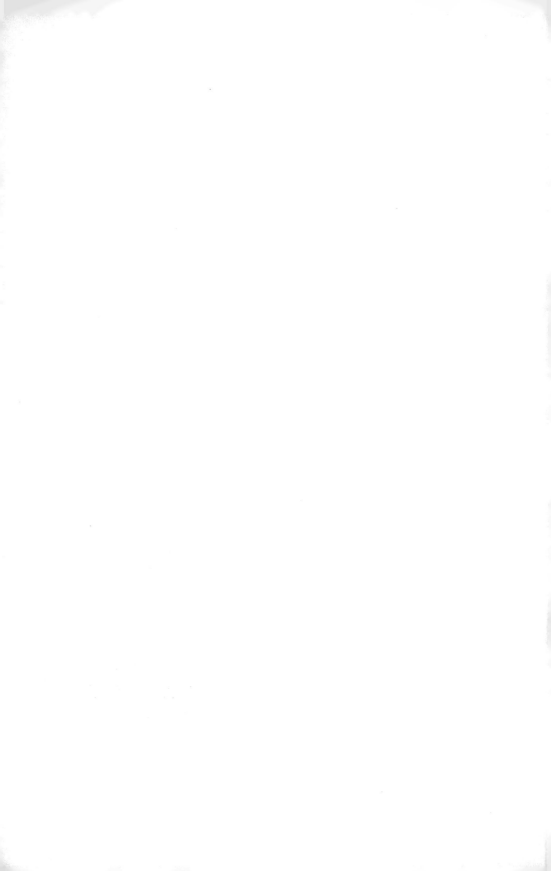

S·U·R·V·I·V·O·R·S

OF

CHILDHOOD CANCER

Assessment and Management

EDITED BY

Cindy L. Schwartz, M.D.
Associate Professor of Oncology and Pediatrics
Johns Hopkins Oncology Center
Baltimore, Maryland

Wendy L. Hobbie, R.N., M.S.N.
Assistant Professor of Clinical Nursing
University of Rochester Medical Center
Rochester, New York

Louis S. Constine, M.D.
Associate Professor of Radiation Oncology and Pediatrics
University of Rochester Medical Center
Rochester, New York

Kathleen S. Ruccione, R.N., M.P.H.
Director of Advanced Oncology Nursing and Psychosocial Programs
Children's Hospital of Los Angeles
Los Angeles, California

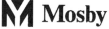 **Mosby**

St. Louis Baltimore Boston Chicago London Madrid Philadelphia Sydney Toronto

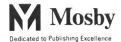

Dedicated to Publishing Excellence

Publisher: George Stamathis
Editor: Laurel Craven
Associate Developmental Editor: Wendy Buckwalter
Project Manager: Linda Clarke
Project Coordinator: Veda King
Designer: Renée Duenow
Manufacturing Supervisor: Karen Lewis

Printed in the United States of America
Composition by Carlisle Communications
Printing/binding by Maple Vail-York

Mosby–Year Book, Inc.
11830 Westline Industrial Drive
St. Louis, Missouri 63146

Library of Congress Cataloging in Publication Data

Survivors of childhood cancer:
   assessment and management/edited by Cindy L. Schwartz . . . [et al.].
      p. cm.
   Includes bibliographical references and index.
   ISBN 0-8016-6521-3
     1. Tumors in children—Treatment—Complications. I. Schwartz,
Cindy L.
    [DNLM: 1. Neoplasms—infancy & childhood. 2. Neoplasms—
complications. 3. Neoplasms—therapy. 4. Antineoplastic Agents—
adverse effects. QZ 266 S963 1994]
   RC281.C4S95 1994
   618.92'994—dc20
   DNLM/DLC
   for Library of Congress   93-42565
                                                            CIP

94 95 96 97 98 / 9 8 7 6 5 4 3 2 1

Contributors

David Abramson, M.D.

Clinical Professor of Ophthalmology, Cornell University Medical Center, New York Hospital, New York, NY

Julie Blatt, M.D.

Associate Professor of Pediatrics, Division of Hematology-Oncology, The Children's Hospital of Pittsburgh, Pittsburgh, PA

W. Archie Bleyer, M.D.

Head, Division of Pediatrics, Chairman, Department of Pediatrics, and Mosbacher Chair in Pediatrics, The University of Texas M.D. Anderson Cancer Center, Houston, TX

Paul Carpenter, Ph.D.

Associate Professor of Oncology in Psychiatry (Psychology) and Pediatrics, University of Rochester Medical Center, Rochester, NY

J. Robert Cassady, M.D.

Professor and Head, Department of Radiation Oncology, University of Arizona School of Medicine, Tucson, AZ

Edward Clark, M.D.

Professor of Pediatrics and Chief of Pediatric Cardiology, University of Rochester Medical Center, Rochester, NY

Louis S. Constine, M.D.

Associate Professor of Radiation Oncology and Pediatrics, University of Rochester Medical Center, Rochester, NY

Jay Cooper, M.D.

Director, Division of Radiation Oncology, New York University Tisch Hospital, New York, NY

Giulio D'Angio, M.D.

Professor of Radiation Oncology, Radiology, and Pediatric Oncology, University of Pennsylvania School of Medicine, Philadelphia, PA

Bernadine Donahue, M.D.

Assistant Professor of Radiology, Division of Radiation Oncology, New York University Medical Center, New York, NY

Judith G. Fenton, R.N., M.S.N., P.N.P.

Department of Pediatrics, University of Pennsylvania School of Medicine, Philadelphia, PA

Jean H. Fergusson, C.R.N.P., Ed.D.

Assistant Professor and Practitioner of Pediatric Oncology, University of Pennsylvania School of Medicine and Children's Hospital of Philadelphia, Philadelphia, PA

Edward Halperin, M.D.

Associate Professor, Department of Radiation Oncology, Duke University Medical Center, Durham, NC

Steven D. Handler, M.D.

Associate Director of Otolaryngology, Department of Pediatric Otolaryngology, Children's Hospital of Philadelphia and University of Pennsylvania School of Medicine, Philadelphia, PA

Ruth Heyn, M.D.

Professor Emeritus of Pediatrics, Division of Pediatric Hematology/Oncology, University of Michigan Medical School, Ann Arbor, MI

Wendy L. Hobbie, R.N., M.S.N.

Assistant Professor, Clinical Nursing, and Coordinator, Follow-Up Clinic, Division of Pediatric Hematology/Oncology, University of Rochester Medical Center, Rochester, NY

Barbara Hoffman, J.D.

Adjunct Faculty, Seton Hall University School of Law, Newark, NJ, and General Counsel, National Coalition for Cancer Survivorship

Patricia Hollen, Ph.D., R.N.

Assistant Professor of Nursing, University of Rochester Medical Center, Rochester, NY

Deborah Karl, M.S.

Clinical Instructor and Special Educator Coordinator, Hematology/Oncology Educational Liaison Program, University of Rochester Medical Center, Rochester, NY

T. S. Lawrence, M.D., Ph.D.

Associate Professor of Radiation Oncology, Director of Cancer Biology, Division of Radiation Oncology, University of Michigan Medical School, Ann Arbor, MI

Carla LeVant, B.S.W., M.S.W.

Social Worker, Division of Pediatric Hematology/Oncology, University of Rochester Medical Center, Rochester, NY

Brigid Leventhal, M.D.

Professor of Oncology and Pediatrics and Director, Clinical Research Administration, The Johns Hopkins Hospital, Baltimore, MD

Robert B. Marcus, Jr., M.D.

Professor of Radiation Oncology and Pediatrics, Department of Radiation Oncology, University of Florida Health Science Center, Gainesville, FL

Lawrence Marks, M.D.

Assistant Professor of Radiation Oncology, Department of Radiation Oncology, Duke University Medical Center, Durham, NC

Sandra McDonald, M.B., Ch.B

Assistant Professor, Department of Radiation Oncology and Pediatrics, University of Rochester Medical Center, Strong Memorial Hospital, Rochester, NY

Bryan McGrath, M.D.

Orthopedic Oncology Fellow, Department of Orthopaedics, University of Florida Health Science Center, Gainesville, FL

Anna Meadows, M.D.

Professor of Pediatrics, University of Pennsylvania School of Medicine; Director, Division on Oncology, Children's Hospital of Philadelphia, Philadelphia, PA

Cyril Meyerowitz, D.D.S.

Professor and Chair, Department of Clinical Dentistry, University of Rochester Medical Center, Strong Memorial Hospital, Rochester, NY

Ida Moore, R.N., D.N.S.

Associate Professor, College of Nursing, University of Arizona School of Medicine, Tucson, AZ

Deborah Neigut, M.D.

Assistant Professor of Pediatrics, Division of Pediatric Gastroenterology, The Children's Hospital of Pittsburgh, Pittsburgh, PA

Kathy O'Conner, R.N., M.N., C.P.N.

Clinical Nurse Specialist, Department of Pediatric Hematology/Oncology, University of Florida Health Science Center, Gainesville, FL

Roger J. Packer, M.D.

Professor of Neurology and Pediatrics, The George Washington University School of Medicine; Chairman, Department of Neurology, Children's National Medical Center, Washington, DC

Howard Panken, B.A.

Computer Consultant,
Rochester, NY

R. Beverly Raney, M.D.

Professor of Pediatrics, Division of Pediatrics, and Chief, Non-Neural Solid Tumor Section, University of Texas M.D. Anderson Cancer Center, Houston, TX

J.M. Robertson, M.D.

Department of Radiation Oncology, University of Michigan Medical School, Ann Arbor, MI

Leslie Robison, Ph.D.

Associate Professor, Department of Pediatrics, University of Minnesota Medical School, and Division of Epidemiology, University of Minnesota School of Public Health, Minneapolis, MN

Philip Rubin, M.D.

Professor of Radiation Oncology, Department of Radiation Oncology and Pediatrics, University of Rochester Medical Center, Strong Memorial Hospital, Rochester, NY

Kathleen S. Ruccione, R.N., M.P.H., C.P.O.N.

Assistant Professor, UCLA School of Nursing; Director of Advanced Oncology Nursing and Psychosocial Programs, Children's Hospital of Los Angeles, Los Angeles, CA

Jean Sanders, M.D.

The Fred Hutchinson Cancer Research Center, Seattle, WA

Mark Scarborough, M.D.

Assistant Professor, Department of Orthopaedics, University of Florida Health Science Center, Gainesville, FL

Cindy L. Schwartz, M.D.

Associate Professor of Oncology and Pediatrics, Associate Director for Clinical Activities, Pediatric Oncology Division, Johns Hopkins Oncology Center, Baltimore, MD

Camille Servodidio, R.N.

Lecturer in Ophthalmology, Cornell University Medical Center, New York Hospital, New York, NY

Richard Severson, Ph.D.

Assistant Professor, Division of Epidemiology, University of Minnesota School of Public Health, Minneapolis, MN

Charles Sklar, M.D.

Associate Attending and Associate Professor of Pediatrics, Cornell Medical College and Department of Pediatrics, Memorial Sloan-Kettering Cancer Center, New York, NY

Angel Torano, M.D.

Associate Professor, Department of Radiation Oncology, Duke University Medical Center, Durham, NC

Susie C. Truesdell, P.A.

Physician's Assistant, Division of Pediatric Cardiology, University of Rochester Medical Center, Rochester, NY

To the memory of those children
for whom our knowledge was insufficient;

To those children
who have been cured but must approach adult life
with the residua of treatment;

And in memory of Brigid Gray Leventhal
mentor and friend to a generation of pediatric oncologists
who dedicated her career to improving the duration
and quality of life for children
with malignancies.

Acknowledgments

The creation of this book has required the efforts of many. First and foremost we would like to thank our spouses (Howard, Danny, and Sally) and our children (Jaffa, Adam, Tali, Jonathan, Sarah, Alysia, Joshua, and Daniel) who have given up family time to allow us to prepare this book. We hope that our combined efforts will improve the lives of affected children and families. It is by watching our growing children that we can fully understand the importance of the task at hand.

Our excitement and satisfaction in composing a book that addresses what we consider to be a critical need is possible only because of the efforts of the clinicians and scientists who have developed our knowledge about late effects. Beyond this, we are deeply indebted to our personal mentors: Harvey Cohen, Brigid Leventhal, Jean Fergusson, Anna Meadows, Sarah Donaldson, and Philip Rubin. Harvey J. Cohen's vision and support of a program dedicated to providing comprehensive care and investigating the effect of treatments was essential. We would also like to thank the community organizations in Rochester that have provided so much for the care of children with cancer, in particular Camp Good Days and Special Times, for supporting our clinic for long-term survivors, and CURE, for providing support for the educational liaison.

The quality of this book is also dependent on the authors who gave their time to write sections of this book. Dolores DiCesare and Michelle Abraham were invaluable in typing portions of the manuscript and coordinating the communications necessary to gather the information into one text. We would also like to thank the editors at Mosby–Year Book, Inc. for their assistance and advice.

Finally, we must thank the children (our patients) for their willingness to help us understand the effects of therapy on their lives. From them, we learn on a daily basis the medical and psychosocial consequences of cure. They inspire us to continue striving for better treatments for childhood cancer.

Cindy L. Schwartz
Wendy L. Hobbie
Louis S. Constine
Kathleen S. Ruccione

Contents

Introduction and Historical Perspective

Giulio J. D'Angio

"Cure is not enough" has become the unofficial motto of pediatric oncology. Such a slogan would have been met with cynicism and derision, if not outrage, had it been proposed a few decades ago. At that time, all children with leukemia died within weeks. Mutilating surgery and high-dose radiation therapy (RT) were all that were available in the desperate and often futile efforts to cure children with solid tumors. Most of these children died within a few months, and the deleterious late consequences of the treatments that were employed seldom had time to develop. In any case, they were considered secondary, as the main emphasis was properly placed on survival. This is epitomized perhaps in the approach taken by the late Sir Stanford Cade. His policy was to irradiate the primary tumor in children with osteogenic sarcomas. They were observed for 6 months to determine whether metastases would develop. Parents were told to consider themselves lucky if an amputation could be offered their child after this period of observation. Loss of a limb was to be considered good fortune! One can only imagine the anguish of mothers and fathers confronted by this cruel paradox. Worries regarding the long-term consequences of limb ablation were subordinated, but nonetheless present, in the highly charged emotions churning during the months of waiting. What about the adult such a child would become? Handicapped, a survivor of a dread disease that could recur, would he or she be able to make his or her way in society and in the marketplace? The ability to keep up with peers, employability, insurability, and marriageability all were highly questionable. They remain so today, even though the probability of cure for the malignant diseases of childhood now stands at better than 65% (Fig. I-1).

This success is a tribute to multimodal care utilizing surgery, chemotherapy, and RT. Surgical attempts to cure cancer antedate recorded history. The same can certainly be surmised for medications, but effective drugs have been developed only in the last 50 years or so.[1] It is interesting, in view of the recently discovered efficacy of platinum-containing drugs, that compounds used 100 or more years ago were often based on metals. In this century, lead colloids used with RT in the 1920s were believed to improve RT responses.[14,16] These were perhaps the first attempts to combine the two modalities. Subsequent trials have used a wide range of agents, some simple (e.g., distilled water) and others based on sophisticated rationales (e.g., halogenated pyrimidines).[3,8] Medical pioneers in the early years of this century had already identified that RT—then considered the "breakthrough" treatment to

TRENDS IN SURVIVAL FOR CHILDREN UNDER AGE 15, SELECTED SITES OF CANCER, 1960 - 1987

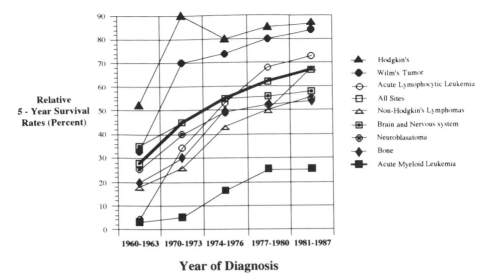

Year of Diagnosis

control cancer—had undesirable side effects on the young. One of the earliest radiobiologic experiments was conducted by Perthes.[10] He found that irradiated chick wings did not grow like their untreated counterparts. This and similar observations alerted physicians to an important side effect of any antimitotic treatment: interference with normal growth and development. Screening for these and other side effects on various organ systems therefore became routine in the evaluation of new anticancer chemical compounds as they were developed. Farseeing investigators like Schulte warned 50 years ago that adverse effects might occur from drug-RT interactions.[13] It was through serendipity, however, that such interactions became recognized.[5,7]

These observations were being made as the modern era of pediatric oncology dawned and the team effort became established. Surgeons, radiation therapists, and chemotherapists working together brought their skills to the bedside. The benefits of the combined care that evolved have been written large in the list of successful battles fought against pediatric cancers. The three modalities complement each other in bringing tumors under both local and systemic control. At the same time, they complement each other in producing side effects. Awareness of this double-edged sword has given rise to the correct concept that both early and late effects of treatment can often be attributed to combined treatment effects rather than to any single modality. It was also logical to explore the value of combinations of drugs having different toxicities and modes of action.[9,11] Many of these combinations are very effective, such as mechlorethamine, Oncovin, prednisone, and procarbazine

(MOPP) for the treatment of Hodgkin's disease.[6] Unexpected late adversities have sometimes been the price for success, however. The leukemogenesis attributed to MOPP is an example.[2] Much clinical research has therefore been conducted over the past 20 years or so to devise better means of controlling cancer while minimizing complications. The major goal of therapy remains cure, but it is also important to ensure as much as possible that the cured patient will be sound in brain and body. This is part of the concept of "total care."

These concerns were shared by pediatric oncologists in many lands. They soon appreciated that the word "cured" was not synonymous with "life" in the full meaning of that word. The long-term neuropsychologic well-being as well as the somatic health of the survivor became a focus of attention.[15] Also very much a part of total care is the concern for the psychosocial and emotional welfare of the entire family. When a child develops cancer, it is often siblings who suffer the most and longest-lasting psychic trauma.[12] Support for the entire family and an understanding that siblings may feel neglected, if not abandoned, must be part of the total management plan. The health of the family unit must be preserved. There is the future family unit to be considered, too. This is the one that will be established by the long-term survivors, for whom insurability and employability are major concerns. It is clear that difficulties are still encountered in the marketplace despite considerable progress made in this area in recent years.[17] Continuing pressure on legislatures and the business community is needed if this state of affairs is to improve.

Pediatric oncologists and their colleagues understand these problems very well. Children grow up, however, and outgrow the pediatric clinic. Where will they receive the needed supervision and follow-up? It is extremely difficult to involve health care workers who look after adults.[4] They are not familiar with the forms of childhood cancer and their treatments. This is understandable because patients have different problems and needs. There is therefore a distinct role for the specially trained nurses working with physicians and other health professionals as a team in a dedicated "late effects" clinic. If the clinic is based in a pediatric institution, compliance is best attained when the clinic is relatively isolated. Teenagers and young adults must feel comfortable in the environment and not part of a "kiddie clinic," which some find objectionable. Ultimately, however, information is best carried forward by the cured person. It is therefore important that relevant data in convenient formats be provided each patient in sufficient detail at an appropriate age. The patient will then be able to provide accurate information concerning treatments received and the late complications that might ensue. The risks of delayed adversities often are small, but nonetheless real. The well-informed patient can be a help to health caretakers in detecting these problems before they become insuperable, and thus assure that the ultimate goal is achieved. A book such as this one will prove an extremely valuable resource. It will be helpful not only for patients and late effects teams, but also for gynecologists, internists, medical oncologists, and others who will be caring for those adults who were cured of cancer when they were children.

REFERENCES

1. Burchenal JH: *The historical development of cancer chemotherapy.* In Kuemmerle HP et al, editors: *Clinical chemotherapy,* New York, 1984, Thieme-Stratton.

2. Cimino G et al: Second primary cancer following Hodgkin's disease: updated results of an Italian multicentric study, *J Clin Oncol* 9:432-437, 1991.

3. D'Angio GJ: *Pediatric tumors.* In Madhu J et al, editors: *Chemoradiation: an integrated approach to cancer treatment,* Philadelphia, 1993, Lea & Febiger.

4. D'Angio GJ: The child cured of cancer: a problem for the internist, *Semin Oncol* 9:142-149, 1982.

5. D'Angio GJ et al: Potentiation of x-ray effects by actinomycin-D, *Radiology* 73:175-177, 1959.

6. DeVita VT et al: Curability of advanced Hodgkin's disease with chemotherapy. Long-term follow-up of MOPP-treated patients at the National Cancer Institute, *Ann Intern Med* 92:587, 1980.

7. Donaldson SS et al: Adriamycin activating a recall phenomenon after radiation therapy, *Ann Intern Med* 81:407-408, 1974 (letter to the editor).

8. Kligerman MM: *The role of combination radiation and chemotherapy,* Proceedings of the Conference on Research on the Radiotherapy of Cancer, American Cancer Society 147-157, 1961,

9. Li MC et al: Effect of methotrexate therapy upon choriocarcinoma and chorioadenoma, *Proc Soc Exp Biol Med* 93:361-366, 1956.

10. Perthes G: Ueber den Einfluss der Roentgen-Strahlen auf epithelial Gewebe insbensondere auf das Carcinom, *Arch Klin Chir* 71:955-1000, 1903.

11. Ross GT et al: Sequential use of methotrexate and actinomycin D in the treatment of metastatic choriocarcinoma and related trophoblastic diseases in women, *Am J Obstet Gynecol* 93:223-229, 1965.

12. Schuler D et al: Psychosocial problems in families of a child with cancer, *Med Pediatr Oncol* 13:173-179, 1985.

13. Schulte G: Erfahrungen mit neuen cytostatischen Mittein bei Haemoblastosen und Carcinomen und die Abgrenzung ihrer Wirkungen gegen Roentgentherapie, *Z Krebsforsch* 58:400, 1952.

14. Ullmann HJ: Combination of colloidal lead and irradiation in cancer therapy, *JAMA* 89:1218-1222, 1927.

15. Ullmo D et al: Traumatisme cérébral traumatisme psychique? Etude de 47 enfants atteints de médulloblastome et de leur devenir, *Arch Fr Pediatr* 35:559-570, 1978.

16. Wood FC: Effects of combined radiation and lead therapy, *JAMA* 89:1216-1218, 1927.

17. Zevon MA et al: Adjustment and vocational satisfaction of patients treated during childhood or adolescence for acute lymphoblastic leukemia, *Am J Pediatr Hematol Oncol* 12:454-461, 1990.

Overview

Cindy L. Schwartz
Louis S. Constine
Wendy L. Hobbie

One in 600 children develops a malignancy, and 1 in every 1000 young adults will be a survivor of childhood cancer. Although long-term survivors of childhood cancer should be members of the mainstream of society, they often have complex psychosocial and physical problems that require understanding, evaluation, and management by concerned knowledgeable caretakers. Many survivors see their pediatric oncologists on an occasional basis after completing therapy, but primary care is managed by pediatricians, family practitioners, and internists. These caretakers should have an understanding of the treatment regimen and consequent injury to normal tissues to adequately evaluate and treat the problems that may arise, particularly those that can be modulated by interventions.

The goal of this book is to assist caretakers in providing optimal care for the long-term survivors of childhood cancer. The initial chapters comprise a three-pronged tool for determining which specific late effects of therapy might exist. In addition, the reader will be directed to relevant areas of the book for future understanding of particular problems.

Chapter 1 is a compilation of algorithms that describe common pediatric malignancies. For a given tumor, the common treatments are noted, as well as their late effects and screening methodologies. A physician caring for a patient with Wilms' tumor can look up this tumor and find that treatment may include various therapeutic modalities, including chemotherapy (vincristine, actinomycin D, and doxorubicin), radiation therapy, and surgery. These algorithms will assist the physician who is not well versed in the treatment of pediatric cancer to determine potential late effects in the individual patient and appropriate screening methodologies. Treatments do change over the years. The algorithms were designed to include therapeutic regimens that were used extensively in the past 25 years. Patients may not have received all of the treatments listed (especially with low-stage tumors) or may have received additional therapies (especially with resistant tumors). Nonetheless, these charts should provide an easy method for a primary caretaker to determine organs at risk in his or her patient.

In Chapter 2, Facilitated Assessment of Chronic Treatment Effects, symptoms that may be attributable to the long-term effects of cytotoxic therapy are listed. If a patient's presenting symptom is a cough, one can readily see that it may be due to the cardiac or pulmonary toxicity of either radiation therapy or chemotherapy. The reader then can examine the appropriate organ chapters (Cardiac [Chapter 8] and

Pulmonary [Chapter 9] to further understand these effects, their risk factors, and possibilities for management and detection. In perusing these charts, the practitioner should be aware that they list only the treatment-related causes of these symptoms. Not included under cough, for example, are asthma and pneumonia, which may occur but are not due to the cancer treatment.

Also in Chapter 2 are charts detailing the injuries that can occur in each organ system and outlining suitable evaluations and management options. In these charts, the late effects are listed followed by the causative treatments, signs and symptoms, screening and diagnostic tests, and management and intervention. For example, if the patient appears to have pulmonary problems, the caretaker can determine whether the observed symptoms and signs may have been caused by the treatments received.

After the physician uses these tools to determine the likely side effects, the organ chapters that follow will be of great benefit in analyzing the degree of risk for a given patient and in helping the physician to understand the pathophysiologic basis of the late effect, the clinical presentation, the methods of screening and detection, and the potential interventions. Therefore, the book should be used in a systematic manner beginning with the disease-specific, symptom-specific, and organ-specific charts and using those charts in determining which organ chapters should be perused. An additional chapter comprehensively describes the multiple effects attributable to a bone marrow transplant.

The subsequent chapters focus on the psychosocial aspects of the care of long-term survivors, including social adjustment, legal rights, and genetic risks within the immediate family and to the patient.

The final sections of this book will be of benefit to those who are intending to establish their own dedicated clinics for survivors of childhood cancer. Our recommendations incorporate the methodologies used at the University of Rochester in which there is a systematic approach to the evaluation of long-term side effects. Cases are discussed prior to the patients' clinic visits by the pediatric and radiation oncologists and the nurse practitioner to determine potential late effects. The patient is then seen and screening tests are performed to detect subclinical injury in normal tissues that are at risk. Overt injuries are evaluated and interventions offered. In this chapter, the respective roles of members of the multidisciplinary team (physicians, nurses, and psychosocial specialists) are analyzed. For those planning clinical investigations, the statistical section will help in devising research efforts that lead to reliable data.

Knowledge in this field is constantly accruing, and late side effects may be discovered that are not currently recognized. Therefore, any unusual clinical symptomatology noted in a long-term survivor should be evaluated with consideration of the physiologic effects of the treatments to normal tissues. Although this manual may not describe every possible complication that may arise, we hope it will enable caretakers to understand the etiology of late effects and to think systematically about the risks when evaluating an individual patient.

1

Algorithms of Late Effects by Disease

Cindy L. Schwartz
Wendy L. Hobbie
Louis S. Constine

This book begins with algorithms that should facilitate entry into the subsequent text. By locating the tumor type, information may be accessed from the algorithms regarding standard tumor therapies, more common late effects, and methods of detection. Since the algorithms are relatively inclusive, not all patients will have received all therapies. Availability of the treatment record can assist in the determination of potential risks and in streamlining screening procedures.

Clinical acumen of the health care professional cannot be replaced by these algorithms because an occasional patient may have received unusual therapies or show rare or currently unrecognized effects. Instead, these recommendations should be used as guidelines to potential risks. Information provided in the organ chapters will deepen the medical provider's understanding of the pathophysiology, manifestations, and methods of detecting late effects.

Listed below are abbreviations that are commonly used in the algorithms.

ACS	American Cancer Society
ALL	Acute lymphoblastic leukemia
ANLL	Acute nonlymphocytic leukemia
ARA-C (HD)	Cytosine arabinoside (high dose)
BMT	Bone marrow transplant
BP	Blood pressure
BUN	Blood urea nitrogen
CA	Carcinoma
CBC	Complete blood cell count
CCNU	Chloroethyl cyclohexyl nitrosourea
Cr	Creatinine
CrCl	Creatinine clearance
CXR	Chest radiograph
DTIC	Dacarbazine
ECHO	Echocardiogram
EKG	Electrocardiogram
FSH	Follicle-stimulating hormone
GFR	Glomerular filtration rate

GU	Genitourinary
HD	Hormone dependent
HiB	Hemophilus influenzae type B (vaccine)
H/P	Hypothalamic/pituitary
IT	Intrathecal
LFTs	Liver function tests
LH	Luteinizing hormone
PFTs	Pulmonary function tests
PO4	Phosphate
6-TG	Thioguanine
TSH	Thyroid-stimulating hormone
UA	Urinalysis
VP-16	Etoposide

ALL

Radiotherapy

- Cranial
  - Educational assessment q yr.
  - neurocognitive testing-baseline, q 2-3 yrs.
  - Dental exam at age 5
  - Monitor for precocious puberty
  - Growth curve q yr. (q 6 mo. - age 10-12 yrs.)
  - Bone Age at ~9 yrs. then q yr. to puberty
  - Eye Exam q yr. (cataracts)
- Spinal
  - Free T4, TSH q yr. x 10 (hypothyroidism)
  - Growth curve q yr.
  - Sitting / Standing height
- Testicular
  - Testes exam, LH, FSH,
  - testosterone (gonadal failure)
- Abdomen
  - LH, FSH, estra/testos (>12 yr.)
  - semen analysis (gonadal failure)

Chemotherapy

- Vincristine
- Methotrexate
  - (IT, HD) educational assessment q yr.
  - neurocognitive testing - baseline, q 2-3 yrs.
  - LFT's q yr (hepatic fibrosis)
- 6-mercaptopurine
  - LFT's q yr (hepatic fibrosis)
- L-asparaginase
- Prednisone
- Cyclophosphamide
  - LH, FSH, estra/testos (>12 yr.)
  - semen analysis (gonadal failure)
  - Urinalysis q yr. (hematuria/bladder CA)
- Doxorubicin
  - EKG, ECHO q 3 yrs. (cardiomyopathy)
- VP-16
  - Peripheral neurologic exam (? neurotoxicity)
  - CBC q year (secondary leukemia)
- ARA-C (HD)
  - Neurologic Exam (ataxia)

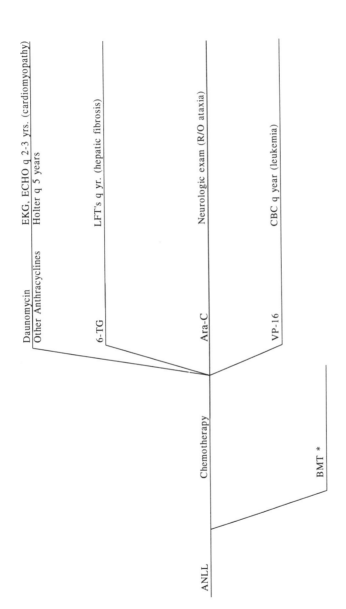

ANLL

Chemotherapy

Daunomycin — EKG, ECHO q 2-3 yrs. (cardiomyopathy)
Other Anthracyclines — Holter q 5 years

6-TG — LFT's q yr. (hepatic fibrosis)

Ara-C — Neurologic exam (R/O ataxia)

VP-16 — CBC q year (leukemia)

BMT *

* See Chapter 15 for follow-up after transplantation.

Brain Tumor

Surgery

Radiotherapy
- Cranial
  - Educational assessment q yr.
  - neurocognitive testing-baseline, q 2-3 yrs
  - Dental panorex at age 5 (root hypoplasia)
  - Eye exam q yr. (cataracts, optic nerve damage)
  - LH, FSH, estra/testos, prolactin (age >12 yrs, pubertal delay, precocious puberty, ↓libido)
  - Growth curve q yr. (q 6 mo. - age 10-12 yrs.)
  - Bone age, GH stimulation
  - Free T^4, TSH q yr. x 10 (hypothyroidism-1°, 2°)
- Spinal
  - Growth curve q yr.
  - Sitting / Standing height
  - UA q yr. (hematuria)

Chemotherapy
- Cyclophosphamide
- Nitrogen Mustard
  - CBC q yr. (marrow damage / leukemia)
  - LH, FSH, estra/testos (>12 yr.)
  - semen analysis (gonadal failure)
- CCNU
  - CXR, PFT's q 3-5 yrs. (Fibrosis)
- Vincristine
- Procarbazine
  - LH, FSH, estra/testos (>12 yr.)
  - semen analysis (gonadal failure)
- Dexamethasone
  - Osteoporosis
- VP-16
  - CBC q year (leukemia)
- Cisplatin
  - Mg q yr. (↓Mg : tubular dysfunction)
  - Cr q yr., CrCl baseline (↓ GFR)
  - Audiogram q 5 yr. (high frequency loss)

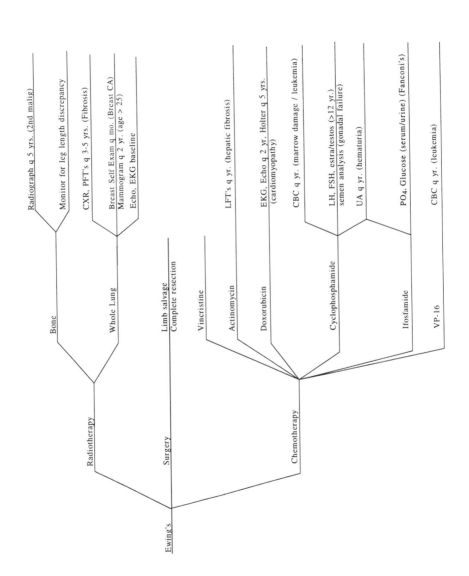

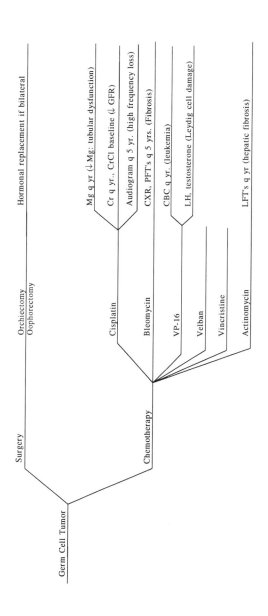

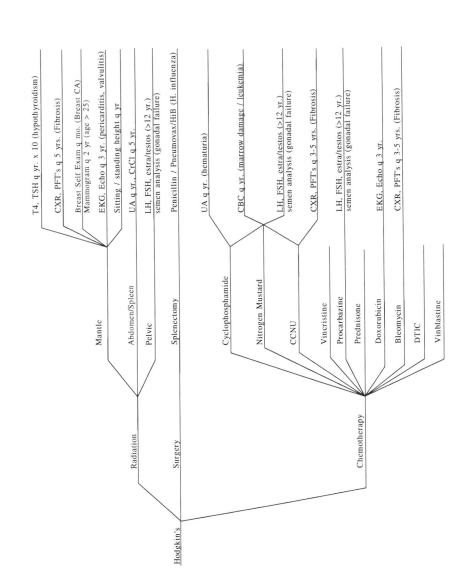

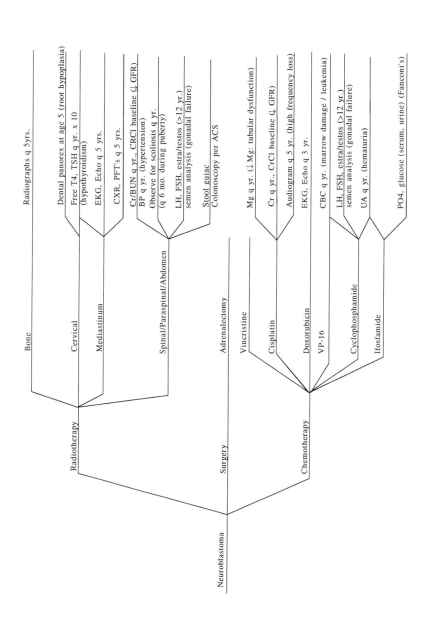

Neuroblastoma

Radiotherapy
- Bone — Radiographs q 5 yrs.
- Cervical — Dental panorex at age 5 (root hypoplasia)
  - Free T4, TSH q yr. x 10 (hypothyroidism)
- Mediastinum — EKG, Echo q 5 yrs.
  - CXR, PFT's q 5 yrs.
- Spinal/Paraspinal/Abdomen
  - Cr/BUN q yr., CRCl baseline (↓ GFR)
  - BP q yr. (hypertension)
  - Observe for scoliosis q yr. (q 6 mo. during puberty)
  - LH, FSH, estra/testos (>12 yr.) semen analysis (gonadal failure)
  - Stool guiac
  - Colonoscopy per ACS

Surgery
- Adrenalectomy

Chemotherapy
- Vincristine
- Cisplatin
  - Mg q yr. (↓ Mg: tubular dysfunction)
  - Cr q yr., CRCl baseline (↓ GFR)
  - Audiogram q 5 yr. (high frequency loss)
- Doxorubicin — EKG, Echo q 3 yr.
- VP-16 — CBC q yr. (marrow damage / leukemia)
- Cyclophosphamide
  - LH, FSH, estra/testos (>12 yr.) semen analysis (gonadal failure)
  - UA q yr. (hematuria)
- Ifosfamide — PO4, glucose (serum, urine) (Fanconi's)

NHL

Radiotherapy

- **Cranial**
  - Educational assessment q yr.
  - neurocognitive testing-baseline, q 2-3 yrs.
  - Dental panorex at age 5.
  - Monitor for precocious puberty
  - Growth curve q yr. (q 6 mo. - age 10-12 yrs.)
  - Bone Age at ~9 yrs. then q yr. to puberty
  - Eye Exam q yr. (cataracts)

- **Mediastinum**
  - Breast Self Exam q mo. (Breast CA)
  - Mammogram q 2 yr. (age > 25)
  - CXR, PFT baseline
  - EKG, ECHO baseline q 5 yrs.
  - Free T4, TSH x 1 (hypothyroidism)

- **Abdomen**
  - Stool guiac q yr.
  - Colonoscopy per ACS
  - LFT's q yr. (hepatic fibrosis)
  - Cr q yr., CrCl baseline
  - LH, FSH, estra/testos (>12 yr.)
  - semen analysis (gonadal failure)
  - UA q yr. (hematuria)

Chemotherapy

- **Cyclophosphamide**
  - CBC q year (marrow damaged / leukemia)
- **Vincristine**
- **Methotrexate**
  - LFT's q yr. (hepatic fibrosis)
- **6-mercaptopurine**
- **Prednisone**
- **Doxorubicin**
  - EKG, ECHO q 3 yrs. (cardiomyopathy)
- **ARA-C (HD)**
  - Neurologic Exam (R/O ataxia)

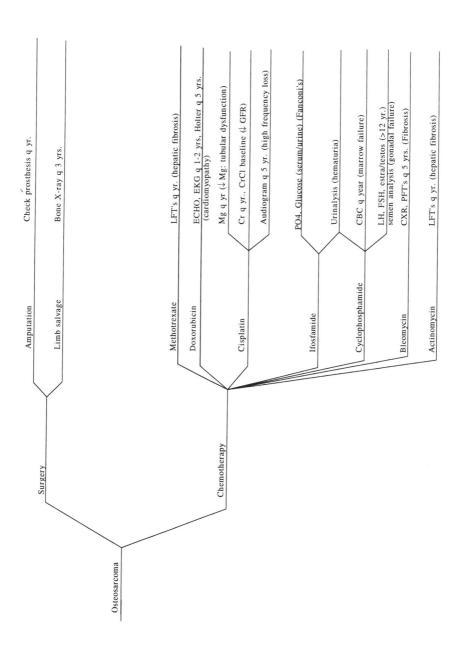

Rhabdomyosarcoma

Radiotherapy

Orbit, Ear, Pharynx
- Eye Exam q yr. for cataracts (Orbital Rhabdo)
- Audiogram (Ear Rhabdo)
- H/P axis evaluation (Growth, LH, FSH, estra/testos Free T4, TSH)
- Sinus evaluation prn

Cranial
- Dental panorex (age 5) - root hypoplasia
- Educational assessment q yr. neurocognitive testing-baseline, q 2-3 yrs
- Monitor for precocious puberty
- Growth curve q yr. (q 6 mo. - age 10-12 yrs.)
- Bone Age at ~9 yrs. then q yr. to puberty
- Eye Exam q yr. (cataracts)

Neck
- Free T4, TSH q yr. x 10 (hypothyroidism)

Thorax
- CXR, PFT baseline
- EKG, ECHO q 5 yrs. (cardiomyopathy)

Abdomen
- LFT's q yr. (hepatic fibrosis)
- Evaluate for scoliosis q yr. until mature
- Stool guiac, colonoscopy per ACS
- BP, UA, CR, BUN q yr. (↓GFR, proteinuria)

Pelvis/GU
- LH, FSH, estra/testos
- semen analysis (gonadal failure)

Extremity
- Radiograph q 5 yrs.

Surgery

Chemotherapy

Vincristine

Actinomycin
- LFT's q yr. (hepatic fibrosis)

Doxorubicin
- EKG, ECHO q 3 yrs. (cardiomyopathy)

Cyclophosphamide
- LH, FSH, estra/testos semen analysis (gonadal failure)
- CBC q year (leukemia)
- Urinalysis q yr. (hematuria/bladder CA)

Ifosfamide
- PO4 , glucose (serum/urine) (Fanconi's)

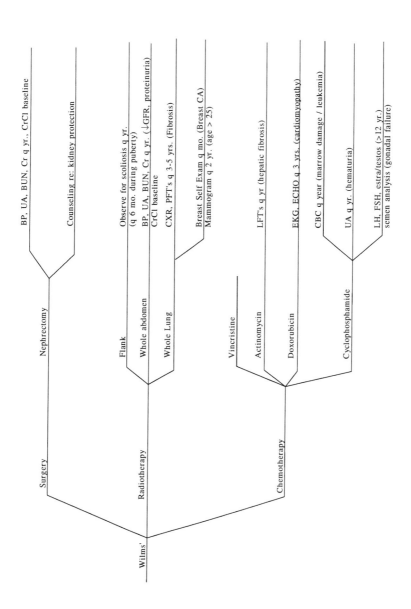

Wilms'

Surgery
  Nephrectomy
    BP, UA, BUN, Cr q yr., CrCl baseline
    Counseling re: kidney protection

Radiotherapy
  Flank
    Observe for scoliosis q yr.
    (q 6 mo. during puberty)
  Whole abdomen
    BP, UA, BUN, Cr q yr. (↓GFR, proteinuria)
    CrCl baseline
  Whole Lung
    CXR, PFT's q 3-5 yrs. (Fibrosis)
    Breast Self Exam q mo. (Breast CA)
    Mammogram q 2 yr. (age > 25)

Chemotherapy
  Vincristine
  Actinomycin
    LFT's q yr (hepatic fibrosis)
  Doxorubicin
    EKG, ECHO q 3 yrs. (cardiomyopathy)
    CBC q year (marrow damage / leukemia)
  Cyclophosphamide
    UA q yr. (hematuria)
    LH, FSH, estra/testos (>12 yr.)
    semen analysis (gonadal failure)

2

Facilitated Assessment of Chronic Treatment by Symptom and Organ Systems

Louis S. Constine
Wendy L. Hobbie
Cindy L. Schwartz

This chapter contains two sets of charts. The first section, Signs and Symptoms, lists in alphabetical order patient symptoms that may be late consequences of cancer therapies. The organ system to which the symptom can be attributed is listed, allowing the reader to refer to the relevant chapter in this book for further information. Treatments that increase the likelihood of an effect are shown in the column entitled Things to Consider.

The second section of this chapter consists of evaluation charts by organ system. A physician or nurse caring for a patient with cardiac symptomatology, for example, can review the cardiac chart and find the common late effects, causative treatments (chemotherapy, radiation, surgery), the signs and symptoms, screening and diagnostic tests, and appropriate management and intervention. If further information is needed, the appropriate organ chapter will provide a more detailed discussion of pathophysiology, clinical manifestations, detection and screening, and management and intervention.

The use of these charts in conjunction with the algorithms of chapter 1 will provide an easy method for the health care provider to plan the evaluation of his or her patient and to access the more comprehensive chapters that follow. Abbreviations used within this section are included in the glossary at the end.

Signs and Symptoms

Symptoms	Organ System	Late Effect	Things to Consider
Abdominal pain, distension	GI	Fibrosis—small or large intestine Gastritis, Enteritis, Ulceration, Luminal narrowing, Fistula, Obstruction (strictures)	Abdominal/pelvic RT (>45 Gy), especially after Act-D, Doxo Laparotomy
	Hepatic	Chronic hepatic damage	Hepatic RT, Mtx, 6MP
	Neuroendocrine	Hypothalamic dysfunction (↓ACTH)	Cranial RT (H/P axis)
Alopecia (see Hair)			
Amenorrhea (see Oligomenorrhea)			
Anemia	Hemopoietic	Hypofunctional marrow 2° leukemia	CT, RT to large area of BM, BMT Alkylators, Epipodophyllotoxins
	GI	Esophageal varicies Malabsorption Ulceration, Perforation	Abdominal RT, Hepatic resection (massive)
	GU	Bladder—hemorrhagic cystitis Renal→↓ GFR	Bladder RT/CPM/Ifos Renal RT, cisplatin, BCNU/CCNU
Anorexia (see Eating)			
Aphasia	CNS	Cerebrovascular accident CNS necrosis Secondary brain tumor	RT to brain Cranial RT, H/O leukemia

Symptom	System	Complication	Cause/Treatment
Arm pain (see Chest pain)	Cardiac	Atherosclerotic heart disease	Thoracic RT
Arrhythmia	Cardiac	Conduction system damage	Thoracic RT/anthracyclines
	Thyroid	1° hyperthyroidism	Cervical/thoracic RT
Ascites	GI/hepatic	Chronic liver damage	Hepatic RT 6MP, Mtx, BCNU/CCNU
Ataxia	CNS	Cerebellar dysfunction	Cranial RT/Ara-C
		SMN	Cranial RT, H/O leukemia
Azotemia	Renal	Renal damage	Renal RT, especially if Act-D, Doxo Cisplatin, BCNU/CCNU, Ifos
Bladder (also see Hematuria; Urinary incontinence)	GU	SMN—bladder CA	Bladder RT, CPM, Ifos
Breathlessness (see Cyanosis)			
Bone pain	Musculoskeletal	Pathologic fracture	Skeletal RT (>50 Gy) (especially if H/O biopsy)
		Slipped capitofemoral epiphysis	Hip RT (>25 Gy at age <5 years)
		Osteoporosis (see Infertility)	Steroids
		Osteonecrosis	
		Joint (hip, shoulder)	RT >40 Gy
		Long bone	RT >60 Gy

Continued.

Signs and Symptoms—cont'd

Symptoms	Organ System	Late Effect	Things to Consider
Breast Hypoplasia Nodules Fibrosis	Integumentary	Hypoplasia (lack of development) SMN Fat atrophy, subcutaneous fibrosis	Thoracic RT (>10-20 Gy) Thoracic RT Thoracic RT (>40 Gy)
Bruising	Hemopoietic Hepatic	2° leukemia Chronic liver damage	Alkylators, epipodophyllotoxins Abd RT, 6MP, Mtx
Cardiomegaly	Cardiac	Cardiomyopathy Pericarditis	Cardiac RT/anthracycline Cardiac RT
Chest pain	Cardiac GI	Pericardial damage Cardiomyopathy Coronary artery disease Esophageal stricture/erosion	Cardiac RT Cardiac RT/anthracycline Cardiac RT Esophageal/thoracic RT (especially if Act-D, Doxo) Chronic candidal esophagitis
Coagulopathy (see Bruising)			
Cold intolerance	Thyroid Neuroendocrine	1° hypothyroidism 2°, 3° hypothyroidism	Cervical/thoracic RT Thyroidectomy Cranial RT (H/P axis)
Conjunctiva Injection Hemorrhage Telangiectasia Adhesions Pain Photophobia	Eye	Conjunctival damage	Eye/orbital RT

Symptom	Organ system	Effect	Treatment/etiology
Cough	Pulmonary	Fibrosis	Thoracic RT, Bleo, BCNU/CCNU (mtx, CPM)
	Cardiac	Valvular injury	Cardiac RT
		Congestive heart failure	Thoracic RT/anthracycline
Constipation	GI	Intestinal fibrosis	Abdominal RT
	Thyroid	1° hypothyroidism	Cervical/thoracic RT
			Thyroidectomy
		2°, 3° hypothyroidism	Cranial RT (H/P axis)
Contractures	Musculoskeletal/integumentary	Fibrosis of joint, subcutaneous tissue	Extremity RT
			Chronic GVHD (post BMT)
Cor pulmonale	Pulmonary	Fibrosis	Thoracic RT (>25 Gy hemithorax)
Cyanosis	Pulmonary	Fibrosis	Thoracic RT
			Bleo, BCNU/CCNU (CPM, Mtx)
	Cardiac	Cardiac damage (multiple etiologies)	Thoracic RT, anthracyclines
Dementia	CNS	Leukoencephalopathy	Cranial RT, mtx, Ara-C
Defecation	GI	Perirectal fibrosis	Rectal/pelvic RT (>50 Gy)
Pain, straining			
Reduced stool caliber			
Sensation of incomplete evacuation			
Diarrhea	GI	Malabsorption	Abdominal RT
	Thyroid	Hyperthyroidism	Cervical (thyroid) RT
Dysphagia	GI	Esophageal stricture, erosion	Thoracic RT (>50-60 Gy) (especially if doxo)

Continued.

Signs and Symptoms—cont'd

Symptoms	Organ System	Late Effect	Things to Consider
Dyspareunia	GU	Small vaginal vault	Vaginal RT (prepubertal)
	Ovary	Dry vagina (↓estrogen)	Ovarian RT, alkylators
	Neuroendocrine	Dry vagina (↓estrogen)	Cranial RT (H/P axis)
Dyspnea (see Cyanosis)			
Eating			
↑Appetite	Neuroendocrine	Hypothalamic dysfunction	Cranial RT (H/P axis)
	Thyroid	1° hyperthyroidism	Cervical/thoracic RT
↓Appetite	Neuroendocrine	Hypothalamic/pituitary dysfunction (↓ACTH or TRH)	Cranial RT (H/P axis)
	Thyroid	1° hypothyroidism	Cervical/thoracic RT Thyroidectomy
Ecchymosis (see Bruising)			
Edema	Cardiac	Cardiac damage (multiple etiologies)	Thoracic RT, anthracyclines
	Integumentary, musculoskeletal	Lymphatic damage	Pelvic, extremity surgery or extremity RT (>40 Gy whole limb)
	GU	Renal damage	Abd RT
Emesis (see Nausea)			
Esophageal varices	GI/hepatic	Liver damage	Abdominal RT (especially if Act-D), massive hepatic resection 6MP, Mtx

Symptom	Organ system	Effect/injury	Cause
Exophthalmos	Thyroid	1° hyperthyroidism	Cervical/thoracic RT
Extremity shortening	Musculoskeletal	Growth plate injury	Extremity RT (>20 Gy)
Eye ↓Extraocular motion Dryness Pain (*also see* Conjunctiva, Vision, Photophobia)	Eye Eye, orbit	Muscle injury Lacrimal gland, conjunctiva Cornea, ciliary body, scleral damage	Surgery Eye, orbital RT (>40 Gy), 5FU Eye RT
Fatigue	Psychosocial GI Cardiac Neuroendocrine Thyroid Hemopoietic Pulmonary GU	Emotional depression Malabsorption Cardiac damage 2°, 3° hypothyroidism 1° hypothyroidism Anemia Pulmonary fibrosis Renal impairment	H/O cancer Abdominal RT Thoracic RT, anthracyclines Cranial RT (H/P axis) Cervical RT/thyroidectomy BM RT (>40 Gy large volume), BMT Thoracic RT, Bleo, BCNU/CCNU Renal RT, CDDP, Ifos, BCNU/CCNU
Finger clubbing	Pulmonary	Fibrosis	Thoracic RT, Bleo, BCNU/CCNU
Foot drop	Peripheral nervous system	Peripheral neuropathy	VCR, CDDP, VP-16
Fractures	Musculoskeletal GU Gonadal	Skeletal damage Osteoporosis Renal Fanconi syndrome Osteoporosis (↓Estrogen)	RT, especially after bone biopsy Steroids Ifos, CDDP Ovarian RT, alkylators
Friction rub	Cardiac	Pericardial damage	Thoracic RT

Continued.

Signs and Symptoms—cont'd

Symptoms	Organ System	Late Effect	Things to Consider
Gait abnormality	Musculoskeletal	(see Scoliosis) Slipped capitofemoral epiphysis	Hip RT (>25 Gy, at age <5 yrs)
	Peripheral nervous system	(see Foot drop)	
	CNS	Leukoencephalopathy, necrosis Myelitis	Cranial RT, Mtx Spinal cord RT (Thoracic, abd RT)
Gallop rhythm	Cardiac	Cardiomyopathy	Thoracic RT, anthracyclines
Growth Retardation	Neuroendocrine	Hypothalamic/pituitary damage (↓GH)	Cranial RT (H/P axis)
(also see Puberty)	Thyroid	1° hypothyroidism	Cervical RT, thyroidectomy
	Musculoskeletal	Skeletal	Skeletal RT (>20 Gy)
	GU	↓GFR, Renal Fanconi syndrome	Cisplatin, ifos, renal RT
	GI	Malabsorption	Abd RT
Hair Alopecia Dry, brittle	Integumentary	Hair follicle damage	Cranial RT (>40 Gy)
	Thyroid	1° Hypothyroidism	Cervical/Thoracic RT
	Neuroendocrine	2°, 3° Hypothyroidism	Cranial RT
Headache	CNS	SMN Cerebrovascular accident	Cranial RT, H/O leukemia Cranial RT
	GU	Renal impairment (hypertension) or renal artery stenosis	Renal RT, especially after doxo, Act-D
	Eye	Retinal, iris damage	Eye RT (>45 Gy)

Symptom/Sign	Organ system	Condition	Treatment
Heart Murmur, gallop Distant heart sounds	Cardiac	Valvular damage, congestive heart failure Pericardial tamponade	Thoracic RT, anthracyclines
Heat intolerance	Thyroid	1° hyperthyroidism	Thoracic RT
Hematemesis	GI/hepatic	Chronic fibrosis/esophageal varices	Hepatic RT (> 40 Gy)
Hematochezia (*see* Abdominal pain)			
Hematuria	GU	Hemorrhagic cystitis	Bladder RT, CPM, Ifos
Hemorrhoids	GI/hepatic	Chronic liver damage	Abd RT, Mtx, 6MP, blood transfusion (viral hepatitis)
Hepatomegaly	GI/hepatic	Chronic liver damage	Abd RT, Mtx, 6MP, blood transfusion (viral hepatitis)
Hip pain (*see* Bone pain, Scoliosis)			
Hoarseness (*see* Voice)			
Hot flashes (*see* Infertility)			
Hypertension	GU	Renal damage, hypoplasia, artery stenosis	Renal RT, CDDP, abdominal surgery
Hyperpigmentation (*see* Skin)			

Continued.

Signs and Symptoms—cont'd

Symptoms	Organ System	Late Effect	Things to Consider
Impotence or ↓Ejaculate	GU Neuroendocrine Testes	Prostate hypoplasia or absence Hyperprolactinemia, ↓testosterone Testicular failure	Pelvic RT or surgery Cranial RT (H/P axis) Testicular RT ($>$25 Gy) Alkylators
Incontinence or Urinary frequency	GU	Bladder fibrosis	Pelvic RT, CPM, Ifos
Incoordination	CNS Peripheral nervous system	SMN Neuropathy	Cranial RT Vincristine, VP-16, CDDP
Infertility	Neuroendocrine Gonadal	Hypothalamic/pituitary damage (↓gonadotropins, ↓TRH, ↑prolactin) Germ cell damage or ovarian/ testicular failure	Cranial RT (H/P axis) Gonadal RT Alkylators
Jaundice	GI/hepatic	Chronic liver damage	Abd RT, Mtx, 6MP
Lactation Increased Decreased	Neuroendocrine Integumentary	Hyperprolactinemia Breast hypoplasia	Cranial RT (H/P axis) Thoracic RT
Learning disability (see Neurocognitive)			
Lethargy (see Fatigue)			

Libido (decreased)	Neuroendocrine	Hyperprolactinemia ↓Testosterone, estrogen	Cranial RT (H/P axis)
	Gonadal	Testicular/ovarian failure	Testicular/ovarian RT, alkylators
Malabsorption (*see* Abdominal pain)			
Melena (*see* Abdominal pain)			
Mouth Dryness, thick saliva Mucosal ulceration Exposed jaw bone	Head/neck	Salivary gland atrophy Mucosal injury Osteoradionecrosis	Head/neck RT (>40 Gy) (>50 Gy) Surgery/dental extraction + RT
Muscular Weakness Atrophy	Neuroendocrine CNS (including spinal cord) or peripheral nerve Musculoskeletal	↓ACTH Neurologic damage Muscle injury or hypoplasia	Cranial RT (H/P axis) Cranial-peripheral RT (>50 Gy) or spinal cord RT (>45 Gy) Muscle RT (>20 Gy, hypoplasia) (>50-60 Gy, atrophy)
Nausea	GI Neuroendocrine Eye CNS	(*see* Abdominal pain) ↓ACTH Iritis, glaucoma SMN, necrosis	Abd RT Cranial RT (H/P axis) Eye RT Cranial RT
Nevi (*see* Skin)			

Continued.

Signs and Symptoms—cont'd

Symptoms	Organ System	Late Effect	Things to Consider
Neurocognitive deficit	CNS	CNS damage/ leukoencephalopathy	Cranial RT, Mtx (IT, HD)
Neurologic deterioration	CNS	CNS damage/ leukoencephalopathy	Cranial RT, Mtx (IT, HD)
		SMN	Cranial RT H/O leukemia Neurofibromatosis Nevoid basal cell cancer syndrome
	Spinal cord	Cerebro-vascular accident	Cranial RT
		Myelitis	Spinal cord RT (>45 Gy) (also *Thoracic, Abdominal RT*)
Neuropathy—peripheral	Peripheral nerves	Nerve damage	RT (>50 Gy) Vinca alkaloids, cisplatin, VP-16
Odynophagia (*see* Dysphagia)			
Oligomenorrhea	Neuroendocrine, gonadal (*see* *Infertility*)		
	Thyroid	1° hypothyroidism	Thoracic RT
Orbital asymmetry	Skeletal	Hypoplasia	Orbital RT
Orthopnea (*see* Cyanosis)			
Osteoporosis (*see* Infertility)			

Symptom	Organ system	Condition	Treatment
Pallor (*see* Anemia, Fatigue)			
Palpitations (*see* Arrhythmia)			
Paradoxical pulse	Cardiac	Pericardial damage	Thoracic RT
Paresis (*see* Neurologic deterioration)			
Paresthesias	CNS	Myelitis	Spinal cord RT (>45 Gy) (including Thoracic, Abdominal RT)
	Peripheral nerves	Nerve damage	RT (>55 Gy)
Petechiae (*see* Bruising)			
Photophobia	Eye	Retinitis, iritis, lacrimal apparatus injury, corneal ulceration, glaucoma	Eye RT (>45 Gy)
Pleural effusion (*see* Jaundice)			
Pregnancy Premature delivery	GU	Uterine fibrosis	Pelvic RT
Proteinuria (*see* Renal)			
Pruritis	GI	Chronic liver damage	Abdominal RT, Act-D, 6MP, Mtx

Continued.

Signs and Symptoms—cont'd

Symptoms	Organ System	Late Effect	Things to Consider
Puberty Delayed	Neuroendocrine	Hypothalamic/pituitary dysfunction	Cranial RT (H/P axis)
	GU Thyroid	Ovarian/testicular failure 1° hypothyroidism	Gondal RT, alkylators Cervical RT, thyroidectomy
Accelerated	Neuroendocrine	Hypothalamic/pituitary dysfunction	Cranial RT (H/P axis)
Rales (*see* Cyanosis)			
Renal dysfunction (e.g., ↓creatinine clearance, Fanconi syndrome = ↓serum phosphate acidosis) (*also see* Hypertension, Hematuria, Fracture, Growth, Anemia, Dyspnea, Fatigue)	GU	↓GFR Tubular dysfunction—↓Mg Fanconi syndrome	Renal RT, cisplatin, Ifos Cisplatin Ifos
Scoliosis, kyphosis	Musculoskeletal	Vertebral body asymmetry Pelvic/hip/leg asymmetry Abdominal musculature hypoplasia, loss	Thoracic, abdominal/pelvic, extremity RT (>20 Gy) Hemiabdominal RT, surgery
Scotoma	Eye (CNS)	Optic nerve damage	Posterior orbital RT (>45 Gy)

Seizures	Renal	↓Mg wasting (tubular dysfunction)	Renal RT, CDDP
	CNS (*see* Neurologic deterioration)		
Sensory changes (*see* Paresthesias)			
Skin			
Fibrosis, telangiectasia Growths, pigmented, nevi	Integumentary	Skin damage, SMN	RT
Dryness	Integumentary	Sweat gland injury	RT (>40-50 Gy)
Hyperpigmentation, indurated plaque	Integumentary	Melanogenesis	RT
			Bleo, BCNU/CCNU, CPM, Act-D, Mtx, HU
Dryness	Thyroid	(*see* Cold intolerance)	
Spasticity (*see* Neuro Deterioration)			
Splenomegaly	Hemopoietic	SMN	Alkylators
	Hepatic	Chronic liver damage	Abdominal RT
Stools			
Hematochezia	GI	Anal fissure	Abdominal/rectal RT
Melena		Esophageal varices, ulceration, perforation	Thoracic/Abdominal/pelvic RT
Loose, watery		Intestinal, rectal mucosal damage	

Continued.

Signs and Symptoms—cont'd

Symptoms	Organ System	Late Effect	Things to Consider
Sweating (*see* Heat/cold intolerance) Decreased	Integumentary	Sweat gland hypoplasia	RT to involved area
Syncope (*see* Arrhythmia)			
Tachycardia (*see* Arrhythmia)			
Tachypnea (*see* Cyanosis)			
Tearing	Eye	Lacrimal duct stenosis	Eye RT, 5FU
Teeth Agenesis, stunting, tapered roots, delayed eruption	Head and neck	Tooth germ damage	Head and neck RT (>20 Gy)
Malocclusion	Skeletal	Mandibular or maxillary maldevelopment	
Caries	Head and neck, salivary	Tooth or salivary gland damage	Salivary gland RT (>40 Gy)
Telangiectasia (*see* Skin)			
Testicular atrophy, hypoplasia (*see* Infertility)			

Symptom	Organ	Effect	RT
Thyroid Nodules Hypoplasia Enlargement	Thyroid	SMN Thyroid fibrosis 1° hyperthyroidism	Thyroid RT
Tremors (*see* Thyroid)			
Trismus	Head/neck	Joint fibrosis	Head/neck RT (>60 Gy)
Urinary Infections Decreased stream (*also see* Hematuria) Incontinence (*also see* Paresthesia)	GU	Fibrosis of ureter, bladder, urethra	Abdominal/pelvic RT
Vaginal dryness, bleeding (*see* Dyspareunia)			
Venous distension (*see* Cardiomegaly)			
Vision Blurred	Eye	Ocular damage—lens, conjunctivae, retina	RT
Field cuts	CNS CNS	Optic nerve damage Occipital lobe, optic nerve damage	

Continued.

Signs and Symptoms—cont'd

Symptoms	Organ System	Late Effect	Things to Consider
Voice			
Hoarseness	Head and neck	Hypoplasia of vocal cords	Cervical RT (> 45 Gy)
	Thyroid	Hypothyroidism (1°, 2°, 3°)	Cervical RT, cranial RT
High and thin	Head and neck	Hypoplasia of vocal cords	Cervical RT (>30 Gy)
Vulva	GU	Soft tissue damage	Vulvar RT
Atrophy, fibrosis			
Introital stenosis			
Weakness			
(*see* Muscle weakness)			
Weight			
Gain	Neuroendocrine	Hypothalamic injury	Cranial RT (H/P axis)
Loss (*see* Growth)	SMN	SMN/recurrence	RT, alkylators
Xerostomia			
(*see* Mouth dryness)			

Evaluation of Patients at Risk for Late Effects: CNS Effects

Late Effects	Causative Treatment			Signs and Symptoms	Screening and (Diagnostic Tests)	Management and Intervention
	Chemotherapy	Radiation	Surgery			
Neurocognitive deficit	High-dose IV Mtx IT Mtx	>18 Gy	Resection of CNS tumor	Difficulty with: Reading Language Verbal/non-verbal memory Arithmetic Receptive and expressive language Decreased speed of mental processing Attention deficit Decreased IQ Behavior problems Poor school attendance Poor hand-eye coordination	Neurocognitive testing: Psychoeducational Neuropsychologic	Psychoeducation assistance

Continued.

Evaluation of Patients at Risk for Late Effects: CNS Effects—cont'd

| Late Effects | Causative Treatment | | | Signs and Symptoms | Screening and (Diagnostic Tests) | Management and Intervention |
	Chemotherapy	Radiation	Surgery			
Leukenceph-alopathy	Mtx: IT or IV IT Ara-C	>18 GY		Seizures Neurologic impairment *Compare with premorbid status	CT/MR scan baseline and symptoms	Symptom management: Muscle relaxant Anticonvulsants Physical therapy Occupational therapy
Focal necrosis	Mtx: IT or high-dose IV BCNU, CDDP	>50 Gy (especially with >21 Gy daily fraction)	Resection of tumor	Headaches Nausea Seizures Papilledema Hemiparesis/other focal findings Speech, learning, and memory deficits	CT/MR scan baseline, prn symptoms PET or SPECT scan	Steroid therapy Debulking of necrotic tissue

Large-vessel stroke		>60 Gy		Headache Seizures Hemiparesis Aphasia Focal neurologic findings	CT scan/MRI Arteriogram	Determined by specific neurologic impairment
Blindness	Intraarterial BCNU, CDDP	RT (optic nerve chiasm, occipital lobe)	Resection of tumor	Progressive visual loss	Ophthalmic evaluation Visual-evoked response	Visual aids
Ototoxicity	CDDP	>50 Gy (middle/inner ear)		Abnormal speech development Hearing	Audiogram baseline prn symptoms	Speech therapy Hearing aid
Myelitis		>45-50 Gy	Spinal cord surgery	Paresis Spasticity Altered sensation Loss of sphincter control	MRI	Steroids Physical therapy Occupational therapy

Evaluation of Patients at Risk for Late Effects: Peripheral Nervous System Effects

Late Effects	Causative Treatment			Signs and Symptoms	Screening and (Diagnostic Tests)	Management and Intervention
	Chemotherapy	Radiation	Surgery			
Peripheral neuropathy	VP-16, VCR CDDP	60 Gy		Generalized weakness Localized weakness Lack of coordination Tingling and numbness	Annual neurologic examination	Protecting affected area from excess heat or cold exposure Physical therapy Occupational therapy

Evaluation of Patients at Risk for Late Effects: Neuroendocrine

Late Effects	Causative Treatment			Signs and Symptoms	Screening and (Diagnostic Tests)	Management and Intervention
	Chemotherapy	Radiation	Surgery			
Growth hormone deficiency		>18 Gy to H/P axis	Tumor in region of H/P axis	"Falling off" of growth curve Inadequate growth velocity Inadequate pubertal growth spurt	Annual stadiometer height (q 6 mo at age 9-12 yr) Growth curve Bone age at 9 yr, then q yr to puberty (Insulin stimulation test and pulsatile GH analysis)	Growth hormone therapy Delay puberty with GnRH agonist
ACTH deficiency		>40 Gy to H/P axis	Tumor in region of H/P axis	Muscular weakness Anorexia Nausea Weight loss Dehydration Hypotension Abdominal pain Increased Pigmentation (skin, buccal mucosa)	Cortisol (a.m.) baseline, prn symptoms (Insulin—hypoglycemia; metapyrone stimulation tests)	Hydrocortisone

Continued.

Evaluation of Patients at Risk for Late Effects: Neuroendocrine—cont'd

Late Effects	Causative Treatment			Signs and Symptoms	Screening and (Diagnostic Tests)	Management and Intervention
	Chemotherapy	Radiation	Surgery			
TRH deficiency		>40 Gy H/P axis	Tumor in region of H/P axis	Hoarseness Fatigue Weight gain Dry skin Cold intolerance Dry brittle hair Alopecia Constipation Lethargy Poor linear growth Menstrual irregularities Pubertal delay Bradycardia Hypotension	Free T_4, T_3, TSH baseline, q 3-5 yr	Hormone replacement with thyroxine Anticipatory guidance regarding symptoms of hypothyroidism
Precocious puberty (especially females)		>20 Gy to H/P axis	Tumor in region of H/P axis	Early growth spurt False catch-up Premature sexual maturation: Female: Breast development and pubic hair before 8 yr and menses before 9 yr	Height, growth curve q yr Bone age q 2 yr until mature (LH, FSH, estradiol or testosterone) (Pelvic ultrasound, GnRH-stimulation testing)	GnRH agonist

Gonadotropin deficiency: Male	>40 Gy to hypothalamic region	Tumor in region of hypothalamus	Delayed/arrested/absent pubertal development: Lack of or diminished: Pubic and axillary hair Penile and testicular enlargement Voice change Body odor Acne Testicular atrophy (softer and smaller) Failure to impregnate	Male: Testicular/penile growth and pubic hair before 9-9.5 yr	LH, testosterone q 3-5 yr (GnRH testing)	Testosterone replacement

Evaluation of Patients at Risk for Late Effects: Neuroendocrine—cont'd

Late Effects	Causative Treatment			Signs and Symptoms	Screening and (Diagnostic Tests)	Management and Intervention
	Chemotherapy	Radiation	Surgery			
Gonadotropin deficiency: Female		>40 Gy to hypothalamic region	Tumor in region of H/P axis	Delayed/arrested/ absent pubertal development including: Breasts Female escutcheon Female habitus Vaginal estrogen effect Body odor Acne Changes in duration, frequency, and character of menstruation (less cramping)	Tanner stage LH, FSH, estradiol q 3-5 yr GnRH-stimulation tests	Anticipatory guidance regarding symptoms of estrogen deficiency Hormone replacement Early intervention may prevent: Osteoporosis Atherosclerosis

| Hyper-prolactinemia | >40 Gy H/P axis | Tumor in region of H/P axis | Estrogen deficiency: Hot flashes Vaginal dryness Dyspareunia Low libido Infertility *If not on birth control pills | Prolactin-level baseline, then prn symptoms | Dopamine agonist (bromocriptine) |
| | | | Female Menstrual irregularities Loss of libido Infertility Galactorrhea Hot flashes Osteopenia Male Loss of libido Impotence Infertility | | |

Evaluation of Patients at Risk for Late Effects: Ophthalmology

Late Effects	Causative Treatment			Signs and Symptoms	Screening and (Diagnostic Tests)	Management and Intervention
	Chemotherapy	Radiation	Surgery			
Lacrimal glands: Decreased tear production	5FU	>50 Gy		Dry, irritated red eye Foreign-body sensation Positive fluorescein staining	Penlight/slit lamp exam Fluorescein staining	Tear replacement Occlude lacrimal puncta Education regarding avoiding rubbing lids when puncta plug is intact
Lacrimal duct: Fibrosis	5FU	>50 Gy		Tearing	Ophthalmic exam	Dilation of duct
Eyelids: Ulceration		>50 Gy		Blepharitis Bleeding/crusted lesion Previous infections	Physical exam	Topical/oral steroids Skin balm Teach: Lid hygiene Radiosensitizing drugs
Telangiectasia		>50 Gy		Enlarged, tortuous blood vessels Pigmentary changes	Slit lamp/penlight exam Open and closed eyelid exam	UV protection Avoid trauma, harsh soaps and lotions

	Dose	Findings/Symptoms	Evaluation	Treatment
Conjunctiva: Necrosis	Radioactive plaque therapy	Dry, irritated eye; Foreign-body sensation	Slit lamp/penlight exam; Fluorescein stain	Steroids/antibiotic drops
Scarring	>50 Gy	Irregular, rough conjunctival surface; Telangiectasia		Tear replacement (resolves spontaneously)
Subconjunctival hemorrhage	>45 Gy	Irritated eye; Foreign-body sensation; Dry, irregular conjunctival surface		Patching; Tear replacement
Sclera: Thinning	>50 Gy	May be asymptomatic; Dry eyes; Foreign-body sensation; Grey, charred, blue sclera	Slit lamp/penlight exam	Antibiotic drops; Avoid trauma; Protective glasses
Cornea: Ulceration	>45 Gy	Pain; Foreign-body sensation; Decreased VA; Photosensitivity	Slit lamp/penlight exam; Fluorescein staining	Tear replacement; Antibiotics; Soft bandages; Soft contact lens; Surgery; Ophthalmology

Continued.

Evaluation of Patients at Risk for Late Effects: Ophthalmology—cont'd

Late Effects	Causative Treatment			Signs and Symptoms	Screening and (Diagnostic Tests)	Management and Intervention
	Chemotherapy	Radiation	Surgery			
Neovascularization		>50 Gy		Increased tearing Increased vessels surrounding edge of cornea	Slit lamp exam	Same as *Ulceration*
Keratinization		>50 Gy		Decreased corneal sensation Photosensitivity Fluorescein staining	Slit lamp exam Fluorescein staining	
Edema		>40 Gy		Decreased visual acuity Hazy cornea	Penlight/slit lamp exam: White, opaque cornea	
Lens: Cataract	Steroids (incidence varies with dose)	>8 Gy (single dose) >10-15 Gy (frac-tionated)		Decreased visual acuity Opaque lens	Direct ophthalmoscopic exam Decreased red reflex Slit lamp/penlight exam: Opaque lens	Prevention by shielding during treatment Surgical removal Educate regarding UV protection

Iris:					
Neovascularization		>50 Gy		May be asymptomatic New blood vessels in iris (rubeosis) Blood in anterior chamber Different colored irises	Slit lamp/penlight exam	Steroid drops
Secondary glaucoma				Eye pain, headache, nausea/vomiting, decreased peripheral vision, increased IOP	Measure ocular pressure	Beta blocker drops Atropine Diamox
Atrophy		>50 Gy		Decreased iris stroma at pupillary margin	Slit lamp/penlight exam	Photocoagulation

Continued.

Evaluation of Patients at Risk for Late Effects: Ophthalmology—cont'd

Late Effects	Causative Treatment			Signs and Symptoms	Screening and (Diagnostic Tests)	Management and Intervention
	Chemotherapy	Radiation	Surgery			
Retina: Infarction		>50 Gy		Blanched white cotton spots; Decreased visual acuity; Decreased visual field; Blurred vision (central or peripheral); Blood vessels: Yellow fluid; Bleeding	Visual acuity; Visual field (confrontation computerized or Amslergrid); Direct and indirect ophthalmoscope exam; Fundus photography	Steroids; Photocoagulation; Education regarding avoiding ASA and bleeding precautions
Exudates		>50 Gy		Thin, incompetent vessels; Tortuous, enlarged vessels		
Hemorrhage		>50 Gy				
Telangiectasia		>50 Gy				
Neovascularization		>50 Gy				
Macular edema (VA and VF)		>50 Gy		Blister of fluid in the macula		
Optic neuropathy		>50 Gy	Tumor resection	Pale optic disc; Abnormal pupillary responses	Visual evaluation	Visual aids

Evaluation of Patients at Risk for Late Effects: Head and Neck

Late Effects	Causative Treatment			Signs and Symptoms	Screening and (Diagnostic Tests)	Management and Intervention
	Chemotherapy	Radiation	Surgery			
Xerostomia (decreased salivary gland function)		>40 Gy and >50% of gland must be radiated		Decreased salivary flow Dry mouth Altered taste perception Dental decay Candida (thrush)	Dental examination Salivary flow studies Attention to early caries, periodontal disease	Encourage meticulous oral hygiene Saliva substitute Prophylactic fluoride Dietary counseling regarding avoiding fermentable carbohydrates Nystatin for oral candidiasis Pilocarpine
Intranasal scarring		>40 Gy		Chronic rhinosinusitis Nasal discharge Postnasal drip Facial pain Headache	Inspection of mucosa Nasopharyngoscopy	Decongestants Drainage procedures Antibiotics prn

Continued.

Evaluation of Patients at Risk for Late Effects: Head and Neck—cont'd

Late Effects	Causative Treatment			Signs and Symptoms	Screening and (Diagnostic Tests)	Management and Intervention
	Chemotherapy	Radiation	Surgery			
Epilation		>40 Gy		Thinning of hair Alopecia	Examination	Wigs Compensatory hair styling
Fibrosis		>40 Gy		Pain Constriction Facial asymmetry Limitation of jaw motion (TMJ fibrosis)	Examination	Prevention of infection (especially after trauma) "Stretching" exercises of TMJ
Osteonecrosis		>50-60 Gy (or interstitial radiation)	Tooth extraction	Ulcers/necrosis	Examination	Symptomatic care
Abnormal facial growth		>30 Gy		Facial asymmetry Hypoplastic development of orbit, maxilla, mandible	Examination	Prosthetic devices Surgical repair

			Surgery		Examination	Surgical repair
Craniofacial deformity						
Abnormal tooth and root development	(VCR, Act-D, CPM, 6MP, PCZ, HN$_2$)	≥1 Gy Generally ≥10 Gy can destroy developing roots		Enamel appears pale Teeth appear small, uneven Malocclusion	Dental exam q 6 months with attention to early caries, periodontal disease, and gingivitis, and Panorex/bite-wing radiographs baseline (age 5-6)	Careful evaluation prior to tooth extraction, endodontics, and orthodontics Fluoride Antibiotics prn risk of infection (e.g., trauma)
Chronic otitis		≥40-50 Gy		Dryness and thickening of canal and tympanic membrane Conductive hearing loss Perforation of TM	Otoscopic exam Audiometry	Antibiotic therapy Decongestants Myringotomy PE tubes Preferential seating in school Amplification
Sensorineural hearing loss	Cisplatin	≥40-50 Gy Cranial RT enhances the platinum effect		High frequency hearing loss (bilateral) Tinnitus Vertigo	Conventional pure tone audiogram baseline and then q 2-3 yr Bilateral, symmetrical, irreversible	Preferential seating in school Amplification

Continued.

Evaluation of Patients at Risk for Late Effects: Head and Neck—cont'd

Late Effects	Causative Treatment			Signs and Symptoms	Screening and (Diagnostic Tests)	Management and Intervention
	Chemotherapy	Radiation	Surgery			
Decreased production of cerumen		≥30-40 Gy		Hard and encrusted cerumen in canal Hearing impairment Otitis externa	Examination of canal	Periodic cleaning ear canal Cerumen-loosening agents Otic drops for otitis externa Keep ear dry: Ear plugs Drying solution
Chondritis		≥50 Gy		Cauliflower ear	Inspection of auricle	Antibiotics Surgical repair (Reconstruction may be hampered by poor blood supply)
Chondronecrosis		≥60 Gy				

Evaluation of Patients at Risk for Late Effects: Thyroid

| Late Effects | Causative Treatment | | | Signs and Symptoms | Screening and (Diagnostic Tests) | Management and Intervention |
	Chemotherapy	Radiation	Surgery			
Overt hypothyroidism (Elevated TSH, decreased T₄)		>20 Gy to the neck, cervical spine >7.5 Gy TBI (total body irradiation)	Partial or complete thyroidectomy	Hoarseness Fatigue Weight gain Dry skin Cold intolerance Dry brittle hair Alopecia Constipation Lethargy Poor linear growth Menstrual irregularities Pubertal delay Bradycardia Hypotension	Free T₄, TSH annually up to 10 years postradiation or if symptomatic Plot on growth chart	Thyroxine replacement Anticipatory guidance regarding symptoms of hyperthyroidism/ hypothyroidism
Compensated hypothyroidism (Elevated TSH, normal T₄)		Same as *Overt hypothyroidism*	Same as *Overt hypothyroidism*	Asymptomatic	Same as *Overt hypothyroidism*	Thyroxine to suppress gland activity

Continued.

Evaluation of Patients at Risk for Late Effects: Thyroid—cont'd

Late Effects	Causative Treatment			Signs and Symptoms	Screening and (Diagnostic Tests)	Management and Intervention
	Chemotherapy	Radiation	Surgery			
Thyroid nodules		Same as *Overt hypothyroidism*		Same as *Overt hypothyroidism*	Same as *Overt hypothyroidism* Physical exam Ultrasound (or technetium ^{99}m scan) baseline and then prn symptoms	Thyroid scan Biopsy/resection
Hyperthyroidism Decreased TSH, elevated T_4		Same as *Overt hypothyroidism*		Nervousness Tremors Heat intolerance Weight loss Insomnia Increased appetite Diarrhea Moist skin Tachycardia Exophthalmus Goiter	Same as *Thyroid nodules* T_3, antithyroglobulin, antimicrosomal antibody baseline, then prn symptoms	Refer to endocrinologist PTU, Propranol ^{131}I Thyroidectomy

Evaluation of Patients at Risk for Late Effects: Cardiac

Late Effects	Causative Treatment			Signs and Symptoms	Screening and (Diagnostic Tests)	Management and Intervention
	Chemotherapy	Radiation	Surgery			
Cardiomyopathy	Anthracycline >300 mg/m^2 >200 mg/m^2 and RT to mediastinum High-dose CTX (BMT) (Possibly Ifos)	>35 Gy >25 Gy and Anthracyclines		Fatigue Cough Dyspnea on exertion Peripheral edema Hypertension Tachypnea/rales Tachycardia Cardiomegaly (S3/S4) Hepatomegaly Syncope Palpitations Arrhythmias	EKG, ECHO/RNA and CXR baselines, q 2-5 yr (depending on risk factors) Holter monitor and exercise testing baseline, prn symptoms and after high cumulative anthracycline dose (>300 mg/m^2)	Diuretics Digoxin Afterload reduction Antiarrhythmics Cardiac transplant Education regarding risks of: Isometric exercises Alcohol consumption Drug use Smoking Pregnancy Anesthesia
Valvular damage (Mitral/tricuspid aortic)		>40 Gy		Weakness Cough Dyspnea on exertion New murmur Pulsating liver	ECHO and CXR (baseline), q 3-5 yr then prn symptoms	Penicillin prophylaxis for surgery/dental procedures

Continued.

Evaluation of Patients at Risk for Late Effects: Cardiac—cont'd

Late Effects	Causative Treatment			Signs and Symptoms	Screening and (Diagnostic Tests)	Management and Intervention
	Chemotherapy	Radiation	Surgery			
Pericardial damage		>35 Gy		Fatigue Dyspnea on exertion Chest pain Cyanosis Ascites Peripheral edema Hypotension Friction rub Muffled heart sounds Venous distension Pulsus paradoxicus	EKG (ST-T changes, decreased voltage), ECHO, CXR baseline, q 3-5 yr	Pericardial stripping
Coronary artery disease		>30 Gy		Chest pain on exertion (radiates to arm/neck) Dyspnea Diaphoresis Pallor Hypotension Arrhythmias	EKG q 3 yrs Stress test (consider thallium scintigraphy) baseline, q 3-5 yr or prn symptoms	Diuretics Cardiac medications Low-sodium, low-fat diet Conditioning regimens

Evaluation of Patients at Risk for Late Effects: Pulmonary

| Late Effects | Causative Treatment | | | Signs and Symptoms | Screening and (Diagnostic Tests) | Management and Intervention |
	Chemotherapy	Radiation	Surgery			
Pulmonary fibrosis	Bleo, CCNU, BCNU, (CPM), (Mtx), (Mitomycin), (Vinca alkaloids)	Pulmonary RT >10 Gy Risk increases with doses, larger volume irradiated, and younger age		Fatigue Cough Dyspnea on exertion Reduced exercise tolerance Orthopnea Cyanosis Finger clubbing Rales Cor pulmonale	Baseline CXR and O_2 saturation, PFT including DLCO, then q 3-5 yr or prn	Refer to pulmonary Steroid therapy Prevention: Avoidance of smoking Avoidance of infections: Influenza vaccine Pneumovax After bleomycin: Avoid FiO_2 > 30% intraoperatively and postoperatively Avoid excessive hydration

Evaluation of Patients at Risk for Late Effects: Gastrointestinal

Late Effects	Causative Treatment			Signs and Symptoms	Screening and (Diagnostic Tests)	Management and Intervention
	Chemotherapy	Radiation	Surgery			
Enteritis	Act-D, doxo, enhance RT effect	>40 Gy	Abdominal surgery enhances RT effect	Abdominal pain Diarrhea Decreased stool bulk Emesis Weight loss Poor linear growth	Height and weight q yr Stool guaiac q yr CBC with MCV q yr Total protein & albumin q 3-5 yr (Absorption tests, vitamin B_{12} level, and contrast studies)	Dietary management Refer to gastroenterologist
Adhesions		RT enhances effect	Laparotomy	Abdominal pain Bilious vomiting Hyperactive bowel sounds	Abdominal radiograph	NPO Gastric suction Adhesion lysis

Fibrosis: Esophagus (stricture)	Doxo and Act-D (RT enhancers)	>40-50 Gy	Abdomen	Dysphagia Weight loss Poor linear growth	Height and weight q yr CBC q yr (BA swallow/endoscopy prn)	Esophageal dilation Antireflux surgery
Fibrosis: Small intestines		>40 Gy	Abdomen	Abdominal pain Constipation Diarrhea Weight loss Obstruction	Height and weight q yr CBC with MCV q yr Serum protein and albumin q 3-5 yr (Upper GI, small bowel biopsy)	High-fiber diet Decompression Resection Balloon dilation
Fibrosis: Large intestine, colon		>40 Gy	Abdomen	Abdominal colic Rectal pain Constipation Melena Weight loss Obstruction	Height and weight q yr Rectal exam Stool guaiac q yr Lower GI Colonoscopy Sigmoidoscopy	Stool softeners High-fiber diet

Evaluation of Patients at Risk for Late Effects: Hepatic

Late Effects	Causative Treatment			Signs and Symptoms	Screening and (Diagnostic Tests)	Management & Intervention
	Chemotherapy	Radiation	Surgery			
Hepatic Fibrosis/cirrhosis	Mtx Act-D 6MP 6TG	>30 Gy	Massive resection	Itching Jaundice Spider nevi Bruising Portal hypertension: Esophageal varices Hemorrhoids Hematemesis Encephalopathy	Height and weight q yr CBC, retic, platelets q yr LFTs q 2-5 yr (Hepatitis screen) (Liver biopsy) (Endoscopy)	Hepatitis screen (hepatitis A, B, C/CMV) Diuretics Liver transplant Varices: Sclerosis Vascular shunting

Evaluation of Patients at Risk for Late Effects: Ovarian

Late Effects	Causative Treatment			Signs and Symptoms	Screening and (Diagnostic Tests)	Management and Intervention
	Chemotherapy	Radiation	Surgery			
Ovarian failure	CPM, PCB, bus, BCNU, CCNU, Ifos	4–12 Gy Tolerance decreases with increasing age	Oophorectomy or oophoroplexy	Delayed/arrested/ absent pubertal development including: Breasts Female escutcheon Female habitus Vaginal estrogen effect Development of body odor and acne Changes in duration, frequency, and character of menses (cramping) Estrogen deficiency: Hot flashes Vaginal dryness Dyspareunia Low libido Infertility	Tanner stage LH, FSH, estradiol: 1) Age 12 years 2) Failure of pubertal development 3) Baseline when fully mature 4) PRN symptoms Assess basal body temperature (mid-cycle elevation suggests ovulation) (DHEAS for failure of development)	Hormone replacement (estrogen) Anticipatory guidance regarding symptoms of estrogen deficiency and early menopause Alternate strategies for parenting Early intervention (hormone replacement) may prevent: Osteoporosis Atherosclerosis

Evaluation of Patients at Risk for Late Effects: Testicular

Late Effects	Causative Treatment			Signs and Symptoms	Screening and (Diagnostic Tests)	Management and Intervention
	Chemotherapy	Radiation	Surgery			
Germ cell damage: Oligospermia/ azospermia	CPM, HN$_2$ CCNU/ BCNU, PCB, Ifos	>1–6 Gy	Orchiectomy or surgical manipulation	Testicular atrophy (softer and smaller) Failure to impregnate	Tanner stage Inquire regarding previous sperm banking Determine testicular size and consistency LH, FSH, testosterone: 1) For failure of pubertal development 2) Baseline when sexually mature 3) For failure to impregnate (repeat q 3 yr for possible recovery) Analysis of sperm at maturity or for failure to impregnate (repeat q 3–5 years to assess recovery)	Instruct: Testicular self-examination Anticipatory guidance regarding germ-cell damage Infertility counseling: Alternate strategies for fathering

Leydig cell damage: Testosterone deficiency	CPM VP-16 >24 Gy to the testes (direct or scattered from pelvis) Orchiectomy	Delayed/ arrested/ absent pubertal development: Pubic and axillary hair (female hair pattern) Lack of penile and testicular enlargement Voice change Body odor and acne Testicular atrophy (softer & smaller)	LH and testosterone at: Age 13 years Failure of pubertal development Baseline, if sexually mature Changes in libido or sexual performance	Testosterone replacement Anticipatory guidance regarding testosterone deficiency

Evaluation of Patients at Risk for Late Effects: Genitourinary

Late Effects	Causative Treatment			Signs and Symptoms	Screening and (Diagnostic Tests)	Management and Intervention
	Chemotherapy	Radiation	Surgery			
Glomerular dysfunction	CDDP			Asymptomatic or Fatigue Poor linear growth Anemia Oliguria	Annual: Blood pressure Height, weight Hemoglobin/ hematocrit Urinalysis Creatinine, BUN Creatinine clearance baseline and q 3 yrs	Low-protein diet Dialysis Renal transplant
Hypoplastic kidney/renal arteriosclerosis		20-30 Gy 10-15 Gy with chemo		Fatigue Poor linear growth Hypertension Headache Edema (ankle, pulmonary) Albuminuria Urinary casts Hepatomegaly	Same as *Glomerular dysfunction*	Same as *Glomerular dysfunction*

Tubular dysfunction	CDDP Ifos		Seizures ($\downarrow$Mg) Weakness ($\downarrow$Po$_4$) Glycosuria Poor linear growth	Same as *Glomerular dysfunction* and Mg, Po$_4$ (24 hour urine for Ca, Po$_4$)	Mg supplement Po$_4$ supplement
Nephrotic syndrome		20-30 Gy	Proteinuria Edema	Urinalysis q yr Blood pressure q yr (Serum protein, albumin, Cr, BUN) (24 hr urine for protein, Cr)	Low-salt diet Diuretics
Bladder: Fibrosis or Hypoplasia (reduced bladder capacity)	CPM Ifos	>30 Gy prepubertal >50 Gy postpubertal	Urgency Frequency Dysuria Incontinence (nocturia) Pelvic hypoplasia	Urinalysis q yr (cystoscopy, IVP/US; volumetrics)	Exercises to increase bladder capacity Surgical referral

Continued.

Evaluation of Patients at Risk for Late Effects: Genitourinary—cont'd

Late Effects	Causative Treatment			Signs and Symptoms	Screening and (Diagnostic Tests)	Management and Intervention
	Chemotherapy	Radiation	Surgery			
Hemorrhagic cystitis	CPM Ifos	(RT enhances chemotherapy effect)		Hematuria Frequency Urgency Dysuria Bladder tenderness	Urinalysis q yr— R/O UTI, renal calculi (Cystoscopy if hematuria on 2 exams)	Transfusion Antispasmotics Formalin Counsel regarding risk of bladder cancer
Prostate		40-60 Gy (lower doses inhibit development; higher doses cause atrophy)		Decreased volume of seminal fluid Hypoplastic or atrophied prostate	Examination of prostate gland Semen analysis × 1 (Ultrasound)	Counsel regarding: possible infertility due to inadequate seminal fluid Monitor prostate (exam, ? prostate- specific antigen)

Vagina: Fibrosis/ diminished growth	(Act-D, doxo enhance RT effect)	>40 Gy		Painful intercourse Vaginal bleeding Small vaginal vault	Pelvic exam (possibly under anesthesia) baseline, during puberty and prn symptoms	Dilations Reconstructive surgery Potential need for cesarean section
Uterus: Fibrosis/ decreased growth		>20 Gy (prepubertal) >40-50 Gy (postpuberal)		Multiple spontaneous abortions Low birth-weight infants Small uterus	Pelvic Baseline, puberty, then annually	? Endometrial bx Counsel regarding pregnancy
Ureter: Fibrosis		>50-60 Gy		Frequent UTIs Pelvic hypoplasia Hydronephrosis	Urinalysis q yr (Uretherogram)	UTI prophylaxis
Urethra: Strictures		>50 Gy	GU	Frequent UTIs Dysuria Stream abnormalities	Urinalysis q yr (Voiding cystogram)	UTI prophylaxis Surgical intervention

Evaluation of Patients at Risk for Late Effects: Musculoskeletal

Late Effects	Causative Treatment			Signs and Symptoms	Screening and (Diagnostic Tests)	Management and Intervention
	Chemotherapy	Radiation	Surgery			
Muscular hypoplasia		>20 Gy (growing child) Younger children more sensitive	Muscle loss or resection	Asymmetry of muscle mass when compared with untreated area Decreased range of motion Stiffness and pain in affected area (uncommon)	Careful comparison and measurement of irradiated and unirradiated areas Range of motion	Prevention: Good exercise program: Range of motion Muscle strengthening

Spinal abnormalities: Scoliosis Kyphosis Lordosis Decreased sitting height	For young children, RT to hemiabdomen or spine (especially hemivertebral) 10 Gy (minimal effect) >20 Gy (clinically notable defect)	Laminectomy	Back pain Hip pain Uneven shoulder height Rib humps or flares Deviation from vertical curve Gait abnormalities	Standing and sitting height at each visit and plot on chart (stadiometer) During puberty examine spine q 3-6 months until growth is completed and then q 1-2 yr Spinal films baseline during puberty, then prn curvature (COBB technique to measure curvature)	Refer to orthopedist if any curvature is noted, especially during a period of rapid growth

Continued.

Evaluation of Patients at Risk for Late Effects: Musculoskeletal—cont'd

Late Effects	Causative Treatment			Signs and Symptoms	Screening and (Diagnostic Tests)	Management and Intervention
	Chemotherapy	Radiation	Surgery			
Length discrepancy		>20 Gy		Lower back pain Limp Hip pain Discrepancy in muscle mass and length when compared with untreated extremity Scoliosis	Annual measurement of treated and untreated limb (completely undressed patient to assure accurate measurements) Radiograph baseline to assess remaining epiphyseal growth Radiographs annually during periods of rapid growth	Contralateral epiphysiodesis Limb-shortening procedures

			Biopsy			
Pathological fracture		>40 Gy		Pain Edema Ecchymosis	Baseline radiograph of treated area to assess bone integrity, then prn symptoms	Prevention Consider limitation of activities (e.g., contact sports) Surgical repair of fracture; may require internal fixation
Osteonecrosis	Steroids	>40-50 Gy (more common in adults)		Pain in affected joint Limp	Radiograph, CT scan prn symptoms	Symptomatic care Joint replacement
Osteocartilaginous exostoses		RT		Painless lump/mass noted in the field of radiation	Radiograph baseline and prn growth of lesion	Resection for cosmetic/functional reasons Counsel regarding 10% incidence of malignant degeneration
Slipped capito-femoral epiphysis	High-dose steroids	>25 Gy (at young age)		Pain in affected hip Limp Abnormal gait	Radiograph baseline to assess integrity of the treated joint(s), then prn symptoms	Refer to orthopedist for surgical intervention

Evaluation of Patients at Risk for Late Effects: Integumentary/Breast

Late Effects	Causative Treatment			Signs and Symptoms	Screening and (Diagnostic Tests)	Management and Intervention
	Chemotherapy	Radiation	Surgery			
Alopecia		>40 Gy		Area of hair loss involving the scalp, eyelashes, or eyebrows	Examination	Wig management
Hyper-pigmentation: Skin Nails	Bleo, Bus, DTIC	>30 Gy		Hyperpigmentation bands: vertical or horizontal	Examine skin and nails	Cosmetic intervention only
Increased benign or malignant melanocytic nevi		RT		Increased numbers of pigmented nevi in the field of radiation	Examine skin at each clinic visit Photograph involved areas to follow accurately	Refer to dermatologist for close follow-up for malignant changes: Biopsy of suspicious lesions
Basal cell carcinoma		RT		Lesion	As above	Excisional biopsy

Hypoplasia of soft tissue	(Effect enhanced by: Act-D Doxo)	>20 Gy (developing child)		Decreased elasticity Decreased tissue volume Local inability to sweat Dryness	Annual examination of skin elasticity and volume	Avoid sun exposure Use sunscreen in treated area Moisturizers
Telangiectasia	As above	>40 Gy	Surgery	Progression of *Hypoplasia* symptoms Skin appears tight with woody texture Spidery pattern of small blood vessels	Annual examination of skin for progression	Same as *Hypoplasia* Avoid trauma
Skin fibrosis/ necrosis	As above	>40 Gy	Surgery	Progression of *Hypoplasia* symptoms Contractures Discoloration of tissue	Same as *Telangiectasia* Examination for tissue breakdown	Must be in the care of a dermatologist— may require surgery
Hypoplasia of breast tissue		>10 Gy Pubertal breast very sensitive		Reduced breast tissue Failure to lactate in treated breast	Annual breast examination Mammography q 2 yr (age 25-50), annually after age 50	Teach BSE Anticipatory guidance regarding: Breast nodules Impaired lactation

Glossary of Terms Used in Systems Charts
Chemotherapy

ABVD	Adriamycin, bleomycin, vincristine, actinomycin-d
Act-D	Actinomycin-d
Ara-C	Cytosine arabinoside
BCNU	1, 3-Bis [2 chloroethyl-1 nitrosourea]
Bleo	Bleomycin
Bus	Busulfan
CCNU	1, -[2-Chloroethyl-3-cyclohexyl-1-nitrosourea]
CDDP	Cisplatin
CPM	Cyclophosphamide
Doxo	Doxorubicin
DTIC	Dimethyl triazine imidazole carboxamide
Dnm	Daunomycin
HN_2	Nitrogen mustard
HU	Hydroxyurea
Ifos	Ifosfamide
IT	Intrathecal
Mtx	Methotrexate
PCB, PCZ	Procarbazine
VCR	Vincristine
VP-16	Etoposide
5FU	5-Fluorouracil
6MP	6-Mercaptopurine
6TG	6-Thioguanine

Other Terms

Abd	Abdominal
ACTH	Adrenocorticotropic hormone
ASA	Aspirin
B/P	Blood pressure
BA	Barium swallow
BM	Bone marrow
BMT	Bone marrow transplant
BSE	Breast self-examination
BUN	Blood urea nitrogen
Ca	Calcium
CBC	Complete blood count
CMV	Cytomegalovirus
CNS	Central nervous system
CO_2	Carbon dioxide
Cr	Creatinine
CT	Computed tomography
CXR	Chest radiograph
DHEA	Dehydroepiandrosterone
DLCO	Diffusing capacity for carbon monoxide (pulmonary)
ECHO	Echocardiogram
EEG	Electroencephalogram
EKG	Electrocardiogram

Other Terms—cont'd

FiO_2	Fractional inspired oxygen
FSH	Follicular-stimulating hormone
FS	Fractional shortening
GFR	Glomerular filtration rate
GI	Gastrointestinal
GU	Genitourinary
GVHD	Graft-versus-host disease
Gy	Grey (measure of radiation)
GH	Growth hormone
GnRH	Gonadotropin releasing hormone
HD	High dose
H/O	History of
H/P axis	Hypothalamic-pituitary axis
IOP	Intraocular pressure
IQ	Intelligence quotient
IT	Intrathecal
IV	Intravenous
IVP	Intravenous pyelogram
LFT	Liver function tests
LH	Luteinizing hormone
MCV	Mean corpuscle volume
Mg	Magnesium
MRI	Magnetic resonance imaging
NPO	Nothing by mouth
PET scan	Positron emission tomography
PFT	Pulmonary function test
Po_4	Phosphate
PRN	As needed
PTU	Propylthiouracil
QTc	Corrected QT interval
RNA	Radionuclear angiography
R/O	Rule out
RT	Radiation therapy
SMN	Second malignant neoplasm
SPECT	Single photon emission computed tomography
T_3	Triiodothyronine
T_4	Thyroxine
TBI	Total-body irradiation
TMJ	Temporomandibular joint
TSH	Thyroid-stimulating hormone
TRH	Thyrotropin-releasing hormone
U/A	Urinalysis
US	Ultrasound
UTI	Urinary tract infection
UV	Ultraviolet light
VA	Visual acuity
VF	Visual field
WBC	White blood count

3

Adverse Effects of Cancer Treatment on the Central Nervous System

Ida M. (Ki) Moore
Roger J. Packer
Deborah Karl
W. Archie Bleyer

The damaging effects of radiation and chemotherapy on the developing central nervous system (CNS) were described by Price and colleagues in the 1970s. These investigators reported histologic changes that included mineralizing microangiopathy, subacute necrotizing leukomyelopathy, and leukoencephalopathy in children who died following treatment for acute lymphoblastic leukemia (ALL).[24,25] Since then, a large number of children successfully treated for leukemia and brain tumors have demonstrated a spectrum of neuropsychologic deficits and neuroanatomic abnormalities. The purpose of this chapter is to review the normal development of the CNS and to outline the pathophysiology, clinical manifestations, diagnosis, and management of the late CNS toxicities associated with the treatment of childhood cancer.

PATHOPHYSIOLOGY

Normal CNS Development

By the end of the first trimester, the neural tube has formed from the neural plate (dorsal induction), and the cerebral hemispheres have formed from the rostral end of the neural tube (ventral induction).[31a] Neurotoxic events during this period cause major structural anomalies to the brain such as anencephaly, myeloschisis (failure of the neural plate to form a complete tube; cleft spinal cord), and the development of encephaloceles. Neuronal proliferation and migration occur primarily between the second and fifth months of gestation.[14] The brain forms in an inside-out manner, with stem cells located in the subependymal zone lining the ventricles. The stem cells give rise to both glial and neuronal cells, which migrate peripherally along radial pathways, differentiating as they migrate to their target positions. Disruption in the proliferation and migration of neuronal and glial cells during this critical period of development causes significant brain malformations, such as polymicrogyria (numerous small convolutions); lissencephaly (convolutions of the cerebral cortex are not developed, and brain is usually small); pachygyria (moderate reduction in the number of sulci of the cerebrum, resulting in excessive size of the gyri); neuronal heterotopia (displacement or misplacement); and, possibly, foci of neoplasia. Glial multiplication and differentiation begin early in the prenatal period and continue for months after birth and at a low level for many years.[14] Although dendritic arborization of neurons peaks 4 to 6 months after birth, it also continues into adult life.

Myelination of the CNS is somewhat easier to quantify.[14] Myelination begins near the end of the first trimester and continues at a somewhat slower rate for decades thereafter.[14] The rate of myelination is highest during the first months after birth. The effects of anticancer agents on these delicate processes are poorly understood; however, they probably underlie the major pathophysiology of radiation- and chemotherapy-induced neurologic damage. The toxic effects of radiation and, to a lesser extent, chemotherapy on myelin development can be grossly imaged with neuroimaging techniques, including computed tomography (CT) and magnetic resonance imaging (MRI). Concomitant with the gross and microscopic anatomic events that occur in the CNS throughout life, there are ongoing physiologic and neurochemical changes. An understanding of how chemotherapy and radiotherapy alter these changes is lacking.

Cytotoxic Effects of Therapy

Radiation. Cancer treatment during childhood may cause neurologic damage ranging from focal necrosis of the gray and white matter to neuronal dropout without obvious histologic change. Experiments using single high doses of radiation demonstrate a variety of changes, dependent on the time interval following irradiation.[6] Up to 20 weeks following a single fraction of radiation in 24-month-old monkeys, only minimal scattered astrocytic or microglial reactions can be seen. However, after 24 weeks a breakdown in neural tissue is more evident, with focal areas of myelin destruction and associated proliferation and degeneration of astrocytes, microglia, and oligodendroglia. Vascular changes including endothelial cell loss, proliferation, and occlusion may also be seen during this phase, with an associated disruption of the blood-brain barrier.[35] Regional cerebral blood flow may be impaired not only within the irradiated area, but also in areas outside this volume.

Fractionated radiotherapy—using multiple low doses of radiation—causes a different pathophysiology.[6] Minute foci of white matter necrosis are the most frequent lesions, the outcome of which is dependent on the total dose and volume of irradiation and the length of time after irradiation. After small doses of irradiation, complete healing occurs; after high doses, widespread brain destruction may occur. Associated with these areas of necrosis are significant vascular abnormalities that include occlusion of vessels and hyperplastic endothelial cells in adjacent capillaries. In animal studies, age plays a significant role in the occurrence and ultimate effects of irradiation. Younger animals demonstrate earlier and more dramatic findings, which probably is of great clinical significance.

Three basic mechanisms of delayed CNS destruction have been hypothesized.[6] Damage to capillary endothelial cells is one possible mechanism. The pathophysiologic evidence supporting this hypothesis includes alterations of capillary wall permeability and structure with resultant alterations in cerebral blood flow. A second possible mechanism of radiation-induced injury is primary damage to glial cells, especially the oligodendroglia cells.[6] Such damage is manifested initially as transient demyelination, with more severe injury characterized as abnormal glial proliferation. This hypothesis is supported by evidence of focal white-matter destruction in the absence of obvious vascular alterations. A third hypothesis of radiation-induced injury suggests that delayed damage results from an autoimmune reaction to antigens released from damaged glial cells.[6]

The effects of radiation on neuronal differentiation, including dendritic formation and synaptogenesis, are poorly understood. Clearly, these processes are altered by irradiation, and it is conceivable that some chemotherapeutic agents also disrupt these intricate interactions; however, experimental studies documenting the effects of radiation or chemotherapy on neuronal circuitry and other functions, such as cell elimination, are lacking.

Chemotherapy. The pathophysiology of chemotherapy-induced CNS injury is less well delineated than that caused by radiation therapy. Methotrexate can cause white-matter destruction, the extent of which is related to the total dose and route of drug exposure.[4] Concomitant radiotherapy increases the likelihood of methotrexate-induced leukoencephalopathy. The timing of methotrexate delivery and irradiation may be of importance, as toxicity is more severe when methotrexate is given after rather than before radiotherapy. Prior irradiation may cause disruption of the blood-brain barrier, allowing more methotrexate to leak into the brain.

The use of more intensive drug-delivery schedules in an attempt to overcome the blood-brain barrier has made some drugs that were previously thought to be relatively nontoxic quite damaging. BCNU and cisplatin may (rarely) cause focal leukoencephalopathy after intraarterial infusion, as well as visual dysfunction due to direct retinal damage.[8] Methotrexate, CCNU, and ifosfamide used at high doses can cause significant neurologic abnormalities. The pathogenesis of the chemical-induced neurologic sequelae is even less well understood than the mechanisms of radiation toxicity. In addition to glial and capillary cell death, neurotransmitter dysfunction has been postulated as a possible mechanism of damage.

Clinical evidence clearly shows an increased susceptibility of the developing CNS to radiation- and possibly chemotherapy-induced damage, as compared with the CNS of older individuals.[4] However, there is no upper age limit above which the CNS is spared, as adults can be shown to have intellectual compromise following standard doses of whole-brain irradiation. In both children and adults, there is a wide individual variation in the susceptibility to neurologic sequelae of cytotoxic therapy.

CLINICAL MANIFESTATIONS

Clinical Manifestations of Radiation Neurotoxicity

The effects of cranial irradiation on the CNS are most commonly divided into acute, subacute, and delayed effects (Table 3-1).[19]

Table 3-1
Radiation-related Neurotoxicity

Type	Timing	Etiology	Syndrome	Symptoms and Signs
Acute	During or immediately after RT	Peritumoral edema	Increased intracranial pressure	Worsening focal signs; headache; vomiting; nausea
Subacute	Weeks to 3 months after RT	Transient demyelination (? oligodendroglia dysfunction)	Somnolence	Somnolence lasting days to weeks; anorexia
			Myelitis	Paresthesia down spine
			Endocrinologic	Growth failure; hypothyroidism; hypogonadism
			Neurocognitive	School difficulties; memory loss; retardation
Chronic	Months to years after RT	Vasculitis; oligodendroglial dysfunction; autoimmune etiology	Radionecrosis	Focal deficits; seizures; symptoms of increased intracranial pressure
			Large vessel occlusion	Focal deficits; seizures
			Mineralizing microangiopathy	Focal deficits; seizures; headaches
			Myelopathy	Paraparesis; quadriparesis; bowel and bladder dysfunction
			Peripheral neuropathy	Cranial nerve palsies; autonomic dysfunction; weakness

Acute and subacute clinical manifestations of radiation therapy (RT). The acute effects of therapeutic irradiation are rare and are related to high fractional doses. They are thought to result from edema within and remote to the irradiated area and may be a consequence of reactivity of the tumor to treatment.[8] Symptoms include headaches, seizures, and vomiting. Treatment is supportive, and care must be taken to differentiate acute effects of irradiation from possible progressive tumor growth. This may be especially difficult in the case of diffuse infiltrating midline lesions.

Subacute sequelae of irradiation are poorly understood. The most common is the so-called somnolence syndrome, which tends to occur 3 to 9 weeks after completion of whole-brain irradiation.[4,8] It is believed to be due to irradiation-induced oligodendroglia cell dysfunction with inhibition of myelin production; however, this remains unproven. Children experiencing the somnolence syndrome initially become anorexic and irritable; this is followed by increased sleepiness for days to weeks. The somnolence has varied in degree from mild tiredness to a sleep requirement of more than 20 hours per day. Although the syndrome is generally thought to be self-limited, long-term neurologic sequelae, such as school difficulties and seizures, developed in a higher percentage of children who had the somnolence syndrome than in a similarly treated group of patients who did not develop this complication.[7]

Transient radiation myelopathy is another time-limited syndrome occurring shortly after cervical radiotherapy.[4,8] Patients with this condition tend to develop electric shock sensations (Lhermitte's sign) down the spine and into the arms or legs upon neck flexion. Both forms of subacute toxicity may be ameliorated by steroid therapy.

Late clinical manifestations of RT. Delayed effects of RT on the CNS tend to be more varied and of greater significance than early effects. Numerous neuropsychologic studies of children with acute leukemia and brain tumors conducted over the past 15 to 20 years have revealed that treatment of the CNS with RT (and chemotherapy) is frequently associated with cognitive deficits. Although the early studies were limited by retrospective designs and the lack of control groups, recent prospective studies incorporating more rigorous designs with control of confounding variables provide convincing evidence that many children who have been successfully treated for cancer subsequently experience persistent cognitive deficits. These deficits occur in the following areas: general intelligence and age-appropriate developmental skills; academic achievement in reading, language, and arithmetic; visual and perceptual motor skills; nonverbal and verbal memory; receptive and expressive language; and attention.[10,12,20,26,30] Many of the deficits may be mediated by a deleterious effect on the speed of information processing. The incidence and magnitude of the deficits are influenced by pretreatment, treatment, and posttreatment parameters.

Pretreatment parameters. Age at the time of CNS treatment has been identified as a significant parameter for determining risk of cognitive deficits. Children treated before the age of 5 to 6 years, and especially before the age of 3 years, are at greater risk for cognitive impairments than those treated after the age of 8 to 10 years. Furthermore, the severity of the cognitive deficits, as evidenced by lower IQ scores, is generally greater in children treated at younger ages. In a recent study of 48 children, the greater the total radiation dose and the younger the child at time of irradiation, the greater the decline in intelligence scores.[29]

The sex of the child is another important parameter when estimating the risk of cognitive impairments. Girls treated for acute leukemia with 18 to 24 Gy of cranial radiation in combination with intrathecal methotrexate experience more severe neurotoxicity in terms of global depression of cognitive functions (i.e., IQ scores) than boys.[32] High-dose intravenous (IV) methotrexate administered once during remission induction increased the risk of IQ loss for girls. Performance on measures of language-based academic skills and on rote memory for digit strings does not appear to be influenced by the sex of the child.

Leukemia treatment regimens involving 24 Gy of whole-brain radiation in combination with intrathecal methotrexate have been associated with neuropsychologic sequelae. The dose of cranial radiation in many of the more recent leukemia protocols has been reduced from 24 to 18 Gy in order to reduce neurotoxicity. Although 18 Gy has been found to be equally effective in preventing meningeal leukemia, the effect on neuropsychologic performance has not been thoroughly evaluated. Findings from several studies with relatively small sample sizes are controversial. Some investigators have reported that 24 and 18 Gy are equally neurotoxic[31] and that the cognitive impairments associated with 18 Gy and intrathecal chemotherapy are comparable.[17] More modern treatment regimens often use more intensive systemic therapies that may counteract any benefit of radiation dose reduction. The time interval between treatment and the manifestation of neuropsychologic sequelae may be longer following lower radiation doses.[16]

Posttreatment parameters. One of the most important posttreatment parameters is the length of time since CNS treatment. Neuropsychologic deficits experienced by children with ALL treated with cranial radiation usually do not become fully manifest until approximately 1 to 2 years after irradiation. The time interval between irradiation and cognitive impairments may be shorter for children with brain tumors who receive higher radiation doses. Very little is known about the trajectory of neuropsychologic sequelae associated with the use of intrathecal chemotherapy alone.

Rare late effects of radiation. Radiation necrosis is both rare and disasterous. It occurs in 1% to 5% of patients treated with 5 to 6 Gy of radiation and correlates with higher total or fractional doses of radiation.[27] Pathologic changes are mainly vascular in nature, and at lower doses are generally limited to the white matter. Onset of this syndrome may occur from 3 months to many years after irradiation. The signs and symptoms of radiation necrosis may be confused with those of tumor recurrence. They include headaches and nausea associated with increased intracranial pressure; alterations in the sensorium; seizures; hemiparesis; papilledema; and other focal deficits. Treatment depends on the location of the lesion and the presence of mass effect. Patients with surgically accessible masses may benefit from resection of the necrotic tissues. Patients who respond to steroids may require them indefinitely.

Radiation can produce a spectrum of vascular injury ranging from small vessel vasculitis to large vessel sclerosis, which can result in hemiparesis, aphasia, and other stroke-related symptoms. Large vessel strokes are rare occurrences. Mineralizing microangiopathy and dystrophic calcification occur more commonly after radiotherapy.[24] Deposition of calcium occurs in the walls of small vessels, occasionally with occlusion of lumina with mineralized deposits. Some patients with this complication have been reported to have headaches and seizures, but the association between the pathologic changes and clinical manifestations is unclear.

Other rarer complications, such as cerebellar sclerosis, may occur following irradiation.[34] Cerebellar sclerosis was demonstrated in an autopsy series, and only some of the children with this autopsy finding had clear cerebellar dysfunction. Factors that seemed to be associated with the development of this syndrome include a history of extrinsic cerebellar compression by tumor, chronically increased intracranial pressure, a history of ischemic events, and prior treatment with high-dose methotrexate.

Clinical Manifestations of Chemotherapy Neurotoxicity

Methotrexate. Neurologic complications of chemotherapy have become increasingly prevalent as higher doses of standard chemotherapeutic agents have been used in more dose-intensive fashions.[4]

The clinical spectrum of chemotherapy-induced injury is best defined for methotrexate, but the mechanism of injury is still not fully known.[4] The acute effects of intrathecal methotrexate include radiculitis and arachnoiditis. After high-dose systematic methotrexate, an acute encephalopathy associated with hemiparesis, seizures, aphasias, and altered consciousness may arise as a result of abnormal glucose metabolism or neurotransmitter synthesis.[8] Subacute encephalopathy and myelopathy can occur days to weeks after repeated doses of intrathecal methotrexate.

Chronic methotrexate toxicity may result in leukoencephalopathy with symptoms including dementia, mental dysfunction, pseudobulbar signs, ataxia, spasticity, seizures, coma, and death.[1] It is believed that prior irradiation of endothelial cells compromises the blood-brain barrier and allows for excessive amounts of methotrexate to infuse into the CNS. It has been suggested that the administration of methotrexate prior to irradiation may be less damaging.[2] In one study, children who received preradiation methotrexate were reported to have IQ scores comparable to nonirradiated control groups. Even those at greatest risk for cognitive sequelae (i.e., girls younger than 5 years of age at the time of irradiation) had IQ scores that were 10 to 29 points higher than those who received cranial irradiation and intrathecal methotrexate concurrently.

Other chemotherapy. The CNS effects of conventional doses of other chemotherapeutic agents have been less well delineated (Table 3-2). High-dose chemotherapy or chemotherapy delivered via the intraarterial route or after

Table 3-2
More Common Neurologic Complications Secondary to Chemotherapy (Excluding Methotrexate)

Drug	Acute and Subacute	Chronic
Cytosine arabinoside Intrathecal	Meningitis; seizures; radiculitis; myelitis; brain necrosis (intraparenchymal infusion)	Leukoencephalopathy; myelitis; peripheral neuropathy
IV high-dose	Cerebellar ataxia; encephalopathy	Cerebellar ataxia; ? demyelinating polyneuropathy
5-Fluorouracil	Cerebellar syndrome; encephalopathy	Reversible encephalopathy
Ifosfamide	Encephalopathy; cerebellar ataxia; weakness; cranial nerve dysfunction; seizures	? Encephalopathy
BCNU intraarterial	Focal brain necrosis; blindness; seizures; encephalopathy	Blindness; seizures; encephalopathy; brain necrosis
Intravenous high-dose		
Cisplatin	—	Progressive necrosis
Intraarterial	Encephalopathy; blindness	Blindness; progressive brain necrosis
IV	Increased intracranial pressure; seizures; retrobulbar neuritis	Peripheral neuropathy; ototoxicity*
Vincristine	Muscle cramps; paresthesias; jaw pain; cranial neuropathy; peripheral neuropathy (sensory and motor); autonomic neuropathy; constipation; reversible	Peripheral neuropathy
L-Asparaginase	Metabolic encephalopathy; cerebral vascular accidents due to thrombosis or hemorrhage	Sequelae of cerebral vascular accidents
Procarbazine	Encephalopathy; peripheral neuropathy; ataxia; autonomic neuropathy; psychosis with high dosages	—

*Enhanced by radiotherapy.

blood-brain–barrier disruption has been reported to cause more severe and frequent sequelae.[8] The effects described to date are acute and usually transient. The most frequent syndrome associated with cytosine arabinoside is cerebellar dysfunction consisting of dysarthria, ataxia, and dysmetria.[33] Although cyclophosphamide has not been reported to be neurotoxic, a relatively similar alkylating agent, ifosfamide, can cause significant neurologic toxicity.[23] Symptoms associated with IV infusion of ifosfamide include mental status changes that range from irritability and confusion to coma, cerebellar dysfunction, weakness, cranial nerve dysfunction, and seizures.[23] The mechanism of ifosfamide neurotoxicity is thought to be derived from a neurotoxic metabolite, chloracetalaldehyde, that builds up in the CNS. It is not yet known whether these acute syndromes will be associated with late residual effects.

Both BCNU and cisplatin rarely cause significant neurologic toxicity after IV infusions.[8] However, intraarterial infusion of either drug or high-dose IV infusion of BCNU is reported to cause a severe encephalopathy and leukoencephalopathy.[3,5,28] L-asparaginase rarely causes an acute encephalopathy[8] that has been hypothesized to be related to metabolic aberration. The other major adverse neurologic effect of L-asparaginase is coagulopathy-induced cerebral hemorrhage or thrombosis thought to be due to a rebound effect of L-asparaginase liver toxicity. Again, long-term residua have not been described.

Clinical Manifestations Attributable to Surgery or Tumor

There is limited information about a relationship between the dose of radiation received and the severity of neuropsychologic impairments. Children treated for brain tumors, who traditionally receive over 30 Gy, experience more severe disabilities than do children treated for ALL, who receive 18 to 24 Gy; however, the effects of the tumor and surgery on neural tissues must be taken into consideration.

The site of brain tumors may have a major effect on the severity of cognitive deficits. Children with primitive neuroectodermal tumor (PNET) or medulloblastoma tumors involving the cerebral hemispheres may have cognitive impairments at the time of diagnosis; these deficits tend to become more severe over time. The risk of mental retardation (i.e., IQ less than 70) may be greater if the tumor involves the brain stem[13] or extends to the hypothalamus.[9] One study[13] found that children with tumors of the fourth ventricle had a greater decline in IQ scores than those with tumors involving the third ventricle. There is no convincing evidence that hydrocephalus at diagnosis plays a role in delayed cognitive deterioration.[12]

The association between early postoperative shunting for hydrocephalus in children with brain tumors and neuropsychologic deficits is controversial. Several studies have reported that ventricular size and permanent shunting are not significant correlates or predictors of cognitive outcome.[11,13] Packer and coworkers found that the IQ scores of children with hydrocephalus who required shunting were, on the average, 25 points lower than those of children who did not require shunt placement[21]; however, patients with larger tumors are more likely to need a shunt. Finally, there is modest evidence that children who experience a complicated postoperative course (e.g., postoperative infections) may be at risk for more severe neuropsychologic problems, such as lower IQ scores, than those with an uncomplicated postoperative course.[21]

DETECTION AND SCREENING

Neurocognitive Screening

The basic evaluation of children at risk of neurologic compromise after treatment of the CNS consists of a detailed history and clinical evaluation. Historical information crucial for the determination of the presence and degree of sequelae includes detailed neurodevelopmental appraisals and information concerning school performance. Neurologic evaluation is useful in pinpointing focal neurologic deficits and the presence of rarer CNS sequelae, such as radionecrosis and leukoencephalopathy, but is less useful in the diagnosis of more subtle neurocognitive problems. In the past, much has been made of so-called soft neurologic signs in children with attention and learning problems. These soft signs can alert the clinician to possible problems but have little specificity and in isolation are of no significance. Detailed neurocognitive testing is necessary when such signs are noted after CNS therapy.

Given the frequency of neurocognitive sequelae and their impact on learning, school performance, and occupational opportunity, it is critical to perform prospective, serial neurocognitive assessments for all patients at risk. These include any young child (arbitrarily a child younger than 10 years of age) who has received potentially neurotoxic treatment, as well as any child who has received extensive cranial (especially whole-brain) irradiation, intrathecal medication, or high-dose systemic methotrexate. Baseline testing is mandatory to effectively evaluate the long-term effects of any form of treatment. Many children, especially infants with CNS tumors, have significant neurologic compromise owing to either the tumor or surgery; this must be taken into account when one attempts to determine the detrimental effects of anticancer therapy. The best time to obtain these baseline data is not clear. In theory, children should be tested prior to the initiation of irradiation or any other potentially neurotoxic therapy. Unfortunately, the child tends to be most ill in the pretreatment period. Performance may be transiently poor, resulting in evaluations that are not truly representative of the child's intellectual or neurologic capacity. As an alternative, the baseline evaluation could be conducted following RT (either before or after the somnolence period) and preceding the time when the delayed effects of RT are most likely to become evident. Arbitrarily, such studies have been performed fairly successfully 8 to 12 weeks following RT. In fact, comparison of neurocognitive testing performed immediately before and after RT demonstrates a higher neurocognitive ability in children tested soon after RT.

There are obvious methodologic problems in the study of neuropsychologic function after treatment of cancer. Long, detailed evaluations may provide the best information, but they are stressful for the child and expensive. Financial reimbursement is often lacking, particularly for sequential testing of many children. Prior conceptualization of specific study questions is essential so that important questions may be addressed by the battery. External controls or comparison groups are necessary when neurocognitive testing is being performed partially for study purposes.

The tools used to study patients are crucial in the interpretation of test results. Measures (such as Wechsler scales) that are frequently used to assess levels of intellectual functioning tend to be well standardized. However, more pertinent measures of the child's everyday functioning (attention; individual intellectual subset evaluations; and memory tasks) are less standardized, making interpretation difficult. When one is planning sequential tests, issues concerning "practice effects" become important. Similarly, neurocognitive tests tend to be stressful (as well as expensive) for the parent and the child and cannot be done as frequently as desired.

The major determinant of when testing should be conducted is the reason the test is being performed. If the test is being performed solely for clinical reasons—to assess the needs of the child and help the family and school plan adequate educational needs—the baseline testing may be superfluous and testing can be done on a yearly or biyearly schedule, depending on the clinical situation. However, if testing is being performed as part of clinical research, then baseline evaluations are essential, and much more care must be built into the design of the neuropsychologic investigation. The study questions must be carefully formulated and tests that have established sensitivity and specificity must be used. The use of an appropriate control group and the number of patients available for evaluation must be considered in the project design to ensure sufficient statistical power to address the questions raised and to allow for nonmedical covariates.

Neurophysiologic Testing

The diagnosis of neurologic and neurocognitive compromise secondary to chemotherapeutic agents is highly dependent on the timing of the treatment and assessment, the medical status of the patient, the type of tumor being treated, and the type and amount of therapy given. Knowledge of the effects of the tumor on the nervous system are critical in understanding what may be occurring. A variety of neuroinvestigative studies may be helpful in determining the cause and degree of sequelae but only when the studies are used appropriately.

The backbone of ancillary neurologic investigation is neuroimaging with either CT or MR. Given its greater sensitivity, especially to white-matter damage, MR has essentially supplanted CT in most of these investigations.[2] Occasionally, small areas of calcification found on CT will be missed on MR. Focal neucrosis, atrophy, and diffuse white-matter damage are seen clearly on CT but better on MR. It is possible to crudely separate the types of white-matter damage into categories, such as mild (occasional punctate areas of damage), moderate (large or single areas of damage), or severe (confluent areas of white-matter damage). These criteria correlate grossly with more substantiated types of neurologic damage (e.g., severe impairment in mentation; motor deficits; seizures) but have not been found to be useful in understanding milder degrees of neurocognitive dysfunction.[2] Similarly, although the presence of scattered or even confluent areas of calcification have been associated with more subtle neurologic compromise, such as intellectual dysfunction and headaches, the relationship is variable. Other neuroimaging tools, such as positron emission tomography (PET) and single positron emission computed tomography (SPECT) may aid in the evaluation of treatment-related sequelae.[8] PET scanning is useful for differentiating radiation-induced necrosis (characterized by decreased metabolism) from recurrent malignant tumor (characterized by increased metabolism). PET scanning abnormalities have also been seen following methotrexate-induced brain injury. However, because of the relative unavailability of PET scanning, and the difficulty of obtaining quantitative information when this procedure is used in infants and young children, its role in determining more subtle abnormalities has not been defined.

Neurophysiologic measures have been of limited use in investigation of treatment-related sequelae. Electroencephalographic abnormalities are relatively nonspecific. In patients with the somnolence syndrome, slowing on the electroencephalogram has been correlated with an increased incidence of permanent neurocognitive sequelae.[7] However, this correlation has only been shown in one study and has not been universally reproduced. It was initially hoped that evoked-response measures of the conductivity of neurologic signals within the CNS, such as visual evoked responses and brain stem auditory evoked responses, would help unravel the pathophysiology of treatment-induced sequelae and would provide effective means with which to diagnose and follow patients at highest risk for sequelae. However, studies to date have been disappointing, and although evoked-response tests may be useful in isolated cases, confirmation of their widespread use is not available.

Cerebral spinal fluid myelin basic protein has been shown to be elevated in children with overt leukoencephalopathy, but has not been helpful as a marker of neurologic damage. Measurement of other CNS markers in cerebrospinal fluid, such as neuronal proteins, antineuronal antibodies, and neurotransmitters, has not yet been shown to help in the diagnosis and follow-up of children with subtle neurologic sequelae.

MANAGEMENT OF ESTABLISHED PROBLEMS

School intervention programs to assist children with neuropsychologic impairments focus on early reentry into the school system and development of individualized educational programs. School reentry programs are based on the premise that early return to the school environment minimizes academic problems and facilitates psychosocial adjustment. Remediation of specific cognitive problems requires the expertise of special education professionals. For example, training programs designed to teach the adoption, maintenance, and generalization of memory strategies in other brain-injured populations[15] may be of benefit to children previously treated with radiation therapy or chemotherapy.

Educational Intervention

Early intervention may help prevent or minimize problems with school performance. Under the Public Law 101-476 Individuals with Disabilities Act, all children treated for cancer are entitled to special educational services.[22] Based upon the results and impressions formed during psychoeducational evaluation, the educational liaison may offer specific recommendations for effective interventions to address particular educational concerns. Recommendations must be individualized and frequently include the use of the following: compensatory strategies that utilize the student's learning and performance strengths to circumvent weakness; modifications in the mode of presenting information or in the manner of response; alternate testing arrangements, such as separate administration or extended time; special cues or other recall aides; technologic devices such as a calculator, word processor or "spell checker"; experimental teaching, which measures performance rates across different instructional conditions; curricular modifications; the teaching and monitoring of time management and organizational skills; and other means of accommodating the individual's learning process in the school setting. Special therapies may be recommended, such as speech and language therapy, physical therapy, occupational therapy, counseling, and social skills training. These therapies are offered as "special services" for students involved in special education and are provided by the school system when they are deemed necessary for the student to benefit from an educational program.

Special Educational Needs

If the student has special needs constituting an educational disability that cannot be addressed adequately in the regular education program, the student is eligible for special education. Special education is specially designed instruction, and related services provide a thorough individualized education plan (IEP). The IEP is developed by a specialized, multidisciplinary school-system team and the child's parents, and is implemented in the child's school program, which is overseen by a special education teacher. Appropriate related services provided may include speech and language therapy, counseling, occupational therapy, physical therapy, and the services of a teacher of the hearing impaired or visually impaired, if necessary for the student to benefit from the educational program. Special education services are provided with typical peers, to the extent possible, along a continuum of settings— from having a special educational teacher consult within the regular classroom, to having part-time, supplemental instruction in a special-education class with fewer students and additional personnel in the classroom or residential school.

In conjunction with school staff, the educational liaison can help determine the need for special education and, when necessary, can initiate the referral and planning process. A formalized process for referring, evaluating, planning, and implementing programs for students with special educational needs is mandated by federal law, outlined in the states' education regulations, and implemented by special multidisciplinary teams in the public school systems. Parental consent, participation, and procedural safeguards are an integral part of this process. Although founded upon strong parental participation, the process of obtaining needed special-education services can be both confusing and intimidating for parents. It is critical that the educational liaison be prepared to support and supplement the advocacy efforts of the child's family. This advocacy is necessary to ensure that the student receives appropriate educational services and opportunities.

School systems often lack familiarity with the educational needs of children treated for cancer and especially those experiencing late effects of CNS treatment.

Finally, it is essential that parents and educators be prepared for the possibility of specific neuropsychologic problems. Teachers may be unaware of the child's prior cancer treatment and uninformed about the nature of the cognitive problems, because such problems may not become apparent until months to years after CNS treatment. Therefore, close communication among teachers, parents, and the staff of the treatment center is essential after the child has completed cancer treatment.

REFERENCES

1. Allen JC, Rosen G, Mehta BM: Leukoencephalopathy following high-dose IV methotrexate with leucovorin rescue, *Cancer Treat Rep* 64:1261-1273, 1980.
2. Balsom WR, Bleyer WA, Robinson LL et al: Intellectual function in long-term survivors of childhood acute lymphoblastic leukemia: protective effect of preirradiation methotrexate? "A Children Cancer Study Group study," *Pediatr Oncol* 19:486-492, 1991.
3. Berman IJ, Mann MP: Seizures and transient cortical blindness associated with cisplatin (II) diaminedichloride (PDD) therapy in a thirty-year-old man, *Cancer* 45:764-766, 1980.
4. Bleyer WA, Griffen TW: White matter necrosis, mineralizing microangiopathy and intellectual abilities in survivors of childhood leukemia. In Gilbert MA, Kegan AR, editors: *Radiation damage to the nervous system,* New York, 1980, Raven Press.
5. Bremer AM, Kleriga E, Nguyen TQ et al: Complications associated with intra-arterial BCNU administered in combination with vincristine and procarbazine for the treatment of malignant brain tumors, *J Neurooncol* 2:219, 1984.
6. Caveness WF: Experimental observations: delayed necrosis in the monkey brain. In Gilbert, MA, Kagan, AR, editors: *Radiation damage to the nervous system,* New York, 1980, Raven Press.
7. Ch'ien FT, Aur RJA, Stanger S et al: Long-term neurological implications of somnolence syndrome in children with lymphocytic leukemia, *Ann Neurol* 8:273-277, 1980.
8. Cohen BH, Packer RJ: *Adverse neurologic effects of chemotherapy and radiation therapy.* In Berger BO, editor: *Neurologic aspects of pediatrics,* Boston, 1992, Butterworth-Heinemann, pp. 567-594.
9. Danoff BF, Cowchock FS, Marquette C et al: Assessment of long-term effects of primary radiation therapy for brain tumors in children, *Cancer* 49:1585-1586, 1992.
10. Duffner PK, Cohen ME, Thomas PRM et al: The long-term effects of cranial irradiation on the central nervous system, *Cancer* 56:1841-1846, 1985.
11. Ellenberg L, McComb JC, Siegel SE et al: Factors affecting intellectual outcome in pediatric brain tumor patients, *Neurosurgery* 21:638-644, 1987.
12. Glauser TA, Packer RJ: Cognitive deficits in long-term survivors of childhood brain tumors, *Childs Nerv Syst* 7:2-12, 1991.
13. Hirsh JF, Reiner D, Czernichow P et al: Medulloblastoma in childhood: survival and functional results, *Acta Neurochir (Wien)* 48:1-15, 1979.
14. Holmes GL: Morphological and physiological maturation of the brain in the neonate and young child, *J Clin Neurophysiol* 3:209-238, 1986.
15. Kramer JJ, Engle RW: Teaching awareness of strategic behavior in combination with strategy training: effects of children's memory performance, *J Exp Child Psychol* 2:513-530, 1981.

16. Moore IM, Kramer JH, Wara W et al: Cognitive function in children with leukemia: effect of radiation dose and time since radiation, *Cancer* 68:1913-1917, 1991.
17. Mulhern RK, Wasserman AL, Fairclough D et al: Memory function in disease-free survivors of childhood acute lymphoblastic leukemia given CNS prophylaxis with or without 1800 cGy of cranial irradiation, *Clin Oncol* 6:315-320, 1988.
18. Reference deleted in proof.
19. Packer RJ, Meadows AT, Rorke LB et al: Long-term sequelae of cancer treatment on the central nervous system in childhood, *Med Pediatr Oncol* 15:241-253, 1987.
20. Packer RJ, Meadows AT, Rorke LB et al: Long-term sequelae of cancer treatment on the central nervous system in children, *Med Pediatr Oncol* 15:241-253, 1987.
21. Packer RJ, Sposto R, Atkins TE: Quality of life in children with primitive neuroectodermal tumor (medulloblastoma) of the posterior fossa, *Pediatr Neurosci* 13:169-180, 1988.
22. P. L. 101-476: Individuals with Disabilities Act (formerly Education of the Handicapped Act, P. L. 64-142).
23. Pratt CB, Green AA, Horowitz ME et al: Central nervous system toxicity following the treatment of pediatric patients with ifosfamide/MESNA, *J Clin Oncol* 1986:1253-1261, 1986.
24. Price RA, Birdwell DA: The central nervous system in childhood leukemia: III. mineralizing microangiopathy and dystrophic calcification, *Cancer* 42:717-728, 1978.
25. Price RA, Jamieson PA: The central nervous system in childhood leukemia: II. Subacute leukoencephalopathy, *Cancer* 35:306-318, 1975.
26. Rodgers J, Britton PG, Morris RG et al: Memory after treatment for acute lymphoblastic leukemia, *Arch Dis Child* 67:266-268, 1992.
27. Rottenberg DA, Chernik NL, Deck MDF et al: Cerebral necrosis following radiotherapy of extracranial neoplasms, *Ann Neurol* 1:339-357, 1977.
28. Schold SC, Fay JW: Central nervous system toxicity from high-dose BCNU treatment of systemic cancer, *Neurology* 30:429, 1980.
29. Silber JH, Radcliffe J, Peckham V et al: Whole brain irradiation and decline in intelligence: the influence of dose and age on IQ score, *J Clin Oncl* 10:1390-1396, 1992.
30. Stehbens JA, Kaleih TA, Noll RB et al: CNS prophylaxis of childhood leukemia: what are the long-term neurological, neuropsychological and behavioral effects? *Neuropsychology Review* 2:147-176, 1991.
31. Tameroff M, Saliven R, Miller D et al: Neuropsychological sequelae in irradiated (1800 rads) (r) and 2400 (r) and nonirradiated children with acute lymphoblastic leukemia (ALL) (abstract), *Proc Am Soc Clin Oncol* 3:C 644, 1985.
31a. Volpe JJ: *Dorsal induction and ventral induction.* In Volpe JJ, editor: Neurology of the newborn, Philadelphia, 1987, W.B. Saunders.
32. Waber DP, Tarbell NJ, Kahn CM et al: The relationship of sex and treatment modality to neuropsychologic outcome in childhood acute lymphoblastic leukemia, *J Clin Biol* 10:810-817, 1992.
33. Winkelman MD, Hines JD: Cerebellar degeneration caused by high-dose cytosine arabinoside: a clinico-pathologic study, *Ann Neurol* 14:620-627, 1983.
34. Wiznitzer M, Packer RJ, Rorke LB et al: Cerebellar sclerosis in pediatric cancer patients, *J Neurooncol* 4:353-360, 1987.
35. Wright TL, Bresnan MJ: Radiation-induced cerebrovascular disease in childhood, *Neurology* 25:540-543, 1976.

4

Neuroendocrine Complications of Cancer Therapy

Charles A. Sklar

PATHOPHYSIOLOGY

Overview

The hypothalamic-pituitary axis (HPA) is a highly complex system that allows neurologic and chemical signals from the brain to be translated into endocrine responses. The hypothalamus is connected to various regions of the brain by means of reciprocal neuronal circuits. Owing to these afferent and efferent nerve pathways, the hypothalamus serves as a vital link between distant and diverse regions of the brain. The hypothalamus is also the site of the production of several peptide hormones and biogenic amines that are the predominate regulators of the anterior pituitary hormones (Fig. 4-1). These hypothalamic factors reach the anterior pituitary gland by way of a portal venous system, which is composed of a primary and secondary capillary plexus. The six known anterior pituitary hormones and their major hypothalamic regulatory hormones are listed in Table 4-1.

The hypothalamic regulatory factors generally stimulate the secretion of anterior pituitary hormones, but mixed stimulatory and inhibitory as well as predominant inhibitory controls also occur. A brief summary of the regulation and mechanisms of the anterior pituitary hormones follows.

Growth hormone. Growth hormone (GH) is a single chain polypeptide that contains 191 amino acids. Circulating GH causes bone and soft tissue growth. Most of its growth-promoting effects are mediated through the production of a family of peptide hormones known as insulin-like growth factors (IGFs), with IGF-I being the most GH dependent. GH is secreted episodically with a burst occurring approximately every 4 hours. The predominant pulse of GH takes place during the first 2 hours of nocturnal sleep, coincident with the first episode of slow-wave sleep. The secretory pattern of GH can be affected by a variety of factors including age, sex, pubertal status, body weight, and nutritional status. GH is principally regulated by the hypothalamic hormones GHRH and somatostatin. There is good evidence that the release of GH is due to the coordinated interaction between these two hypophysiotropic hormones. A variety of central and peripheral factors are able to modulate GH release by altering the activity of GHRH or somatostatin. In particular, the alpha-2 adrenergic system and the cholinergic neuronal system play important roles in the control of GH release.

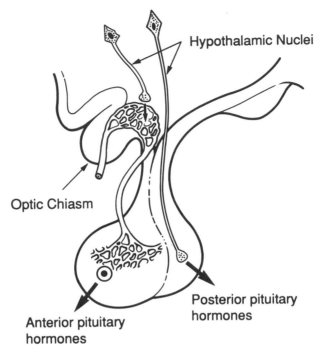

Fig. 4-1. Schematic representation of the hypothalamus and the pituitary gland.

Table 4-1
Anterior Pituitary Hormones and Hypothalamic Regulatory Factors

Pituitary hormone	Hypothalamic factor
Growth hormone (GH)	GH-releasing hormone (+)
	Somatostatin (−)
Prolactin	Dopamine (−)
Luteinizing hormone (LH)	Gonadotropin-releasing hormone (+)
Follicle-stimulating hormone (FSH)	
Thyroid-stimulating hormone	Thyrotropin-releasing hormone (+)
Adrenocorticotropin	Corticotropin-releasing hormone (+)

(+) = stimulatory; (−) = inhibitory.

Prolactin. Prolactin (PRL) is the most recently recognized anterior pituitary hormone. Its structural similarity to GH suggests that both are derived from a common precursor. PRL levels exhibit a diurnal pattern with a slight increase occurring in the early morning. A variety of factors can augment PRL secretion, including stress and the female hormone, estrogen. In the human, the only known physiologic roles for PRL are the induction of lactation and the interruption of ovulation and menstruation during the postpartum period. The primary, if not the sole, hypothalamic factor controlling PRL release is the neurotransmitter dopamine, which tonically inhibits PRL release. Insults to or destructive lesions in or near the hypothalamus, which disturb or destroy normal dopaminergic tone, result in loss of inhibition and hyperprolactinemia. Additional factors that may also play a role in the neuroregulation of PRL release include thyrotropin-releasing hormone (TRH), serotonin, and gamma-aminobutyric acid.

Gonadotropins. The gonadotropins luteinizing hormone (LH) and follicle stimulating hormone (FSH) are glycoproteins that are composed of two subunits — a common alpha subunit and a specific beta subunit that confers both immuno-specificity and functional specificity. These two hormones appear to be stored within and secreted by the same cells within the anterior pituitary gland. The gonadotropins are released in a pulsatile fashion, but the overall pattern of secretion varies according to the pubertal status and sex of the individual. During childhood, the serum concentrations of LH and FSH tend to be very low, with the serum concentrations of FSH being relatively higher. With the onset of puberty, there is a reversal of this pattern, and the serum concentrations of LH are generally greater than those of FSH. In the male, the primary function of LH is to stimulate the Leydig cells within the testes to produce testosterone, and FSH is primarily involved in spermatogenesis. In the female, both gonadotropins are necessary for normal steroidogenesis and normal ovulation. The release of both LH and FSH appears to be under the control of a single hypothalamic factor, gonadotropin-releasing hormone (GnRH). GnRH is released in pulses that are, in turn, responsible for the pulsatile pattern of LH and FSH secretion. The overall pattern of gonadotropin release can be altered by changes in the amount and frequency of GnRH release. Although their exact role is currently unclear, beta-endorphin and dopamine appear to be involved in the regulation of gonadotropin secretion.

Thyroid-stimulating hormone. Thyroid-stimulating hormone (TSH) is a glyco-protein hormone and, similar to LH and FSH, is composed of an alpha and a beta subunit. TSH is secreted in a circadian pattern, with the highest levels occurring at night. TSH binds to specific receptors within the thyroid gland and is the primary regulator of thyroid hormone production. The hypothalamic stimulatory peptide TRH is primarily responsible for the control of TSH release. Both dopamine and somatostatin are capable of inhibiting TSH release, although their precise role in the physiologic regulation of TSH release remains unclear.

Adrenocorticotropin. Adrenocorticotropin (ACTH) is a peptide hormone that is actually cleaved from a precursor hormone known as proopiomelanocortin. ACTH is released in a circadian pattern, with peak serum concentrations being recorded in the early morning and nadir levels occurring near midnight. ACTH is primarily responsible for the stimulation and control of adrenal steroidogenesis. Central control of ACTH release is mediated principally by the hypothalamic corticotropin-releasing hormone (CRH). The peptide hormone vasopressin has the capacity to stimulate ACTH release and can augment the ACTH response to corticotropin-releasing factor (CRF). A host of neurotransmitters including noradrenaline, serotonin, acetylcholine, and histamine may also participate in the regulation of ACTH secretion.

Posterior pituitary. The anatomic and functional relationship between the hypothalamus and the posterior pituitary differs from that previously noted for the anterior pituitary in that the two hormones associated with the posterior pituitary (vasopressin and oxytocin) are actually synthesized by neurons within the hypothalamus. These hormones are subsequently transported along specialized neuronal tracts to the posterior pituitary, where they are stored for later release into the peripheral circulation (Fig. 4-1).

Oxytocin is important in the stimulation of uterine contractions during labor and initiates milk let-down in response to suckling. Vasopressin, the antidiuretic hormone, is responsible for maintaining plasma osmolality by regulating the renal handling of free water.

Therapy-induced Damage to the Hypothalamic-Pituitary Axis

Abnormalities of the HPA are seen commonly after cranial irradiation and irradiation of the face and neck for the treatment of a variety of solid tumors.[17] In general, radiation-induced damage is directly related to the total dose of radiation and to the biologically effective dose, which is determined primarily by the number of fractions and the dose per fraction. Hypothalamic-pituitary dysfunction following radiation therapy (RT) is also time dependent, with the incidence of most problems increasing over time.[9] The age of the patient at the time of treatment may also be important, because there are data suggesting that younger patients are more vulnerable than adults to the damaging effects of radiation. The hypothalamus is more radiosensitive than the pituitary and is more commonly the site of damage, particularly following lower dose (less than 40 to 50 Gy) RT. However, at higher doses of radiation there is evidence for both hypothalamic and anterior pituitary damage.

GH deficiency is the earliest and most consistent neuroendocrine disturbance reported after irradiation of the HPA.[14] Impairment of the other anterior pituitary hormones is much less common and is usually seen in patients treated with higher doses of radiation. At the present time, there are very few data to support the contention that chemotherapeutic agents, either singly or in combination, have the capacity to permanently impair anterior pituitary function. Although certain drugs (e.g., cyclophosphamide, vinca alkaloids, cisplatin) have been associated with transient episodes of inappropriate vasopressin secretion, chronic abnormalities of posterior pituitary function have not been reported following RT or chemotherapy.

CLINICAL MANIFESTATIONS (Table 4-2)

Growth Hormone Deficiency

Growth hormone deficiency (GHD) is the most common and frequently the only pituitary problem noted after cranial irradiation. GHD can be seen following conventional fractionated radiation that exposes the HPA to doses of 18 Gy or more

Table 4-2
Summary of Neuroendocrine Complications

Disorder	Radiation Dose* (Gy)	Diagnostic Studies	Treatment
GH deficiency	≥18-20	1. GH stimulation tests 2. Bone age 3. Frequent sampling for GH (12-24 hours)	Recombinant GH
Gonadotropin deficiency	>30	1. Basal serum concentration of LH, FSH, estradiol, or testosterone 2. GnRH stimulation test	Estrogen/progestin (women) Depot testosterone (men)
Precocious puberty	>10 (?)	1. GnRH stimulation test 2. Estradiol or testosterone concentration 3. Bone age 4. Pelvic ultrasound (women) 5. GH stimulation tests	GnRH agonists plus recombinant GH (if GH deficient)
TSH deficiency	>30	1. Basal serum concentrations T_4, T_3 uptake, TSH 2. TRH stimulation test	L-thyroxine
ACTH deficiency	>30	1. Basal serum cortisol concentration 2. Adrenal stimulation test (e.g., insulin, ACTH)	Hydrocortisone
Hyperprolactinemia	>40-50	Basal serum PRL concentration	Dopamine agonists (e.g., bromocriptine)

GH = growth hormone; TSH = thyroid stimulating hormone; ACTH = adrenocorticotropin; LH = luteinizing hormone; FSH = follicle-stimulating hormone; GnRH = gonadotropin-releasing hormone; TRH = thyrotropin-releasing hormone.
*Based on standard fractionation schedules.

and following total doses as low as 9 to 10 Gy when given in a single dose (e.g., total-body irradiation [TBI]).[14] The greater the dose of radiation, the higher the incidence of GHD and the shorter the time interval between treatment and the development of GHD (Fig. 4-2).[6] Current data suggest that nearly all individuals treated with doses in excess of 35 Gy to the HPA will develop GHD, which generally occurs within the first 5 years after treatment. The clinical ramifications of GHD are most evident in the growing child, with a reduction in growth velocity that is inappropriate for the child's age and stage of puberty, leading to short stature

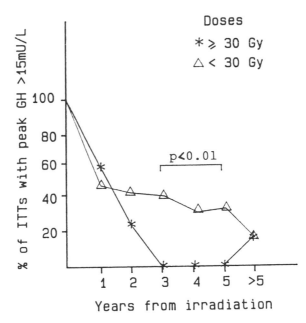

Fig. 4-2.   Percentage of normal GH responses to insulin tolerance testing (ITT) in patients receiving <30 Gy or ≥30 Gy to the HPA. (From Clayton PE, Shalet SM, Price DA: Growth response to growth hormone therapy following craniospinal irradiation, *Eur J Pediatr* 147:597-601, 1988.)

(Fig. 4-3). Although poor linear growth is very common in subjects with GHD, it is neither universal nor always immediately apparent. Several studies suggest that a slowing of growth may not occur for the first year or two after the development of GHD. Fasting hypoglycemia is an additional but rare clinical manifestation of radiation-induced GHD; it is more likely to be seen in a young child who also suffers from additional pituitary deficits (e.g., TSH and ACTH). Although it is not likely to produce clinical symptoms, GHD in the postpubertal individual may be associated with a relative decrease in muscle mass and increase in adipose tissue.[15]

Gonadotropin Deficiency

Complete or partial deficiencies of LH and FSH are encountered primarily in subjects who have been treated with high-dose radiation. Although few studies have evaluated the incidence and evolution of this problem following irradiation during childhood, it can be estimated that irradiation of the HPA with doses of 35 Gy or more causes gonadotropin deficiency in approximately 10% to 20% of individuals within 5 to 10 years.[13] Based on data derived from studies performed in adults, the incidence of gonadotropin deficiency would be expected to increase with time.[9]

Gonadotropin deficiency, when it develops in a young child, will result in failure to enter puberty and primary amenorrhea. Milder forms of the defect may lead to slow or arrested puberty, menstrual irregularities, and secondary amenorrhea. In

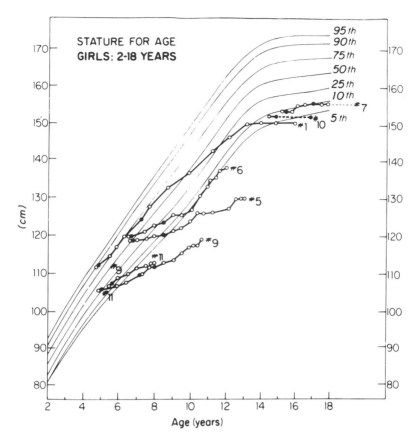

Fig. 4-3.   Composite growth curves in girls following high-dose cranial radiation. The first solid circle represents the time GH therapy was started. The second solid circle represents time therapy was stopped. (From Bajorunas DR et al: Endocrine sequelae of antineoplastic therapy in childhood head and neck malignancies, *J Clin Endocrinol Metab* 50:329-335, 1980.)

adults, lack of normal gonadotropin function can be associated with infertility, sexual dysfunction, and decreased libido. Testicular and ovarian dysfunction can also result from direct injury to the gonads by RT or chemotherapy. Serum gonadotropin concentration is elevated in this situation (see Chapters 11 and 12).

Early Sexual Maturation

Over the past several years it has become apparent that cranial irradiation is associated not only with deficient production of gonadotropins, but also early and precocious puberty in some patient groups.[4,8] This phenomenon, originally described in patients treated with high-dose cranial irradiation for brain tumors, has now been reported following low-dose cranial radiation for acute leukemia and in

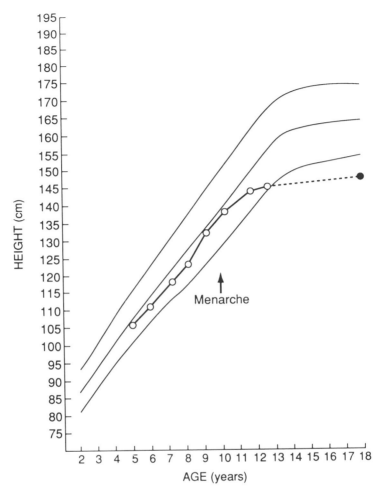

Fig. 4-4.   Growth curve of a girl treated with 24 Gy cranial radiation for acute lymphoblastic leukemia at age 2 years. She experienced menarche at age 10 years, has a bone age of 15 years at age 12 years, and has a predicted adult height (•) of 147 cm (4 ft 10 inches).

patients given low-dose TBI as preparation for a bone marrow transplant. For reasons that are unclear, females are affected more often than males. Several series have shown a direct correlation between age at treatment and age at onset of puberty. The majority of subjects who experience premature sexual maturation have also been found to have GHD.

Precocious puberty is defined as the appearance of breast development in a girl prior to age 8 years and signs of genital development, pubic hair development, and testicular enlargement in a boy prior to age 9 to 9½ years. Additionally, many children will begin their pubertal development at a normal but early age and will progress through puberty at an abnormally rapid rate.[12] These children experience accelerated skeletal maturation, premature epiphyseal fusion, and reduced final height (Fig. 4-4). For those with concomitant GHD, there is an attenuated pubertal growth spurt that results in further loss of growth potential.

Thyrotropin Deficiency

Thyrotropin (TSH) deficiency is relatively rare except in patients who receive high-dose HPA irradiation. There are very few data concerning the incidence of this problem in long-term survivors of childhood malignancies. We have recently reported that following 40 to 50 Gy, two of 36 patients (6%) developed TSH deficiency after a median follow-up of 10 years.[10] One series that evaluated pituitary function in adults irradiated for pituitary tumors found TSH to be the least vulnerable of all the pituitary hormones.[3]

TSH deficiency is often subclinical and does not usually produce serious clinical symptoms. In children, poor linear growth, delayed puberty, excessive weight gain, and lethargy can be seen in individuals with complete TSH deficiency of long duration.

Adrenocorticotropin Deficiency

Complete loss of ACTH secretion leading to adrenal insufficiency is an extremely rare occurrence following therapy for childhood cancer and is most likely to be seen in patients treated with radiation doses of 50 Gy or more.[1]

Clinical manifestations associated with ACTH deficiency include decreased stamina, lethargy, fasting hypoglycemia, and dilutional hyponatremia similar to inappropriate vasopressin secretion.

Hyperprolactinemia

Elevated plasma levels of PRL are well described in patients who have received high-dose radiation (greater than 50 Gy) to the hypothalamus.[1,7] It is seen most commonly in adult women but has been described in both sexes and in all age groups.

Hyperprolactinemia can cause pubertal delay or arrest in children, galactorrhea or amenorrhea in women, and decreased libido and impotence in adult males.

DETECTION AND SCREENING

Growth Hormone Deficiency

Children who have completed treatment for a malignancy that has included RT to the HPA must be closely monitored for evidence of growth failure. Accurate determinations of standing height need to be made at regular intervals (every 3 to 6 months) and the values plotted on standard growth curves. Additionally, sitting heights need to be obtained on all individuals who have received radiation to the spine (e.g., craniospinal, mantle, or TBI). Calculation of the child's growth velocity (cm per year) can be used to detect early deviations in growth, but the data must be derived from observations made at least 6 months apart. For individuals treated with spinal irradiation, growth is best followed by determining changes in leg length (standing height minus sitting height). It is imperative that the height and growth velocity data be viewed in the context of the child's previous growth pattern, current skeletal age (determined by radiograph of hand and wrist), and pubertal status. Therefore, an assessment of the child's stage of pubertal development is an essential part of the follow-up and is as critical as height measurements in monitoring posttreatment growth.

Diagnostic studies should be performed on any child who, once treatment has been discontinued, is growing at a subnormal rate for age *and* pubertal status or who demonstrates deceleration from previous height percentiles. Initial screening should include bone age assessment, thyroid function tests (e.g., thyroxine, TSH, and binding capacity), and routine blood studies to exclude major organ system dysfunction. If the screening studies fail to uncover an explanation for the poor linear growth, GH testing is indicated. The most effective means of evaluating GH secretion in these children remains the subject of much debate. Standard provocative testing with a variety of pharmacologic agents, the traditional means of assessing GH reserve, may be misleading in this population of patients because false-negative results are common, particularly following lower doses of radiation.[2] Although physiologic assessments of GH secretion (frequent sampling over 12 to 24 hours) are the most sensitive and reproducible means of determining an individual's GH status following irradiation of the HPA, such testing is expensive, time consuming, and not generally available outside research centers. A practical solution is initially to perform pharmacologic testing with at least two agents; several workers feel that insulin is superior to other agents because the GH response to hypoglycemia correlates well with the results of physiologic studies.[16] If the GH response to stimulation tests is normal but the patient's growth rate remains abnormal, further assessment using a physiologic study can then be performed.

Luteinizing, or Follicle-Stimulating Hormone Deficiency

In normal children, the onset of puberty occurs by age 13 years in girls and by age 14 to 14½ years in boys. The first signs of sexual maturation in a girl include breast development, greying of the vaginal mucosa, and pubic and axillary hair development. It is important to note that pubic and axillary hair development are due to androgen production; in females, pubic and axillary hair in the absence of breast development may represent isolated adrenarche rather than true puberty. The initial manifestation of puberty in boys is usually testicular enlargement followed by pubic and axillary hair development and phallic development. In many boys treated for a malignancy, testicular size may not be a reliable index of pubertal maturation because both direct gonadal irradiation and a variety of chemotherapeutic agents (e.g., cyclophosphamide, lomustine, cisplatin) cause damage to the seminiferous tubules, which results in reduced testicular volume. If a child fails to demonstrate clinical signs of sexual development by the aforementioned ages, an evaluation for delayed puberty is indicated. Baseline assessment should include a hand radiograph for bone age and basal serum concentrations of LH, FSH, testosterone, or estradiol.

Thyroid function studies need to be conducted on patients who received neck (including spine) irradiation, and a basal serum concentration of PRL should be obtained in patients treated with high-dose radiation to the HPA. Whereas elevated basal serum concentrations of LH and FSH indicate primary gonadal failure, normal or low serum concentrations of gonadotropins suggest LH or FSH deficiency in this clinical setting. A GnRH stimulation test may provide additional, useful clinical information. A similar work up should be undertaken in patients treated with RT to the HPA who develop evidence of arrested pubertal maturation or amenorrhea (primary or secondary).

Precocious Puberty

The appearance of physical signs of puberty prior to age 8 years in a girl or before age 9 years in a boy is considered precocious. Therefore, pubertal staging is mandatory in *all* children following irradiation of the HPA, including the very young. Children with clinical evidence of precocious puberty require a hormonal evaluation to confirm the diagnosis. A bone age assessment and GnRH testing are most critical in the initial evaluation of all children with suspected sexual precocity. Additionally, pelvic ultrasonography is a sensitive and noninvasive method of diagnosing and following girls with premature puberty. Because GHD occurs so commonly in patients with postirradiation precocious puberty, and because the growth impairment may be less obvious in this setting, we routinely perform GH testing on all patients with documented precocious puberty.

Thyroid-Stimulating Hormone Deficiency

Basal plasma concentrations of thyroxine, thyroid hormone–binding capacity (e.g., T3 resin uptake), and TSH levels should be obtained on all patients treated with high-dose (more than 30 Gy) radiation to the HPA. A low or borderline level of thyroxine combined with a normal or low level of TSH is highly suggestive of TSH deficiency. A TRH stimulation test may be helpful in confirming the diagnosis. Patients with normal thyroid studies should be retested on a regular basis. It is important to note that patients who are receiving treatment with the anticonvulsants hydantoin or carbamazepine may have a hormonal profile indistinguishable from patients with TSH deficiency; thyroid function studies should be interpreted with caution in these patients. (Hypothyroidism may also result from primary thyroid injury; see Chapter 7.)

Adrenocorticotropin Deficiency

Routine evaluation of the pituitary-adrenal axis is indicated in patients treated with high-dose radiation to the HPA. Because most tests that directly assess pituitary ACTH reserve (e.g., insulin-hypoglycemia, oral metyrapone) are cumbersome and associated with unpleasant side effects, we generally screen our patients initially by drawing a random cortisol level in the clinic. Random cortisol levels greater than 18 µg/dl indicate normal ACTH function; in these patients, no further testing is indicated. If the random cortisol sample is less than 18 µg/dl, one of several provocative tests would be required in order to establish the status of the ACTH-adrenal axis. Periodic reassessment of ACTH reserve is necessary in patients with normal test results.

Hyperprolactinemia

Determining the serum PRL concentration on samples obtained randomly during a clinic visit is generally adequate for the exclusion of hyperprolactinemia. Periodic retesting is suggested in patients treated with radiation doses greater than 50 Gy to the hypothalamus.

MANAGEMENT OF ESTABLISHED PROBLEMS

Growth Hormone Deficiency

Children with documented growth failure and hormonal evidence of GHD are candidates for GH therapy. The initial reports concerning the efficacy of GH treatment in children following cranial irradiation have been disappointing.[4,5,19] The apparent gains in height have been small — much smaller than gains observed in children with idiopathic GHD. There are many factors that are responsible for the poor response of irradiated patients to GH, including spinal irradiation, early puberty with advanced skeletal maturation, delay in the initiation of GH treatment, and the use of suboptimal dosing schedules of GH in the past. It is anticipated that early initiation of GH therapy combined with the use of more contemporary dosing regimens will result in an improvement in linear growth and an augmentation of final height in these patients. It has been our policy to begin GH therapy in all patients meeting the aforementioned clinical and hormonal criteria once all cytotoxic treatment has been discontinued for at least 1 year. At the present time the maximum dosage and dose schedule for GH administration is not known, but most pediatric endocrinologists use 0.20 to 0.35 mg/kg/week given as a daily subcutaneous injection.

The use of GH in individuals treated for a malignancy raises concerns over the risk of tumor recurrence as a result of the growth-enhancing properties of the hormone. Currently there is no evidence that children treated with GH experience an increased rate of relapse of their primary tumor.[11] Recently, leukemia has been observed to have developed in a small number of individuals after treatment with GH.[18] It is, however, unclear whether treatment with GH is associated with an increased incidence of acute leukemia or if individuals previously treated for acute leukemia are more likely to relapse following treatment with GH. At our center, the uncertainties surrounding this important and disturbing issue are discussed with all the families of prospective GH recipients.

Luteinizing and Follicle-Stimulating Hormone Deficiency

Female patients with complete gonadotropin deficiency require combined therapy with an estrogen and a progestin. Older adolescents and young adult women with partial deficiencies may require only intermittent progestin therapy in order to induce periodic endometrial sloughing. The details of hormonal replacement therapy are beyond the scope of this chapter. It is important that this treatment be supervised by an experienced pediatric endocrinologist or gynecologist.

Males with LH deficiency will require androgen replacement therapy. Currently, most specialists use the depot formulations of testosterone given as an intramuscular injection every 2 to 4 weeks.

Precocious Puberty

Therapy to suppress puberty should be considered in patients with early puberty who have a poor predicted final height or who experience significant psychoemotional stress related to their premature development. GnRH analogs are currently the agents of choice for the treatment of precocious puberty. We have found that the depot formulations, which are given monthly, are very effective and readily accepted by patients and their families. Preliminary data suggest that for patients with coexistent GHD, treatment with a GnRH analog and GH can improve final height prognosis.[3]

Thyroid-Stimulating Hormone Deficiency

Daily thyroxine is the standard therapy for this condition. Dosing is generally based on body weight and age — children between the ages of 3 and 10 years require 3 to 4 μg/kg/day of L-thyroxine, whereas adolescents and young adults usually need 2 to 3 μg/kg/day. Dosages must be individually titrated to achieve serum concentrations of thyroxine within the normal range.

Adrenocorticotropin Deficiency

Replacement therapy for ACTH deficiency consists of hydrocortisone in relatively low doses (10 mg/m^2/day, given once in the morning or divided into two daily doses). Any patient with documented ACTH deficiency will require stress doses (50 to 100 mg/m^2 hydrocortisone equivalents) during febrile illnesses or when undergoing anesthesia for a surgical procedure.

Hyperprolactinemia

Therapy aimed at reducing the level of PRL is most often indicated in young women with amenorrhea or infertility whose basal serum concentration of PRL is elevated. Bromocriptine or related dopamine agonists are the agents of choice.

REFERENCES

1. Bajorunas DR et al: Endocrine sequelae of antineoplastic therapy in childhood head and neck malignancies, *J Clin Endocrinol Metab* 50:329-335, 1980.
2. Blatt J et al: Reduced pulsatile growth hormone secretion in children after therapy for acute lymphoblastic leukemia, *J Pediatr* 104:182-186, 1984.
3. Cara JF, Kreiter ML, Rosenfield RL: Height prognosis of children with true precocious puberty and growth hormone deficiency: effect of combination therapy with gonadotropin releasing hormone agonist and growth hormone, *J Pediatr* 120:709-715, 1992.

4. Clayton PE, Shalet SM, Price DA: Growth response to growth hormone therapy following cranial irradiation, *Eur J Pediatr* 147:593-596, 1988.

5. Clayton PE, Shalet SM, Price DA: Growth response to growth hormone therapy following craniospinal irradiation, *Eur J Pediatr* 147:597-601, 1988.

6. Clayton PE, Shalet SM: Dose dependency of time of onset of radiation-induced growth hormone deficiency, *J Pediatr* 118:226-228, 1991.

7. Constine LS et al: Hyperprolactinemia and hypothyroidism following cytotoxic therapy for central nervous system malignancies, *J Clin Oncol* 5:1841-1851, 1987.

8. Leiper AD et al: Precocious and premature puberty associated with treatment of acute lymphoblastic leukaemia, *Arch Dis Child* 62:1107-1112, 1987.

9. Littley MD et al: Radiation-induced hypopituitarism is dose-dependent, *Clin Endocrinol* 31:361-373, 1989.

10. Oberfield SE et al: *Thyroid and gonadal function and growth of long-term survivors of medulloblastoma/PNET*. In Green DM, D'Angio GJ, editors: *Late effects of treatment for childhood cancer,* New York, 1992, Wiley-Liss.

11. Ogilvy-Stuart AL et al: Growth hormone and tumor recurrence, *Br Med J* 304:1601-1605, 1992.

12. Quigley C et al: Normal or early development of puberty despite gonadal damage in children treated for acute lymphoblastic leukemia, *N Engl J Med* 321:143-151, 1989.

13. Rappaport R et al: Effect of hypothalamic and pituitary irradiation on pubertal development in children with cranial tumors, *J Clin Endocrinol Metab* 54:1164-1168, 1982.

14. Rappaport R, Brauner R: Growth and endocrine disorders secondary to cranial irradiation, *Pediatr Res* 25:561-567, 1989.

15. Salomon F et al: The effects of treatment with recombinant human growth hormone on body composition and metabolism in adults with growth hormone deficiency, *N Engl J Med* 321:1797-1803, 1989.

16. Shalet SM, Clayton PE, Price DA: Growth and pituitary function in children treated for brain tumours or acute lymphoblastic leukaemia, *Horm Res* 30:53-61, 1988.

17. Sklar CA: Growth and pubertal development in survivors of childhood cancer, *Pediatrician* 18:53-60, 1991.

18. Stahnke N, Zeisel HJ: Growth hormone therapy and leukaemia, *Eur J Pediatr* 148:591-596, 1989.

19. Sulmont V et al: Response to growth hormone treatment and final height after cranial or craniospinal irradiation, *Acta Paediatr Scand* 79:542-549, 1990.

5

Ocular Complications Due to Cancer Treatment

David H. Abramson
Camille A. Servodidio

The eye is composed of several tissues that vary greatly in their sensitivity to cytotoxic therapy. This chapter focuses on the acute and long-term side effects of radiation therapy (RT) on all structures of the eye, and discusses the medical and nursing management for each of these side effects (Table 5-1).

ANATOMY OF THE EYE AND ADNEXA

The eyes are the body's organs for vision; they are responsible for converting light to impulse messages and then transporting the messages to the brain for interpretation.[26] The ophthalmic system can be divided into two components. The protective component includes the eyelids and eyelashes, the palpebral and bulbar conjunctiva, the periorbital fat pads, the tissue and surrounding skin, the lacrimal apparatus, and seven orbital bones. The sensory/eyeball component consists of the refractive media (cornea, aqueous humor, lens, and vitreous humor); the muscular components (iris, ciliary body, and extraocular muscles); the sensory components (retina and optic nerve); the vascular layer (choroid); and the fibrous connective tissue layer (sclera).[3,26] Each of these structures will be discussed in this chapter (Fig. 5-1).

EYELIDS AND PERIORBITAL SKIN

Anatomy and Physiology

The anterior portion of the eyelids consists of two folds of loose, elastic skin (upper and lower lids are separated by a space, or palpebral fissure) that protect the eyeball and distribute the tears. Fibrous or cartilaginous tissues called tarsal plates help the eyelid maintain its shape. The upper and lower folds of the posterior portion of the reflected conjunctiva are called fornices. The eyelashes are located on the anterior section of the upper and lower lids and function with the lids to protect the eye.

Three glands are located in the eyelids. The meibomian glands, located on the tarsal plate, secrete the sebaceous or lipid layer for tears, lubricate the lid margin, and prevent tear evaporation when one is awake and during sleep. The glands of

111

Table 5-1
Radiation Effects Involving the Eye

Structure	Acute Effect	Long-Term Effect	Medical Management	Nursing Intervention
Eyelids or periorbital skin	Epilation Erythema Dermatitis	Ulceration Telangiectasia Necrosis	Topical steroids Carrington skin balm	Lid hygiene Ultraviolet protection Educate patient about radiosensitizing drugs Avoid trauma, harsh soaps, and lotion
Conjunctiva	Conjunctivitis Chemosis Ulceration	Necrosis Scarring Subconjunctival hemorrhage ↓ Tear production	Steroid or antibiotic drops Tear replacement patching	Teach administration, dose, side effects of drops
Sclera	Injection	Scleral melting	Antibiotic drops	Teach administration of drops Avoid trauma Encourage protective glasses
Cornea	Corneal Epithelial defects Keratitis ↓ Corneal sensation Myopia	Ulceration Neovascularization Keratinization Edema	Tear replacement Antibiotics Soft contact lens Surgery	Teach administration of drops Preoperative and postoperative teaching
Lens		Cataract Glaucoma	Surgical removal	Patient teaching Ultraviolet protection Preoperative and postoperative teaching

Structure	Effect	Treatment	Nursing intervention
Iris	Iritis	Beta-blocker drops; Steroid drops; Atropine; Diamox; Photocoagulation	Teach administration, dose, and side effects of drops. Teach signs and symptoms of $\uparrow$ intraocular pressure
	Iris neovascularization; Iris atrophy	Steroids; Photocoagulation	Teach patient to avoid ASA. Bleeding precautions. Teach patient administration, dose, and side effects of medications
Retina	Retinal edema; Infarct; Exudates; Hemorrhage; Telangiectasia; Neovascularization; Macular edema; $\downarrow$ VA and VF; Optic neuropathy		
Lacrimal glands	None; $\downarrow$ Tear production	Tear replacement; Occlude lacrimal puncta	Teach administration of medications. Avoid rubbing lids, disturbing plugs
Orbit	None; Retarded bone growth; Osteonecrosis; Orbital infection; Radiation-induced malignancy	Antibiotic therapy; Enucleation	Preoperative and postoperative teaching. Prepare patient for loss of eye

ASA = asprin; VA = visual acuity; VF = visual fields.

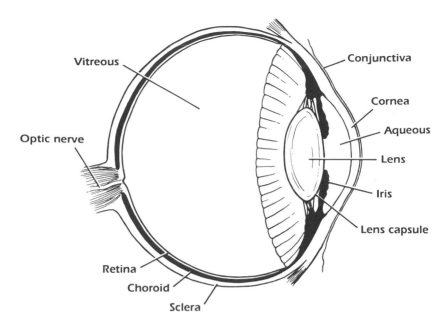

Fig. 5-1. Anatomy of the eye.

Zeis are small, sebaceous glands near the eyelash roots. The glands of Moll are small sweat glands, also near the eyelash roots. The lacrimal puncta are located on the medial canthus of the upper and lower lids and provide an exit orifice for tears produced by the lacrimal system.[3,4,12,35]

Acute Radiation Effects

Epilation, or loss of eyelashes, and erythema are always the first side effects to occur after RT.[19] Usually, the eyelashes will grow back (Fig. 5-2). Erythema can occur within days of the initiation of RT, but it is usually not pronounced until the third week of treatment (generally after doses of at least 20 to 30 Gy); the erythema lasts for a few days. Patient symptoms include redness, peeling, burning, itching, and pain.[32]

The most common acute effect of RT is dermatitis.[38] Dry dermatitis or desquamation and scaling of the irradiated skin can occur after doses of greater than 20 Gy. Moist dermatitis, with exposure of the dermis and serum leakage, can occur after the fourth week of RT following doses of 40 Gy or more fractionated over a 4-week period. Blisters and edema may precede moist dermatitis.[32]

Late Radiation Effects

Late effects of RT to the eyelids include epilation, telangiectasia (enlarged, dilated spidery blood vessels); hyperpigmentation; ectropion (an outward turning of the eyelid); hyperkeratosis; atrophy; necrosis; ulceration; and punctal occlusion — after

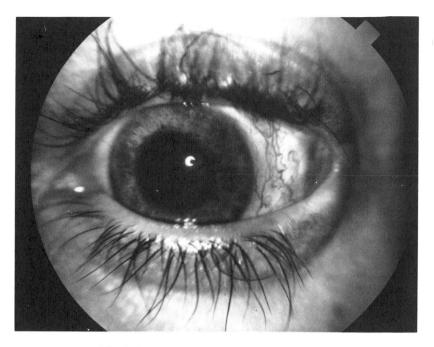

Fig. 5-2.   Epilation, or loss of the eyelashes.

doses ranging from 30 to 60 Gy. Although epilation of eyelashes and eyebrows is an early effect of RT, it can also persist as a late effect, and it may be permanent. Other late effects include hyperpigmentation, which occurs as a result of increased synthesis of melanin approximately 12 months after the completion of RT, and superficial telangiectasia, which occurs 4 to 5 years after the completion of RT.[5,39]

Although rarely seen today, lid deformities such as an ectropion, lid atrophy, or contracture (which occurs when the tarsus is included in the radiation field) are other late effects. Lid necrosis and ulcerations are also rare late effects. These conditions can occur when there is complete destruction of the epidermis (beginning initially as atrophy) or when there has been prior damage of the blood vessels and connective tissue. Time of onset ranges from 2 months to 5 years after treatment. The necrosis or ulceration may be precipitated by infection or intense ultraviolet sun exposure. Destruction or occlusion of the lacrimal punctum may occur when the medial portions of the eyelid are irradiated.[5,19,39]

Medical and Nursing Management

The management for acute radiation effects to the eyelids and periorbital areas can diminish some of the late side effects. Management includes the administration of topical corticosteroid such as 1% hydrocortisone or Carrington skin balm, and punctal probing. Late radiation effects may be remedied by wound debridement, antibiotic therapy, and, rarely, plastic reconstructive surgery. Important nursing interventions include patient teaching about meticulous lid hygiene, encouraging the patient to wear ultraviolet protective sunglasses and sunscreens (with protection of number 15 to 19), and instructing the patient to avoid harsh soaps, lotions, and trauma to the skin.[39] Patients should avoid radiosensitizing drugs such as tetracycline. Written discharge sheets for the patient and family are helpful resources.[16]

CONJUNCTIVA

Anatomy and Physiology

The conjunctiva is the thin, transparent mucous membrane that lines the eyelids and the anterior surface of the sclera.[12] The harmonious relationship between mucin and lacrimal gland production maintains the integrity of the conjunctiva as well as the tearfilm stability.[38] The function of the conjunctiva is to protect the underlying sclera and orbit and to provide moisture to the eye.[12]

The surface of the conjunctiva contains squamous epithelium, goblet cells (which produce the mucin layer of tears), and the sustantia propria.[15] The inner epithelial layer of the conjunctiva is composed of superficial and basal cells.[3]

The accessory lacrimal glands of Krause and Wolfring are located in the conjunctival stroma beneath the superior temporal orbital rim. These glands secrete tears and lysozyme (via the ducts in the upper lid fornix), which in turn protect the conjunctiva and cornea from bacterial invasion.[3,15] At birth, the conjunctiva is sterile, but it is rapidly colonized by saprophytic bacteria. This normal flora protects the eye from more virulent pathogens unless the homeostatic system is compromised.[25]

Acute Radiation Effects

Conjunctivitis, or an inflammation of the conjunctiva, can occur 1 to 3 weeks after the start of treatment; signs include hyperemia, and a clear or purulent discharge.[3,5,15] Chemosis, or edema of the conjunctiva, may occur simultaneously and last for a few days. Duration of these signs may be prolonged when RT doses over 30 Gy are used; then conjunctivitis is complicated by ulceration. There is an increased chance for infection when the conjunctiva becomes ulcerated.[19]

Late Radiation Effects

Late effects of RT to the conjunctiva include prolonged injection, telangiectasia, symblepharon, keratinization, scarring, loss of goblet cells, necrosis, and subconjunctival hemorrhage. With total doses of 30 to 50 Gy, prolonged conjunctival injection and telangiectasia can occur. Injection may occur months after RT and last years, but telangiectasia occurs much later, generally 3 to 6 years after treatment[19] (Fig. 5-3).

Symblepharon, or adhesions from tissue shrinkage and scarring, is another late effect. Symblepharon may lead to limited closure of the eyelids and, hence, dryness of the eye and limited ocular motility.[5,15] Keratinization of the conjunctiva can occur with doses of over 50 Gy and results when the surface epithelium develops

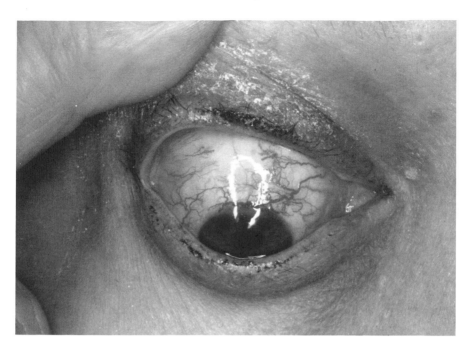

Fig. 5-3.   Telangiectasia of the conjunctival blood vessels.

squamous metaplasia and is transformed into an abnormal, nonsecretory, poorly differentiated dry surface. Tear film becomes unstable owing to radiation-induced loss of goblet cells and mucin deficiency. As a result of this instability, wettability of the tears is poor.[38] Necrosis may occur after radioactive plaque therapy for retinoblastoma patients when the dose to the conjunctiva ranges from 90 to 300 Gy.[37] Subconjunctival hemorrhage is another long-term effect of RT because of the fragility of the telangiectatic blood vessels.[15,19]

Medical and Nursing Management

Antibiotic eye drops are used for prolonged conjunctivitis and for conjunctival ulceration. Corticosteroid ophthalmic drops and ointment are indicated for injection and chemosis. Artificial tears and ointment help replace the moisture lost from damage to goblet cells and keratinization; they also make the eye feel more comfortable.[19] Vitamin A ophthalmic ointment (tretinoin 0.01% or 0.1%) may reverse squamous metaplasia and loss of vascularization from scar formation.[38] Patching the eye or taping the eyelids closed (especially at night) may be helpful for symblepharon. Nursing interventions include patient teaching as to the time, dose, and administration of the eye drops or ointment. Side effects of the drops should also be emphasized (e.g., the side effects of corticosteroid drops include cataracts and glaucoma).[4,35]

CORNEA

Anatomy and Physiology

The cornea is the transparent, avascular anterior portion of the eye that comprises one sixth of the total outer circumference of the eye.[4,35] The function of the cornea is to provide protection for the anterior surface of the eye and to provide two thirds of the refracting power of the eye. The cornea is composed of five layers: the corneal epithelium, Bowman's membrane, the stroma, Descemet's membrane, and the endothelium.[4] The corneal epithelium is the most anterior surface and is continuous with the conjunctiva. Because of the epithelium's ability to regenerate, any damage to this layer heals without scarring. Bowman's membrane is an acellular nonregenerative layer of uniform fibrils that will scar as it heals after injury. The stroma, the thickest layer, comprises 90% of the cornea and consists of collagen fibrils that contribute to the cornea's clarity. Descemet's membrane is an elastic membrane that is the product of endothelial secretion. This membrane is not usually visible on slit lamp (microscopic) examination unless it has been pathologically altered. The endothelium, the innermost layer of the cornea, consists of one single layer of hexagonal cells that acts as a pump mechanism to control the amount of fluid in the cornea and thereby maintains the cornea's transparency. The endothelium does not regenerate; any damage that occurs is permanent and will affect the patient's vision.[4,15,35]

Acute Radiation Effects

The corneal epithelium is directly affected after RT doses of 10 to 20 Gy. Early effects include corneal epithelial defects, acute keratitis, and decreased corneal sensation. When tear production is reduced (after damage to the gland of Krause and Wolfring of the conjunctiva), the cornea will not be properly lubricated, and epithelial defects will be noticed as a result of exposure to air. These defects may persist for months and are best observed with fluorescein stain and a Cobalt blue filter from a slit lamp or from a penlight with a blue filter. Patients may complain of a foreign body sensation and epiphora, or tearing, in the eye.

Keratitis, an inflammation of the cornea, occurs particularly when doses of 50 Gy or more are used to treat the eye. Keratitis may occur in conjunction with conjunctivitis and may last from 4 to 8 weeks.[19] Patients often complain of photophobia when keratitis is present.[35]

Late Radiation Effects

Late RT effects include epithelial desquamation, corneal neovascularization, corneal edema, corneal ulceration, corneal perforation, decreased corneal sensation, and keratinization. Corneal desquamation, or loss of epithelial cells, may persist for months. The irradiated corneal epithelium has a poor capability to heal, despite the growth of new vessels (neovascularization).

If the epithelium continues to erode, ulceration and perforation of the cornea may result. Commonly, these ulcerations are found in the center of the cornea; such ulcerations occur when doses of greater than 40 Gy are used.[2] Because decreased corneal sensation occurs weeks to months after treatment, the child may not complain of pain. Keratinization and scarring result when doses of at least 50 Gy are used and can be more severe with higher doses.[15,19]

Medical and Nursing Management

To lubricate the cornea, artificial tears and ointment can be used. These provide lubrication to the cornea to facilitate epithelial healing. Patching the eye during sleep may also enhance epithelialization. Antibiotic drops and ointment are recommended for keratitis. Infected corneal ulcerations are treated with topical antibiotic drops and ointments. Since the cornea has no blood supply of its own, topical drops and ointment are used as frequently as every 15 minutes to eradicate the infection. Parenteral antibiotics will not be helpful.

Soft contact lenses are sometimes used to promote corneal healing or to decrease corneal edema. Hypertonic tear solutions are also useful for drawing out the excess corneal fluid in corneal edema. Surgical intervention, such as keratoplasty, is required when corneal perforation is pending or apparent. Nursing interventions include teaching the patient the administration, time, dose, and side effects of prescribed ophthalmic drops; providing emotional support for the patient and family; and preoperative and postoperative teaching for surgery when it is indicated. Patients should avoid anything that contributes to the dryness of the eye, such as fans, wind, smoke, and air-conditioning.[22]

LENS

Anatomy and Physiology

The transparent, crystalline, biconvex lens of the eye is formed in utero by infolding ectoderm, the layer that is destined for the epidermis. The encapsulated lens has no nerve or vascular supply after fetal development, is nourished by the aqueous humor and vitreous humor, and is responsible for one third of the refracting power of the eye. The lens lies behind the iris and is suspended by the zonules that are attached to the ciliary body; the lens accommodates by means of the relaxation of the zonules. The anterior portion of the lens is composed of subcapsular epithelium; the lens is completely surrounded by a basement epithelial membrane. Although the central nucleus of the lens is nonmitotic, the preequatorial germinative zone of the lens epithelium is heavy with mitotic activity throughout a person's lifespan. The lens is composed of 65% water and 35% protein.[4,15,35]

Acute Radiation Effects

Within weeks after RT that includes the lens, the patient may complain of a transient myopia that results from edema or increased water content of the lens. This is a rare occurrence.

Late Radiation Effects

A cataract, or an opacity of the lens, is a common long-term consequence of radiotherapy, the occurrence of which depends upon the total dose and fraction-

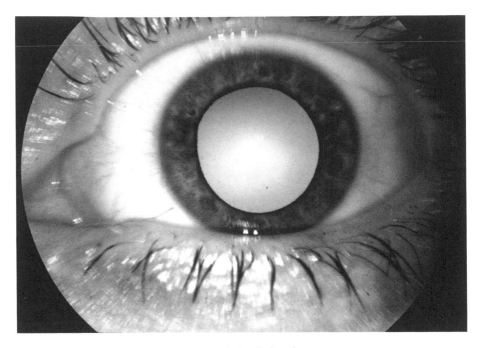

Fig. 5-4. Radiation-induced cataract.

ation.* Because of its ongoing mitotic activity and its inability to remove damaged cells, the lens is the most radiosensitive structure of the eye. Initially, the irradiated epithelial cells of the preequatorial germinative zone are insulted, they stop dividing for 1 to 2 days, and afterward they divide rapidly but produce abortive cells. These abnormal cells migrate to the posterior pole of the lens, fail to elongate, and form a pseudoepithelium of abnormally shaped fibers. These round, often nucleated, bladderlike cells are referred to as "Wedl" cells.[28] The Wedl cells pile up, form fiber layers, and eventually result in a mature, opaque cataract[20] (Fig. 5-4).

Merriam reported that patients who received even one single radiation dose of 200 roentgen (R) later developed lenticular opacities. Patients who received a fractionated dose of 400 R over 3 weeks to 3 months also developed cataracts.[28] Despite fractionation, patients who received more than 1150 R (approximately equivalent to an absorbed dose of 10 Gy) to the lens, always developed cataracts.[19] The latency period for cataract development has been estimated to be 0.5 to 35 years, with an average of 2 to 3 years.[28] The latency period between the radiation exposure and the onset of the cataract is an inverse function of the radiation dose.[28]

Merriam's research also demonstrated that a child's lens is much more sensitive to radiation than an adult's lens and that the potential for cataract formation is greater in children.[28] This increased sensitivity of young lenses seems to be

---

*References 5, 13, 15, 17, 18, 19, 20, 21, 23, 25, 27, 29, 33, 34, 41.

dose-dependent.[28] Some of the flaws from Merriam's paper were that cataract patients were reviewed retrospectively; a wide range of radiation energies (100 to 1200 kVp) was used; dose varied greatly (0.2 to 69 Gy); fractionation varied (one single dose to doses given over 10 years); age varied (from 7 months old to 70 years old); and follow-up was not systemized.

Reports of children treated with different irradiation techniques for retinoblastoma indicate that a total RT dose (fractionated over 3 to 5 weeks) of 8 Gy to 15 Gy will cause cataracts in 6% to 50% of the patients. These cataracts are generally not associated with impaired vision. Higher RT doses will, however, increase the severity of visual impairment from such cataracts.[27,36]

Lappi and co-workers reported that all long-term survivors who were treated with one dose of 10 Gy of total-body irradiation (TBI) for acute lymphoblastic leukemia (ALL) or acute myelogenous leukemia (AML) developed posterior subcapsular cataracts at the end of 3 years. However, because these patients also received high doses of various combinations of chemotherapies, it is hard to exclude the synergistic effects of the chemotherapy in evaluating the cause of the cataracts.[23] Data from Deeg and colleagues emphasize the relevance of dose fractionation to the occurrence of cataracts in the setting of bone marrow transplantation. Less than 20% of patients developed cataracts after 12 to 15.75 Gy in 6 or 7 fractions, in contrast to 80% of patients receiving 10 Gy in a single dose.[14]

Weaver and colleagues showed that whole-brain RT of 24 Gy for prevention of central nervous system (CNS) relapse in ALL patients produced cataracts in 2 of the 16 long-term survivors.[41] The Intergroup Rhabdomyosarcoma Study reported decreased vision from cataract as the most common functional problem of those children treated for orbital tumors with RT and various combinations of chemotherapy.[21]

These described lens changes and cataracts can be viewed by binocular slit lamp microscopy. The first clinical ophthalmic sign of a cataract observed on slit lamp examination is the appearance of dustlike dots noted on the posterior surface of the lens.[20] Later, feathery lines may develop outward from the anterior surface. Finally, the posterior pole becomes opaque and the lens resembles one with a senile cataract.[20] The cataract may also be viewed with the direct ophthalmoscope on a +1.50 setting (the instrument is held approximately 18 inches from the patient) or with a penlight held a few inches from the eye temporally. A distorted or greatly reduced red reflex will be seen when the patient has a dense cataract. The patient's chief complaint will be decreased visual acuity, which is the primary long-term consequence of cataract. The rate of progression of the cataract varies from patient to patient; the cataract may remain stable for years.[19]

Medical and Nursing Management

At the present time, there is no known medical treatment for the prevention or reversal of irradiation-induced cataracts.[19] Prevention of cataracts is best accomplished by fractionation of the RT dose and by lens shielding during treatment.[1] However, there are situations, as in TBI for the treatment of ALL, when the eyes are intentionally left unshielded in order to prevent ocular recurrence of leukemia.[6]

Although surgical removal of the adult or pediatric cataract is rarely mandatory, it may be imperative when the cataract interferes with the patient's ability to carry out activities of daily living. Frequently, it is the patient's (or family's) decision when and if the operation should occur; there is no visual-acuity threshold at which the operation must be performed. Rarely, the lens leaks proteins, causes glaucoma, and necessitates emergency surgery.[15]

Presently, most cataracts in the United States are removed by extracapsular cataract extraction, whereby the anterior capsule, the lens nucleus, and the cortex are removed via a limbal incision. Cataract surgery should occur at least 1 year after RT.[5] Successful surgery is independent of the eye itself; visual results depend upon the child's age when the cataract occurred. If very young children (less than 2 years old) incur a cataract, amblyopia develops and visual results are poor. If the child has normal vision between ages 2 and 6 years, then surgery performed at a later time will be beneficial.[15] The surgery itself is the easy part; compensation for the extracted lens proves to be a challenge for the clinician, the patient, and the family. Although polymethylmethacrylate (PMMA) intraocular lenses are used relatively safely and frequently on adults, there is little long-term follow-up on children who have surgically implanted intraocular lenses.

Contact lenses are also a poor option for children because frequent fittings are necessary, the child loses an average of one lens per week, and the irradiated dry eye may not tolerate the contact lens.[28] A third option is cataract glasses, which, unfortunately, cause a greater magnification in the operated eye and an overall disparity of the visual image.[15] A final, more recently developed technique is epikeratophakia, or corneal transplant. Morgan and co-workers found poor results with epikeratophakia in children with unilateral extracted cataracts. These children were initially diagnosed with rhabdomyosarcoma and were treated with RT and chemotherapy.[30]

Children under 2 years of age who develop monocular cataracts are at risk for amblyopia, or lazy eye. Patching the noncataract eye and forcing the child to see with the cataractous eye can be exhausting, humiliating, and frustrating for both the child and the parents.

Nursing interventions include preoperative and postoperative teaching; the review of antibiotic drop, dose, administration, and side effects; and principles of ultraviolet light protection (sunglasses).

IRIS

Anatomy and Physiology

The iris is a musculovascular diaphragm with a central circular opening called the pupil; it forms the posterior border of the anterior chamber angle.[4,26] The iris stroma is composed of spongy, connective tissue that contains blood vessels, muscle fibers, and pigment cells.[35] The iris is innervated by the involuntary nervous system, and its function is to regulate the amount of light entering the eye. Two muscles found in the iris stroma are the sphincter muscle, which constricts the pupil (parasympathetic nervous system), and the dilator muscle, which dilates the pupil (sympathetic nervous system).[4]

Acute Radiation Effects

Early effects of RT to the iris include an acute iritis (inflammation of the iris) that is due to leakage of protein and cells from the blood vessels in this iris. This iritis is dose-related and can occur after a fractionated dose of greater than 60 Gy over 5 to 6 weeks. The iritis may occur concomitantly with keratitis or corneal ulceration and may be seen on slit lamp examination. Affected patients usually complain of severe photophobia.[5]

Late Radiation Effects

The main long-term effects of RT to the iris include rubeosis iritis (iris neovascularization), posterior synechiae, and iris atrophy. Rubeosis iritis — best seen under the slit lamp — occurs several months to several years after RT with fractionated doses of 70 to 80 Gy over 6 to 8 weeks. Glaucoma may occur when exudates pour into the anterior chamber, the trabecular meshwork becomes clogged with inflammatory cells, and secondary angle closure develops from posterior synechiae (the iris adheres to the lens of the eye). In the past, atrophy of the iris was most often seen more than 3 years after beta-irradiation doses of 170 to 250 Gy. Today, because such high doses are not used, iris atrophy is uncommon.[5]

Medical and Nursing Management

The medical management of iritis includes steroid ophthalmic drops to reduce inflammation and atropine drops to induce cycloplegia to pull the iris away from the lens. Beta-blocker drops and carbonic anhydrase-inhibitors such as acetazolamide may also be used to lower the intraocular pressure. Photocoagulation of the iris is used as a last resort to control the intraocular pressure; this man-made iridotomy provides another outlet through which the aqueous can flow. Nursing interventions include teaching the patient the time and dose of administration of the drops, as well as their side effects. The patient should be taught the signs and symptoms of increased intraocular pressure: headache, eye pain, nausea, and vomiting.

SCLERA

Anatomy and Physiology

The sclera of the eye is the white collagen-fibrous protective layer of the eye. It is 1 millimeter in thickness.[12] The sclera comprises four fifths of the globe, is continuous with the cornea at the limbus anteriorly, and forms the sievelike lamina cribosa posteriorly where the optic nerve exits the eye. The outer surface of the sclera is protected by the episclera — a loose, transparent, vascular tissue.[4,12]

Acute Radiation Effects

The sclera may become injected 2 to 4 weeks after the initiation of RT. This condition is transient and usually resolves on its own.

Late Radiation Effects

The sclera is able to tolerate doses of RT up to 900 Gy from an iodine or cobalt plaque when administered over a 4-day to 1-week period. Thinning, melting, or atrophy of the sclera can occur several years after fractionated RT doses of 20 to 30 Gy helium ion therapy for melanoma. These scleral conditions are uncommon after RT for childhood tumors treated with external beam photons unless extremely high doses are used. When injured, the sclera appears greyish or black and can be viewed with a direct ophthalmoscope or penlight on gross examination. Although scleral perforation can occur, it is rare.[5]

Medical and Nursing Management

Medical treatment for scleral melting can include the administration of aminoglycoside antibiotic drops or tablets when infection occurs. If scleral perforation results, a scleral graft may be necessary. Nursing interventions include teaching the patient the administration and side effects of the drops, and the importance of avoiding trauma and encouraging the patient to use protective glasses for sports and hazard-potential activities.

RETINA AND OPTIC NERVE

Anatomy and Physiology

The function of the retina (the innermost layer of the eye) is to transform light information to the brain for interpretation. The retina is composed of the following 10 layers (from the choroid layer out): 1) the retinal pigment epithelium (RPE), a single layer of cells attached to Bruch's membrane; 2) photoreceptors including rods (twilight vision) and cones (daylight and color vision); 3) external limiting membrane; 4) outer nuclear layer; 5) outer plexiform layer; 6) inner nuclear layer (includes four layers of cell bodies: amacrine, Müller, bipolar, and horizontal cells); 7) inner plexiform layer; 8) ganglion cell layer; 9) nerve fiber layer; and 10) inner limiting membrane (derived from Müller cells).[4,26] The macula, the capillary-free zone that houses the fovea, or area for central vision, is composed of cones and is always located temporal to the optic disc. The peripheral retina is composed mainly of rods.[4]

Acute Radiation Effects Involving the Retina

Although the retina has been reported to be relatively radioresistant, acute injury can occur from irradiation. Transient retinal edema is the main acute effect that can develop during external beam or radioactive plaque therapy; it may be seen several months after treatment with a dose of 20 to 35 Gy fractionated over 2 to 4 weeks or with doses in excess of 50 Gy. This retinal edema usually dissipates in a few weeks.[5,19]

Late Radiation Effects Involving the Retina

Long-term RT effects involving the retina occur 6 months to 3 years or longer after treatment. The retinal injury results from damage to the nutritional blood vessels of the retina and choroid. Radiation retinopathy occurs because of altered vascular supply from obliteration of the retinal vessels and resulting abnormal permeability.[5,19] This may lead to macular edema and macular exudates. Affected patients

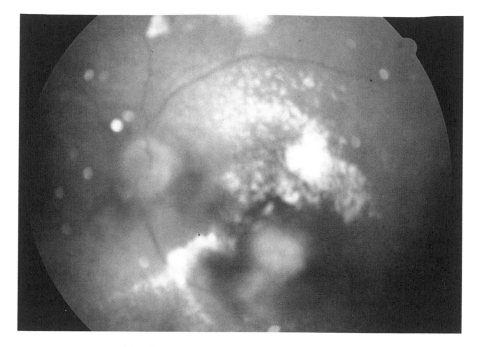

Fig. 5-5.   Radiation retinopathy of the retina.

may complain of blurred central vision or central wavy lines. Neovascularization may result to compensate for the abnormal retinal vessels. These incompetent new retinal vessels leak and bleed, which results in a retinal or vitreous hemorrhage.

Ischemia to the nerve fiber layer of the retina results in infarcts and exudates. Retinal hemorrhages can occur 6 months to many years after RT doses of 30 to 60 Gy fractionated over 3 to 6 weeks.[5] Both total dose and fractionation affect the risk for retinal injury. Whereas most patients treated with greater than 60 Gy in 1.7 to 2.0 Gy fractions will manifest damage, few patients treated with these fractions to 50 Gy or less will suffer damage.[31,40] However, even 35 to 45 Gy can be injurious if daily fraction size is 3.5 Gy or more.[36] Occluded white vessels without any blood flow (ghost vessels) can be seen. Changes in the RPE such as pigmented mottling or atrophy may also be apparent. Other late effects include microaneurysms and telangiectasia (Fig. 5-5). Prolonged vitreous hemorrhage may cause vitreous traction, retinal detachment, and, finally, phthisis bulbi (degenerative shrinkage of the eye). Sometimes enucleation of affected eyes must be performed.[19]

OPTIC NERVE

Late Radiation Effects

Although the optic nerve is composed of relatively radioresistant tissue, optic nerve retinopathy, optic atrophy, neovascularization of the optic disc (the body's mechanism to improve or maintain retinal circulation), and infarcts can occur from 6 months to 2 years after treatment.[5,19] As early as 1933, Stallard documented posterior segment complications from radiation such as RPE changes, exudates, hemorrhages, and optic nerve swelling.[8] Papillitis is frequently associated with radiation retinopathy, and its hallmark signs include disc swelling, peripapillary exudates, and extreme visual loss. Secondary visual loss can also be attributed to optic neuropathy (denoted by disc pallor), ischemic optic neuropathy, and posterior vascular occlusions.[5,19] Brown and co-workers reported optic neuropathy (disc swelling, exudates, hemorrhage, subretinal fluid, and infarcts next to the optic nerve) with total radiation doses of a mean of 125 Gy to the anterior optic nerve (cobalt-60 plaque therapy) and a mean dose of 55 Gy to the optic nerve (external beam radiation).[7] Injury is rare below 50 Gy in 1.8 to 2.0 Gy fractions but common with fractions of greater than 2.5 to 3.0 Gy.[40]

Medical and Nursing Management

Patients may complain of decreased central or peripheral vision as documented by computerized visual fields. Retinal and nerve damage can be viewed with a direct or indirect ophthalmoscope. Fundus photography, or fluorescein angiography, during which a nontoxic dye is injected into a brachial vein to ascertain retinal and choroidal vessel perfusion, may also be helpful to document these long-term effects.

Corticosteroid therapy has been empirically used to ameliorate some of the radiation retinopathy and optic neuropathy. Photocoagulation can be used to seal off some of the leaking blood vessels and to prevent the progression of neovascularization and retinopathy. The authors of this chapter propose that aspirin and aspirin products should be avoided in all patients who have undergone radioactive plaque therapy, as they may precipitate retinal or vitreal bleeding. Finally, in time and without intervention, the hemorrhages of the retina or vitreous may absorb, or macular edema may subside.

Nursing interventions include teaching patients to avoid aspirin products, teaching patients who undergo corticosteroid treatment the relevant side effects, and devising a schedule for tapering the dose.

LACRIMAL GLANDS

Anatomy and Physiology

The lacrimal apparatus consists of the lacrimal glands and their ducts, lacrimal canaliculi, lacrimal sac, and nasolacrimal duct.[12] Each lacrimal gland is located in a fossa behind the temporal superior orbital rim. These glands secrete tears via the 8 to 12 excretory ducts located in the upper lateral aspect of the conjunctival fornix. From the upper fornix, tears travel to the lacrimal sac located in the medial aspect of the eye and exit via the lacrimal puncta of the medial upper and lower lids. The function of the lacrimal gland is to secrete the aqueous layer of tears (water, sodium chloride, and lysozyme) which moisturize and protect the conjunctiva and cornea.[3,4,12]

Acute Radiation Effects

No acute radiation effects to the lacrimal gland are known.

Late Radiation Effects

Atrophy of the gland can occur more than 6 months after treatment with fractionated doses of 50 to 60 Gy over 5 to 6 weeks.[5] This results in decreased tear production and hence a dry eye.

Medical and Nursing Management

Dry eyes are most commonly a result of radiation to the conjunctiva and only partially a result of radiation to the lacrimal gland. The lacrimal gland often cannot be shielded during treatment for retinoblastoma, leukemia, orbital rhabdomyosarcoma, or orbital lymphoma. Medical management includes tear replacement and, less frequently, occlusion of the lacrimal punctum. Nursing interventions include teaching patients the administration, time, dose, and side effects of the drops and instructing the patients to avoid rubbing or pressing on the eye when the puncta plug is in place.

ORBITAL BONES AND TISSUE

Anatomy and Physiology

The orbits are two bony structures located between the cranium and the facial skeleton. The orbital cavity is composed of seven bones: the maxilla, palatine, frontal, sphenoid (greater and lesser wing), zygomatic, ethmoid, and lacrimal bones. The orbital cavities are shaped like quadrilateral pyramids; the orbital apex is where the orbital walls converge.[11] The function of the orbital bones is to protect the eyeball.[3]

Acute Radiation Effects

There are no known acute radiation effects to the orbital bones.

Late Radiation Effects

Orbital RT may cause retarded bone growth, temporal bone suppression, osteonecrosis, purulent orbital infection, phthisical eye (degenerative shrinkage of the eye), soft tissue atrophy, and contracture of the socket years after treatment. The retardation of bone growth is especially noticeable in patients who were treated at a young age with high-dose radiotherapy for bilateral retinoblastoma or for rhabdomyosarcoma. A hollowing of the temporal bone, stunted vertical growth of the orbit, and saddle nose (flattening and shortening of the bridge of the nose) may result[18] (Fig. 5-6). These marked facial deformities can occur years after a dose of 40 to 70 Gy to the orbit fractionated over a 3- to 7-week time period.[5]

Anophthalmic socket syndrome, or soft tissue atrophy and contracture of the socket, has been documented after RT in patients with bilateral retinoblastoma.[29] Osteonecrosis is rare and results only when very high doses of RT are used. The

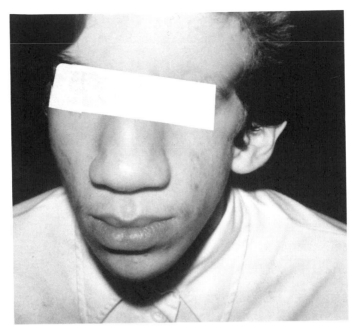

Fig. 5-6.   Temporal bone suppression.

osteonecrosis may or may not be associated with purulent orbital infection. Rarely, the eye may become phthisical. Second nonocular tumors may develop in bone as a long-term consequence of RT.[1]

Medical and Nursing Management

There is no medical treatment to reverse the retardation of bone growth. When osteonecrosis occurs, wound debridement and extensive intravenous antibiotic therapy are required. A phthisical eye may eventually require enucleation. Socket reconstruction is a last resort for poor prosthesis fit due to soft-tissue atrophy or a contracted socket. Nursing interventions include preoperative and postoperative teaching, encouraging patients to ventilate their feelings regarding alteration in body image or loss of body part (enucleation), and preparing the patient for enucleation surgery.

STEROIDS AND THE EYE

Corticosteroid therapy has been associated with the following ocular complications: cataracts, glaucoma, induced uveitis, promotion of herpes virus and fungal infections of the cornea, ptosis, exophthalmos, and enlargement of the pupil. Cataract formation has been described following local or systemic corticosteroid use. These cataracts usually appear in children and adults after several months of daily corticosteroid administration. A posterior subcapsular opacity, which can be viewed by slit lamp microscopy, develops because the lens epithelium contains receptors that have a high affinity for dexamethasone. This relationship has been observed to be dose related; cataracts begin developing when daily doses of over 15 mg of prednisone are taken for 1 year or less. Sometimes the cataracts are arrested or even diminished when the steroid treatment is stopped.[17]

Glaucoma or increased intraocular pressure from repeated steroid use has been widely reported. This relationship is not, however, related to the duration of the exposure, even though the highest pressures develop after several months or years.[18] One third of patients who take daily steroid drops will develop glaucoma within days or weeks. Although systemic steroids can induce glaucoma, this occurs less frequently than with topical steroids. The glaucoma is presumably due to changes in the trabecular meshwork that results in decreased aqueous outflow. Steroid-induced glaucoma does not usually respond as well to standard medical treatment for glaucoma. In most cases, discontinuation of the steroid will decrease the intraocular pressure.[18]

Patients who are treated with steroids for uveitis may develop increased intraocular pressure as a side effect. If the glaucoma is secondary to the uveitis, steroid drops may diminish the inflammation and reduce the intraocular pressure; if the obstruction is due to the uveitis, the intraocular pressure will increase despite steroid therapy. Ptosis of the eyelid may occur with steroid use but is reversible.[18]

Patients need to be informed of the potential side effects from corticosteroid therapy. Verbal and written instruction sheets are helpful. Regular eye examinations are recommended for patients undergoing steroid treatment.

CONCLUSION

The present and future outlook for treatment of childhood cancer is bright and hopeful. Cancers that were once considered fatal and hopeless can today be viewed as "treatable."[10] The current multidisciplinary approach and advanced technologies of RT, chemotherapy, and surgery offer children not only a longer life span, but a life that includes some useful vision.

REFERENCES

1. Abramson DH: The diagnosis of retinoblastoma, *Bull N-Y Acad Med* 64:283-317, 1988.
2. Bessel EM, Henk JM, Whitelock RA: Ocular morbidity after radiotherapy of orbital and conjunctival lymphoma, *Eye* 1:90-96, 1987.
3. Boyd-Monk H: The structure and function of the eye and its adnexa, *JONT* 6:176-183, 1987.
4. Boyd-Monk H, Steinmetz CG: *Nursing Care of the Eye,* Norwalk, Conn, 1987, Appleton & Lange.
5. Brady LW et al: Complications from radiation therapy to the eye, *Front Radiat Ther Oncol* 23:238-250, 1989.
6. Bray LC et al: Ocular complications of bone marrow transplantation, *Br J Ophthalmol* 75:611-614, 1991.
7. Brown GC et al: Radiation optic neuropathy, *Ophthalmology* 89:1489-1493, 1982.

8. Brown GC et al: Radiation retinopathy, *Ophthalmology* 89:1494-1501, 1982.

9. Calman FMB: A symposium on cancer and children: radiotherapy, *Nurs Mirror* 144:56-58, 1977.

10. Campbell A: Tumours of the eye and orbit in childhood, part 2, *Nurs Mirror* 134:26-29, 1972.

11. Cooper WC: A method for volume determination of the orbit and its contents by high resolution axial tomography and quantitative digital image analysis, *Trans Am Ophthalmol Soc* 83:546-609, 1985.

12. Darling V, Thorpe M: *Ophthalmic nursing,* London, 1975, Cassell & Collier Macmillan.

13. Dean G, Alderson M, Maximilien R: Increased risk of cataract patients receiving radiotherapy to the eye: a pilot study, *Br J Radiol* 61:309-311, 1988.

14. Deeg HJ et al: Cataracts after total body irradiation and marrow transplantation: a sparing effect of dose fractionation, *Int J Radiat Oncol Biol Phys* 10:957-964, 1984.

15. Donnenfeld ED, Ingraham HJ, Abramson DH: *Effects of ionizing radiation on the conjunctiva, cornea, and lens* (in press).

16. Eardley A: Radiotherapy: after the treatment's over, *Nurs Times* 82:40-41, 1986.

17. Elliott AJ, Oakhill A, Goodman S: Cataracts in childhood leukaemia, *Br J Ophthalmol* 69:459-461, 1985.

18. Grant WM: *Toxicology of the eye,* Springfield, Ill, 1986, Charles C Thomas.

19. Haik BG, Jereb B, Abramson DH et al: Ophthalmic radiotherapy. In Iliff NT: *Complications in ophthalmic surgery,* New York, 1983, Churchill Livingstone.

20. Hanna C: Cataract of toxic etiology. In Bellows JG, editor: *Cataract and abnormalities of the lens,* London, 1975, Grune & Stratton.

21. Heyn R et al: Late effects of therapy in orbital rhabdomyosarcoma in children. A report from the intergroup rhabdomyosarcoma study, *Cancer* 57:1738-1743, 1986.

22. Hunt L: Dry eye, *Insight* 16:5, 1991.

23. Lappi M, Rajantie J, Uusitalo RJ: Irradiation cataract in children after bone marrow transplantation, *Graefes Arch Clin Exp Ophthalmol* 228:218-221, 1990.

24. Lerman S: *Radiation energy and the eye,* New York, 1980, Macmillan.

25. Limberg MB: A review of bacterial keratitis and bacterial conjunctivitis, *Am J Ophthalmol* 112:2S-9S, 1991.

26. Luckmann J, Sorensen KC: *Medical surgical nursing: a psychophysiologic approach,* Philadelphia, 1980, WB Saunders.

27. McCormick B, Ellsworth R, Abramson D et al: Radiation therapy for retinoblastoma: comparison of results with lens-sparing versus lateral beam techniques, *Int J Radiat Oncol Biol Phys* 15:567-574, 1988.

28. Merriam GR, Worgul BV: Experimental radiation cataract—its clinical relevance, *Bull N Y Acad Med* 59:372-392, 1983.

29. Messmer EP et al: Long-term treatment effects in patients with bilateral retinoblastoma: ocular and mid-facial findings, *Graefes Arch Clin Exp Ophthalmol* 229:309-314, 1991.

30. Morgan KS, Braverman DE, Baker JD: The correction of unilateral aphakia in children treated for orbital rhabdomyosarcoma, *J Pediatr Ophthamol Strabismus* 27:70-72, 1990.

31. Parsons J, Fitzgerald C, Hood C et al: The effects of irradiation on the eye and optic nerve, *Int J Radiat Oncol Biol Phys* 9:609-612, 1983.

32. Radiation therapy, part 8, *Cancer Nurs* 2:233-234, 1979.

33. Radiation therapy: adverse effects, *Nursing* 19:73, 1989.

34. Reifler DM: Radiation sequelae, *CA Cancer J Clin* 36:191-192, 1986.

35. Rooke FCE, Rothwell PJ, Woodhouse DF: *Ophthalmic nursing practice and management,* New York, 1980, Churchill Livingstone.

36. Schipper J, Tan K, vonPeperzeel H: Treatment of retinoblastoma by precision megavoltage radiation therapy, *Radiother Oncol* 3:117-132, 1985.

37. Stannard C et al: The use of iodine-125 plaques in the treatment of retinoblastoma, *Ophthalmic Paediatr Genet* 8:89-93, 1987.

38. Tseng SC: Topical treatment for severe dry-eye disorders, *J Am Acad Dermatol* 15:860-866, 1986.

39. Walder VA: Skin care during radiotherapy, *Nurs Times* 78:2068-2070, 1982.

40. Wara WM et al: Radiation retinopathy, *Int J Radiat Oncol Biol Phys* 5:81-83, 1979.

41. Weaver RG et al: Ophthalmic evaluation of long-term survivors of childhood acute lymphoblastic leukemia, *Cancer* 58:963-968, 1986.

6

Head and Neck

Bernadette Donahue
Cyril Meyerowitz
Steve Handler
Jay Cooper

The head and neck region is affected by treatment of a wide variety of intrinsic and extrinsic tumors. Childhood tumors that can arise within the region (and whose treatment therefore impacts on the structures of the head and neck) include osteosarcomas, rhabdomyosarcomas, Ewing's sarcomas, peripheral neuroepitheliomas (PNETs), juvenile fibrous angiomas, hemangiomas, Burkitt's lymphoma of the jaw, and ameloblastomas. Treatment of the following tumors extrinsic to the region may affect head and neck tissues: central nervous system (CNS) malignancies, Hodgkin's and non-Hodgkin's lymphomas, neuroblastomas, and acute leukemias. The shape of the head and the position of sensitive structures within it may necessitate the inclusion of "normal" head and neck structures in the radiation portals required for therapy of these diseases. Additionally, the head and neck region of children who undergo bone marrow transplantation (BMT) for tumors that may be very distant to this region may experience deleterious late effects of the cytotoxic preparatory regimen (ablative chemotherapy or radiotherapy).

The various normal tissues in a growing child respond to radiation therapy (RT) and chemotherapy in unique fashions. In this chapter, we review the pathophysiology and clinical manifestations of these responses, outline methods for their screening and detection, and suggest interventions that can be used for their management.

PATHOPHYSIOLOGY

Normal Organ Development

The structures of the head and neck region arise from the embryonic branchial arches, which begin to develop early in the fourth week of gestation.[27] Ectoderm, endoderm, and mesoderm, along with migrating neural crest cells and myoblasts, give rise to the specialized structural and functional components of this region. By birth, the skin and mucous membranes, the salivary glands and taste buds, the bones and connective tissue, the deciduous incisor crowns, and the auditory apparatus are all formed.

During the developmental periods of infancy, childhood, and adolescence, the tissues of the head and neck region grow rapidly. It is during this interval that they are most susceptible to the late effects of cytotoxic therapy.

Table 6-1
Development of the Dentition

Tooth	Hard Tissue Formation Begins	Amount of Enamel Formed at Birth	Enamel Completed	Eruption	Root Completed
Primary dentition					
Maxillary					
Central incisor	4 mos in utero	Five sixths	1½ mos	7½ mos	1½ yrs
Lateral incisor	4½ mos in utero	Two thirds	2½ mos	9 mos	2 yrs
Cuspid	5 mos in utero	One third	9 mos	18 mos	3¼ yrs
First molar	5 mos in utero	Cusps united	6 mos	14 mos	2½ yrs
Second molar	6 mos in utero	Cusp tips still isolated	11 mos	24 mos	3 yrs
Mandibular					
Central incisor	4½ mos in utero	Three fifths	2½ mos	6 mos	1½ yrs
Lateral incisor	4½ mos in utero	Three fifths	3 mos	7 mos	1½ yrs
Cuspid	5 mos in utero	One third	9 mos	16 mos	3¼ yrs
First molar	5 mos in utero	Cusps united	5½ mos	12 mos	2¼ yrs
Second molar	6 mos in utero	Cusp tips still isolated	10 mos	20 mos	3 yrs

Permanent dentition

Maxillary

Central incisor	3 - 4 mos	—	4 - 5 yrs	7 - 8 yrs	10 yrs
Lateral incisor	10 - 12 mos	—	4 - 5 yrs	8 - 9 yrs	11 yrs
Cuspid	4 - 5 mos	—	6 - 7 yrs	11 - 12 yrs	13 - 15 yrs
First bicuspid	1½ - 1¾ yrs	—	5 - 6 yrs	10 - 11 yrs	12 - 13 yrs
Second bicuspid	2 - 2¼ yrs	—	6 - 7 yrs	10 - 12 yrs	12 - 14 yrs
First molar	at birth	Sometimes a trace	2½ - 3 yrs	6 - 7 yrs	9 - 10 yrs
Second molar	2½ - 3 yrs	—	7 - 8 yrs	12 - 13 yrs	14 - 16 yrs

Mandibular

Central incisor	3 - 4 mos	—	4 - 5 yrs	6 - 7 yrs	9 yrs
Lateral incisor	3 - 4 mos	—	4 - 5 yrs	7 - 8 yrs	10 yrs
Cuspid	4 - 5 mos	—	6 - 7 yrs	9 - 10 yrs	12 - 14 yrs
First bicuspid	1¾ - 2 yrs	—	5 - 6 yrs	10 - 12 yrs	12 - 13 yrs
Second bicuspid	2¼ - 2½ yrs	—	6 - 7 yrs	11 - 12 yrs	13 - 14 yrs
First molar	at birth	Sometimes a trace	2½ - 3 yrs	6 - 7 yrs	9 - 10 yrs
Second molar	2½ - 3 yrs	—	7 - 8 yrs	11 - 13 yrs	14 - 15 yrs

From Logan and Kronfeld: JADA 20, 1933 (slightly modified by McCall and Schour). Copyright by the American Dental Association. Reprinted by permission.

Growth of the mandible, maxilla, and alveolar ridge takes place from birth to puberty and beyond. The alveolar ridge grows larger and more prominent as teeth erupt. Mandibular growth from the age of 4 years to adulthood is primarily forward, whereas the growth of the maxilla during this time is vertical. Both the maxilla and the mandible undergo substantial growth from birth to 10 years of age, by which time 65% of growth is completed. The remaining growth is completed by 20 years of age. The entire deciduous dentition is completed by the third year. Mineralization of the permanent incisors and first permanent molars starts at birth and continues until the end of the second decade. Table 6-1 summarizes the chronology of development of the dentition. Although the three anatomic components of the ear are fully formed at birth (the auricle and external auditory canal, the tympanic membrane and middle ear, and the inner ear), they continue to grow until they are fully developed by age 5.

Organ Damage and Developmental Effects of Cytotoxic Therapy

The response of tissues to cytotoxic therapy is divided logically into two groups: acute effects and late effects. In a perhaps overly simplistic view, tissues that rapidly or continuously divide are affected by radiation during or shortly after the course of treatment. Cell populations in "late-reacting" tissues are thought to proliferate slowly and may not attempt to divide for months or years after radiation exposure. It is not until they attempt to divide that they die; hence, the gross effects of radiation on these tissues appear to be delayed.[15] It would be misleading to think that no early changes take place in these tissues; in fact, changes likely do occur, but they are not visible with conventional techniques of observation. Although not as well defined, it is likely that late effects of chemotherapy arise in a similar fashion from the effects on slowly dividing cells.

Skin and mucous membranes. The skin and mucosa are composed of rapidly proliferating cells; hence, they manifest reactions early in the course of RT. However, late effects are well documented and primarily result from vascular injury. Histologic studies of irradiated skin suggest that increased vascular permeability leads to deposition of fibrin and subsequent replacement by collagen to form fibrosis in vessel walls and the perivascular interstitial spaces. With the passage of time, increased vascular permeability gives way to decreased vascular perfusion.[30] These effects can result in fibrosis and thinning of vessels, which lead to telangiectasias and atrophy of skin and membranes. Radiation can also stimulate an increase in melanin production leading to permanent darkening of irradiated areas.

Conversely, "cancericidal" doses may destroy melanocytes completely and result in areas of skin that are unable to form pigment.[5] Just as skin and mucosal cells rapidly divide, so do the epithelial cells of the hair follicles. Within an hour of receiving a 5-Gy dose of radiation, mitotic activity of the germinal cells of the hair follicle is interrupted. The more rapidly growing the hair, the more radiosensitive the hair follicle. Higher doses may lead to permanent epilation.

Histologic changes in the mucosa following chemotherapy are variable but are acutely manifested by reddened and ulcerated mucosa occurring 11 to 14 days following the administration of such agents as 5-FU, ara-C, actinomycin D, methotrexate, bleomycin, doxorubicin, vinblastine, and vincristine. The most common changes include epithelial hyperplasia and degeneration of collagen.[21] The buccal and labial mucosa show the highest frequency of histologic changes. In adults, postmortem biopsy specimens have shown that these changes decrease in frequency as time from the last chemotherapy exposure increases, probably reflecting recovery of the mucosa from direct toxic effects of chemotherapy. However, few data are currently available that describe the long-term changes of the mucosa in children exposed to chemotherapy.

Bone and connective tissue. Active bone growth is a characteristic of childhood. Ionizing radiation diminishes the activity and number of osteoblasts while decreasing the vascularity and increasing fibrosis of bone. The most obvious site of radiation injury of bone is at the epiphysis, because this is the main site of potential growth. The number of chondroblasts also decreases, and chondrogenesis is arrested.[37] Normal bone growth can be disturbed, as evidenced by underdevelopment of the flat bones of the head and neck region, the maxilla, or the mandible. Potential effects of radiation on bone also include hypoplasia, deformity, fracture, and necrosis.[29,40] Late-appearing damage of small vessels may lead to difficulty in healing as well as decreased blood supply to adjacent bone.

Growing soft tissues may be similarly affected by radiation. There is an early progressive and sustained deposition of collagen after radiation. The early increase in collagen is possibly due to an inflammatory response and probably reflects enhanced fibroblast proliferation.[25] It may be this fibrosis as well as vascular changes that leads to soft tissue hypoplasia in the growing child exposed to radiation.

Osteoradionecrosis, chondronecrosis, and soft tissue necrosis are occasionally seen as late effects following high-dose radiation exposure. Their occurrence in adults has been documented to be related to dose delivered, rapidity of treatment, and volume irradiated. In the head and neck region, the likelihood of observing necrosis is greater following interstitial implantation of radioactive sources than following external beam teletherapy because of the numerically greater doses used.

Salivary glands and taste buds. Irradiation of the major salivary glands (the parotid, submandibular, and sublingual glands) leads to decreased salivary flow due to atrophy of the secretory cells. Although this response is dose related, dryness of the mouth, alterations in taste, and an increased potential for development of caries are common following cancericidal doses. Serous cells are affected more than mucous cells; the remaining saliva becomes thick and viscous. In adults, permanent pathologic changes can be seen in the glands beginning a few weeks to months following "curative" (more than 50 Gy) irradiation. There is patchy destruction of nearly all acini. The ducts become dilated, surrounded by inflammatory changes, and eventually surrounded by fibrosis.[14] Although serum concentrations of amylase rise during RT, these levels return to normal as treatment continues.[42] The acute effects of chemotherapy on saliva production have been examined,[23] but there is little evidence that cancer chemotherapy has a long-term effect on salivary gland function.

Modification in taste occurs mainly as a result of changes in the oral mucosa and saliva.[24] Patients retain the perception of sweet and salt more readily than that of sour and bitter,[2] which may lead some patients to increase their intake of sugarladen foods, resulting in an environment conducive to caries production. Although the taste buds have been considered to be relatively radioresistant, it has been proposed that some taste alterations may be caused by damage to the microvilli of the taste cells.[10]

Teeth. The effect of radiation on the dentition in children is influenced by the developmental stage of the tooth (Table 6-1), with the most severe disturbances occurring when radiation is given to children younger than 6 years of age.[6,39] These abnormalities include tooth and root agenesis, enamel dysplasias and opacity, incomplete calcification, microdontia, premature apical closure, arrested root development, and abnormal eruption. Studies of the dental effects of cancer chemotherapeutic agents administered independent of radiation,[19,31,33,35,36] have identified malocclusion, enamel hypoplasia, hypodontia, microdontia, enamel opacities, supernumerary teeth, enlarged pulp chambers, altered root development, marked shortening of premolar roots, and thinning of the roots and root constrictions. These abnormalities are thought to occur from the impact of chemotherapy on ameloblasts, odontoblasts, and cementoblasts during development.

Ear. Irradiation of the external, middle, and inner ear is not uncommon in children who have soft tissue sarcomas of the head and neck region or in children who have tumors arising in the brain stem or posterior fossa.

Chronic radiation otitis is the most common otic late effect of radiation. During a typical course of RT, the columnar epithelium lining the middle ear and covering the ossicles desquamates, and the mucosa becomes edematous. After these acute changes resolve, residual fibrosis and permanent scarring may be present. Permanent hearing loss secondary to RT may be due to interference with the conduction pathway, sensorineural abnormalities, or, rarely, necrosis of the ossicle.

The cartilaginous canal acutely responds to therapy by desquamating and forming false membranes, as well as decreasing cerumen production, resulting in hard plugs of wax and desquamated skin. Long-term effects can include stenosis or even necrosis of the cartilage of the canal. Similarly, the cartilage of the external ear can develop chondronecrosis.

Cisplatin, either alone or in combination with other agents, may lead to substantial hearing loss. This effect is related directly to the dose and inversely to the patient's age. Ifosfamide, as a single agent, is not known to be directly ototoxic, but its use prior to platinum appears to potentiate the ototoxicity of cisplatin.[26] Animal studies have shown loss of hair cells over the complete length of the basilar membrane as the likely etiology of hearing loss following platinum exposure.[28,41]

CLINICAL MANIFESTATIONS OF LATE EFFECTS

Skin and Mucous Membranes

Late effects of radiation on the mucosal linings of the upper aerodigestive tract are characterized by paleness and thinning of the epithelium, with loss of mucosal pliability, submucosal induration, and occasionally chronic ulceration and necrosis with exposure of underlying bone or soft tissue. The mucositis and acute inflammation that affect the lining of the oral cavity, the nose, and the paranasal sinuses usually resolve over time. However, several changes may persist to cause chronic problems. Intranasal scarring may interfere with normal nasal mucous production and sinus drainage. The consequence of this alteration in normal nasal physiology is a propensity to recurrent acute and chronic rhinosinusitis. Symptoms of chronic sinusitis include chronic nasal discharge, postnasal drip, nasal obstruction, facial pain, and headache. Because these effects are primarily dose related, children who receive direct radiation to the oral and sinal mucosa for tumors intrinsically involving this region are most at risk. Examples include rhabdomyosarcoma, Ewing's sarcoma or PNETs, osteosarcomas of the mandible or maxilla, and Burkitt's lymphoma of the jaw. Children who receive doses in excess of 40 Gy are most susceptible.

Most children develop some erythema and hyperpigmentation of the skin in the area of radiation during and shortly following treatment. The current use of megavoltage (above 2 MV) radiation, however, has resulted in relative skin sparing, and thus, a decrease in the permanent hyperpigmentation, telangiectasias, atrophy, or dryness that were seen more frequently in the orthovoltage era. These sequelae are now seen only when the skin requires larger radiation doses than are typically given children.

Epilation usually begins after 3 to 4 weeks of radiation administered at 1.8 Gy to 2 Gy per day and may be permanent following total doses greater than 40 Gy.[8] The scalp typically is affected both in the entrance and exit of the beams. Because the loss of hair occurs at the follicle, regrowth is usually not seen until 4 to 6 months after the completion of RT. When hair regrows, the color may be altered secondary to destruction of melanin producing cells. The texture may also be finer.[5] Children at highest risk of experiencing permanent hair loss include those with primary CNS malignancies. The area of permanent epilation is dictated by the site of the primary tumor. For example, children who have medulloblastomas currently receive a dose of 36 Gy to the whole brain and a total of 54 Gy to the posterior fossa; therefore, the most likely area of permanent hair loss will be the area that received the highest dose (i.e., over the posterior fossa). Children who have parameningeal rhabdomyosarcomas who receive doses on the order of 45 Gy to 50 Gy may experience permanent hair loss in the temporal region (depending upon beam arrangement).

Although the use of antineoplastic chemotherapeutic agents (most commonly doxorubicin, cyclophosphamide, or actinomycin) can result in alopecia, this is usually reversible with hair regeneration beginning 1 to 2 months after therapy is discontinued. As with hair regrowth following RT, alteration in the color and texture of the hair may occur.[13]

Bone and Connective Tissue

Bone and soft tissues in the head and neck region are most immediately and obviously affected by surgical procedures that require resection of these tissues as part of the primary surgical management. These surgical procedures can result in craniofacial deformities requiring reconstruction using either synthetic or natural prostheses. The effects of RT or chemotherapy on the bone and soft tissue are seen at a much later date. Long-term effects of RT on the head and neck region include loss of elasticity, constricting fibrosis, soft tissue ulcers, soft tissue necrosis, and osteoradionecrosis. Persons who receive radiation to these regions in childhood are also subject to alterations in the growth of bone and soft tissue.

In 1984, Jaffe reported the maxillofacial abnormalities observed in long-term survivors of childhood cancer at a median of 12 years following treatment (range 2 to 24 years).[19] Forty-five patients had received megavoltage radiation to the maxillofacial region (43 patients had also received chemotherapy including vincristine, actinomycin-D, cyclophosphamide, methotrexate, 6-mecaptopurine, prednisone, procarbazine, or nitrogen mustard in various combinations). The maxillofacial abnormalities noted included trismus, abnormal occlusal relationships, and facial deformities. The most severe deformities were seen in the children who received higher radiation doses at an earlier age. Children who were irradiated for Hodgkin's disease or leukemia had few abnormalities; these children had received median doses of 30 Gy and 24 Gy, respectively. In contrast, children who received radiation for rhabdomyosarcomas received a median dose of 55 Gy. Forty-five percent of these children were found to have trismus; 50% were found to have maxillary and/or mandibular and facial deformities.

Fromm's series of 20 children treated for soft tissue sarcomas of the head and neck supports the concept that growth abnormalities are related to age and dose.[16] All 16 children who were 9 years of age or younger at the time of treatment developed facial growth abnormalities; the 4 children who were over the age of 10 years manifested no abnormality. The degree of deformity appeared to correlate with the dose: the 7 patients classified as "mild" had received doses 40 Gy to 50 Gy, the 4 classified as "moderate" had received 40 Gy to 54 Gy, and the 5 classified as "severe" had received 50 Gy to 60 Gy. Mild and moderate deformities were identified 5.1 and 4.9 years after therapy, respectively, whereas patients who had severe deformities were identified at a median follow-up of 8.6 years. It is therefore possible that some children who had mild or moderate growth abnormalities will go on to manifest severe abnormalities in time.

Sonis, in a study of 97 children with acute lymphoblastic leukemia (ALL) who received chemotherapy and 24 Gy to the cranium, found a 90% incidence of craniofacial abnormalities, primarily mandibular underdevelopment.[39] This probably is explained by the inclusion of the temporomandibular joints and proximal mandible within the radiation portals.

In addition to growth abnormalities, long-term effects on connective tissue and bone may manifest as fibrosis or osteonecrosis, respectively. Two patients in Sonis' series developed fibrosis of the neck that resulted in facial asymmetry, and 3 developed temporomandibular joint fibrosis with limitation of jaw motion.[39]

Osteoradionecrosis in adults is a well-known, although now uncommon, complication of high-dose RT to the head and neck region; it predominantly occurs in the mandible. Risk factors for its development include xerostomia and subsequent trauma, such as dental extractions. There is, however, no literature describing its incidence in children and adolescents.

Chemotherapy alone appears to have little influence on the development of bony or soft tissue abnormalities. Twenty-three children treated at the MD Anderson Cancer Center who received chemotherapy alone for tumors outside the head and neck region manifested no craniofacial abnormalities.[19]

Children at highest risk for developing impaired bone or soft tissue growth include those whose tumors necessitate high-dose radiation because of their types or locations (e.g., brain tumors requiring cranial or craniospinal radiation, the latter with fields that exit through the mouth; soft tissue sarcomas of the head and neck region).

Salivary Glands and Taste Buds

The long-term effects of RT and chemotherapy on the salivary glands and taste buds of children can have profound implications on their dental and nutritional status and thus their overall well-being. Saliva is essential for maintaining oral health. Salivary gland dysfunction may occur when one or more of the major salivary glands is included in a radiation port. Permanent salivary gland damage causes xerostomia that predisposes to dental caries and decay, which in turn can lead to osteoradionecrosis. Even though the taste buds are relatively resistant to radiation, the changes in saliva modify the patient's ability to perceive the taste of food.[24] Increased amounts of sweets are required to satisfy most patients' tastes, leading to increased ingestion of foods high in sugar content, which in turn leads to an environment conducive to the development of caries.

Both the radiation dose and volume of salivary glands exposed are relevant to the likelihood of developing permanent xerostomia in adults. Severe effects are most commonly seen after doses on the order of 50 Gy to 70 Gy. It is likely that xerostomia in children is similarly related to volume and dose.

In 1986, Fromm described 20 children who had soft tissue sarcomas of the head and neck treated from 1972 through 1981.[16] These children were evaluated for deleterious late effects at a median of 5.5 years following RT. All patients had received radiation and combination chemotherapy with vincristine, dactinomycin, and cyclophosphamide; some had received doxorubicin as well. The median age at the time of treatment was 6 years. Eight of 11 parotid glands that had received doses of at least 45 Gy to greater than 50% of the volume failed to secrete saliva thereafter. All glands that received 40 Gy or less retained their ability to secrete.

Although it has been shown that patients treated for acute leukemia with chemotherapy, but no RT, experience alterations in salivary function,[23] data describing permanent damage are not available. However, patients who undergo BMT and receive aggressive chemotherapy (with or without RT) may be at risk for long-term complications. Xerostomia has been noted in the patients with chronic graft-versus-host disease.[1] Although the xerostomia usually resolves within 6 months of onset, it has been seen to persist as long as 1 year later. During this time, these patients are at high risk of developing dental caries.

Children at highest risk of developing long-term xerostomia are primarily those in whom greater than 50% of the parotid tissue receives doses equal to or greater than 40 Gy, for example those with head and neck soft tissue sarcomas. Although children with ALL frequently receive radiation to a cranial field that by necessity treats a portion of the parotids in an attempt to cover the meninges, the parotid volume is relatively small and the doses are usually on the order of 18 to 24 Gy. Therefore, such treatment should not result in permanent xerostomia. Patients who receive craniospinal radiation for medulloblastoma receive doses on the order of 36 Gy to a portion of the parotids and, therefore, are probably at an increased risk. Additionally, for medulloblastoma, the fields used to treat the spine may exit through the mouth, thereby irradiating additional salivary tissue and placing these children at greater risk for altered salivary function. Patients who receive equal to or greater than 40 Gy for Hodgkin's disease, where portions of the parotid, submandibular, sublingual, and minor salivary glands are exposed, have been documented to have flow rate reductions of about 55%.[3]

Teeth

The late effects on the dentition of children who have been treated for malignancies have two etiologies: the cytotoxic effects on the growing tooth buds, and indirect effects resulting from salivary gland damage. As discussed previously, permanent salivary gland damage causes irreversible xerostomia. Even in adults, whose dentition is completely formed, xerostomia results in rampant caries unless appropriate prophylactic measures are taken.

The severity and frequency of long-term dental complications due to RT are related to the type of RT given, the total dose, the size and location of the ports, and the age of the patient. Doses of less than 1 Gy can arrest the growth of tooth buds, and doses greater than 1 Gy can completely destroy buds.[24] Dental abnormalities have been well documented in children who received radiation during tooth and bone development.[4,12,18,34] In Jaffe's series, 37 of the 45 children who received RT to the region developed dental abnormalities.[19] These included root and crown abnormalities in the majority of patients treated for Hodgkin's disease, root and crown abnormalities in the maxillary permanent first molar teeth in 2 of 14 children who received cranial radiation for leukemia, and caries in almost 50% of the children irradiated for head and neck sarcomas. In Fromm's study of children receiving RT for head and neck sarcomas (doses of 40 to 60 Gy), 15 patients received dental evaluations 2 to 10 years after RT (median follow-up 6 years).[16] Fourteen of the 15 experienced root crown defects, radiation caries or absent parotid secretions. Eleven children showed foreshortening or agenesis of their developing teeth; 9 had crown defects as well. Dahloff, in a study of the dental outcome of 16 children treated by BMT (single-dose total body irradiation of 10 Gy and intensive chemotherapy), found impaired root development in all patients.[7]

This included root agenesis, premature apical closure, enamel hypoplasia, and microdontia. Children younger than 6 years of age experienced the most severe and extensive dental abnormalities.

Although the impact of chemotherapy alone on developing dentition has been less well studied, some data suggest adverse outcomes following chemotherapy. In one study comparing 52 children in remission from cancer to 41 of their siblings, the cancer patients who had received chemotherapy alone (or RT distant from the jaw) had significantly more dental abnormalities than their siblings.[31] In this study, there was no difference in caries between the treated and control groups.

In Jaffe's study, 23 children received chemotherapy alone (vincristine, actinomycin-D, cyclophosphamide, methotrexate, 6-mercaptopurine, prednisone, procarbazine, and nitrogen mustard) for tumors remote from the maxillofacial region.[19] Five of these children (22%) developed acquired amelogenesis imperfecta, microdontia of bicuspid teeth, and a tendency toward thinning of roots with an enlarged pulp chamber. Rosenberg evaluated the impact of combination chemotherapy on tooth development in 10 children treated before 16 years of age.[36] A 63% to 84% reduction in premolar root length was found when compared with historical controls. Purdell-Lewis, in a study of the dental health of 45 children who had received chemotherapy during tooth formation, found a very high incidence of disturbed amelogenesis and aesthetically displeasing enamel alterations.[35] Pajari assessed the prevalence of enamel opacities in 37 treated patients and noted a greater incidence of enamel opacities than in a control group, although these opacities were described as mild.[33]

Histologic examination of extracted teeth that were exposed to chemotherapy during developmental periods has shown increased prominence of incremental lines that correlate with chemotherapy exposure, most notably vincristine.[22,45]

Studies of the impact of chemotherapy on the development of dental caries are somewhat equivocal. Some have demonstrated an increase in the frequency of, or susceptibility to, dental caries, while others have shown no difference in patients compared with control subjects. Purdell-Lewis, using "control" data from caries epidemiologic studies, found a higher caries prevalence in 45 children who had received chemotherapy.[35] Pajari obtained control data from randomly selected school children of the same age, sex, and social background and found increased numbers of caries in children treated for cancer.[32] However, Nunn compared 51 children who had received chemotherapy and cranial RT for leukemia with 41 of their siblings and found no significant difference in the incidence of dental caries.[31] Similar results were reported by Maguire.[22] These differences may be explained by variations among the series in treatment regimens, thoroughness of evaluation, and prophylactic care.

Ear

Irradiation of the ears to relatively high doses is not uncommon in children who have malignancies of the head and neck region. Children most likely affected are those treated for parameningeal sarcomas, nasopharyngeal lymphomas, brain stem gliomas, and primary brain tumors that arise in the posterior fossa, such as medulloblastomas and ependymomas. Although many children who have acute leukemia receive irradiation of the cranium (which includes irradiation of the ears), the doses employed are on the order of 18 to 24 Gy and severe late effects are rare.

Chronic otitis is the most common long-term otic sequela associated with high-dose radiation. It typically begins several months after radiation and is characterized by dryness and thickening of the canal and the tympanic membrane. Thickened tympanic membranes do not transmit sound efficiently to the middle ear, leading to a conductive hearing loss. However, radiation-induced deafness appears to be rare. Perforations of the drum also may result from chronic infection and can lead to conductive hearing loss. The dose absorbed by the ear appears to be critical. In Goldwein's series of pediatric patients treated for primary brain tumors, 70% of those receiving doses greater than 50 Gy developed chronic radiation otitis.[17] However, in Fromm's series where the median middle ear dose was 30 Gy, only 1 of 25 children developed a thickened tympanic membrane.[16]

Although children treated with high radiation doses (more than 50 Gy) with older RT techniques (in the 1950s and 1960s) experienced mixed perceptive and conductive hearing losses,[9,20] recent data on children treated with 54 to 60 Gy at St. Jude's hospital revealed normal mean hearing thresholds between 1000 and 8000 Hz; no patient had thresholds less than 25 dB at 500 to 4000 Hz.[26]

The auricle and external ear canal can incur other late effects following high-dose radiation. The cerumen glands present in the lateral portion of the external auditory canal may decrease their production, and the resulting wax becomes hard and encrusted. This can cause hearing impairment as well as trap moisture, which increases the susceptibility to otitis externa. If the radiation dose has been high enough to damage the underlying cartilage of the auricle, chondritis will develop. This can progress to necrosis of the cartilage and may result in permanent disfigurement of the ear (cauliflower ear) and facilitate infection. Shrieve has reported such chondronecrosis in children who had received very high-dose radiation (hyperfractionated to a total of 78 Gy) for primary brain stem gliomas, although its incidence appears rare.[38]

Antineoplastic agents, most notably cisplatin, may produce substantial hearing loss. Ototoxic damage due to platinum results initially in high-frequency loss, followed by damage that can be demonstrated in the conventional pure tone audiogram.[43] Patients may experience tinnitus or vertigo in addition to hearing loss. The hearing loss induced by cisplatin is generally bilateral, symmetrical, and irreversible. The deficit has been shown to be directly related to the dose of platinum and inversely related to the patient's age.[43] Ifosfamide, when given as a single agent, does not appear to be ototoxic, but its administration prior to platinum administration appears to potentiate ototoxicity.[26] The combination of cranial radiation and platinum has an additive effect and may have a synergistic effect as well. McHaney showed that the sequencing of these two modalities may influence the degree of hearing loss.[26] Children who received platinum after prior radiation experienced more profound hearing deficits, as compared with those children whose chemotherapy preceeded RT. Children most at risk of experiencing platinum-based hearing loss include those with primary brain tumors, osteosarcoma, germ cell tumors, and neuroblastoma because these children are most likely to receive platinum as part of their chemotherapy regimen.

DETECTION AND SCREENING

Just as the cure of children who have malignancies is best accomplished by a multidisciplinary approach, the evaluation and treatment of late effects requires the efforts of many specialists.

Children who have received RT and chemotherapy benefit from careful and thorough dental and radiologic examination, the latter including periapical and panoramic views to assess the impact on crown and root development. This is particularly important if children are to undergo orthodontic therapy. With extraction of permanent teeth or movement of teeth, alterations in dental root development might place teeth in substantial jeopardy. As children age, the possibility of periodontal bone loss becomes important. Abnormal root development or shorter roots may predispose a tooth to premature loss. The importance of early recognition of abnormal root development and careful attention to periodontal prophylaxis, such as plaque control and professional cleaning, becomes a particularly important factor in these patients because tooth loss or infection can instigate osteoradionecrosis.

The ramifications of xerostomia on dental health are extremely serious. Assessment of salivary flow rate and appropriate dental prophylaxis in patients with impaired salivary function may help prevent dental caries. Counseling to maximize oral hygiene should be offered. Patients at high risk should be considered for prophylactic fluoride applications using a gel held in contact with the teeth by a tray.[11,44] Alterations in taste may lead to alterations in diet, and patients can be counselled on the importance of dietary control to prevent frequent consumption of fermentable carbohydrates. Frequent visits to the dentist may facilitate detection of increased caries activity, early periodontal diseases, infections, and gingival recession, as well as aid in the assessment of tooth support. Examination of the oral soft tissues may identify ulceration and other abnormalities.

Given the risk of craniofacial abnormalities resulting from radiation effects on bone and soft tissues, screening in children who have received high-dose radiation may identify potential problems with jaw movement.[22] Trismus, crepitus, limited mandibular movement, and abnormal growth associated with the temporomandibular joints may be found.

Routine ear, nose, and throat evaluation, including inspection of the oral mucosa for any signs of ulcers, can be included in the screening process. Indirect and direct laryngoscopy and nasopharyngoscopy can be used to assess the mucosa, as well as to look for evidence of nasal scarring that may interfere with the movement of mucus and normal sinus drainage, leading to recurrent sinusitis. The auricle as well as the skin and soft tissue of the head and neck may show signs of atrophy, fibrosis, or ulceration. Thin skin is particularly susceptible to injury from what would seem to be minor trauma. Because the blood supply to irradiated skin may be impaired, seemingly minor trauma can lead to the development of infection and necrosis. Otoscopic exam can detect impaction of cerumen and tympanic scarring, both of which can lead to conductive hearing loss. The area can also be examined for otitis externa, otitis media, or perforations of the tympanic membrane. Audiometry can be used to assess those children who have received cisplatin or high-dose radiation to the inner ear. Lastly, screening evaluation needs to include evaluation for second malignancies.

MANAGEMENT OF ESTABLISHED PROBLEMS AND REHABILITATION

Oral Cavity

Dental evaluation and treatment of any existing problems (e.g., the repair of caries, extraction of decayed teeth) before initiating cancer therapy minimizes the risk of late effects. However, late effects may still develop. Vigilant attention should be paid to caries, periodontal disease, and gingivitis. If teeth need to be extracted in the postradiation setting, gentle handling is required. Tight sutures should be avoided. Irradiated tissue is susceptible to minor trauma, which may lead to infection and necrosis. However, antibiotics can lessen the risk of infection. Alveolar bone should be evenly trimmed and smoothed so that primary closure is possible. Atraumatic care must be given in the use of endodontics and orthodontics.

Infections as well as caries may result from xerostomia. Patients who have dry mouths may benefit from saliva substitute as well as prophylactic fluoride treatments and appropriate dietary counseling. Fungal infections (which typically are fostered by xerostomia) can be treated with appropriate antifungal medication either topically (swish and swallow) or systemically.

Bone and Connective Tissue

Management of bony or soft tissue abnormalities secondary to altered growth may require dental, orthodontic, and oral surgical therapy as part of a comprehensive rehabilitation program. Surgical procedures and orthodontic and prosthetic intervention must be undertaken with the knowledge that irradiated tissue is more susceptible to trauma and infection and may heal more slowly than expected.

When the muscles of mastication have been involved in the radiation field, edema and fibrosis may result. This can lead to a decrease in patients' ability to open their mouths, which can lead to alterations in nutritional habits and a decrease in oral hygiene, which may result in caries. "Stretching" exercises, in an attempt to minimize microstomia, should be instituted.

Although necrosis of soft tissue or bone infrequently occurs, it can result in major morbidity if not properly managed. Antibiotics may be indicated to help control swelling or suppuration and resultant pain. Care must be taken to avoid trauma that can initiate necrosis, and topical or systemic antibiotics should be considered even for patients with seemingly minor injuries. Conservative management of necrosis is frequently effective; however, if it is not, surgical debridement and removal of the bone or cartilage to control infection may be warranted.

Ears

Chondritis should be managed similarly to other soft tissue or bony damage, with appropriate antibiotics and surgical intervention when necessary. It should be kept in mind that attempts at reconstructing the auricle are hampered by impaired blood supply.

Periodic cleaning of the ear canal may be necessary to remove impacted wax. Cerumen-softening agents may be used to soften or loosen wax. Episodes of otitis externa, which are characterized by discharge from the canal and are associated with ear pain and tenderness, require cleaning of the ear and the use of topical otic drops. Keeping the ear dry is the best way to prevent recurrent bouts. Wearing occluding ear plugs when swimming or washing hair is recommended. A drying solution may be considered as long as the tympanic membrane is intact. Acute otitis media or persistent secretory otitis media may require treatment with antibiotics and decongestants. Myringotomy and placement of pressure-equalizing tubes is required in children who do not respond to conservative medical therapy. If decreased hearing is suspected, complete otologic examination is appropriate. If hearing loss is found, a recommendation should be given for preferential seating at school. Intervention with amplification may be necessary.

CONCLUSION

Surgery, RT, and chemotherapy all play important roles in improving survival despite childhood malignancies. However, they may result in late effects on the structure and function of the tissues of the head and neck region. These effects often are not manifested until years after treatment is completed and therefore necessitate prolonged, vigilant follow-up and monitoring of these patients. Early recognition of complications by a multidisciplinary team can decrease the adverse impact of late effects on the quality of life for survivors.

REFERENCES

1. Berkowitz RJ, Feretti GA, Berg JH: Dental management of children with cancer, *Pediatr Ann* 17:715-725, 1988.
2. Bonanni G and Perazzi F: Variations in taste sensitivity in patients subjected to high energy irradiation for tumors of the oral cavity, *Nucl Radiol* 31:383-397, 1965.
3. Bucker J et al: Preliminary observations on the effect of mantle field radiotherapy on salivary flow rates in patients with Hodgkin's disease, *J Dent Res* 6:518-521, 1988.
4. Burke FJ, Frame JW: The effect of irradiation on developing teeth, *Oral Surg Oral Med Oral Pathol* 47:11-13, 1979.
5. Chahbazian CM: *The skin in radiation oncology.* In Moss WT, Cox JD, editors: *Radiation oncology,* St Louis, 1989, Mosby–Year Book.
6. Dähllof G et al: Effect of chemotherapy on dental maturity in children with hematological malignancies, *Pediatr Dent* 11:303-306, 1989.
7. Dähllof G et al: Disturbances in dental development after total body irradiation in bone marrow transplant recipients, *Oral Surg Oral Med Oral Pathol* 65:41-44, 1988.

8. Deutsch M: Radiotherapy in the management of childhood brain tumors, Norwell, 1990, Kluwer.

9. Dias A: Effects on the hearing of patients treated by irradiation in the head and neck area, *J Laryngol Otol* 80:276-287, 1966.

10. Donaldson SS: Nutritional consequences of radiotherapy, *Cancer Res* 37:2407-2413, 1977.

11. Dreizen S et al: Prevention of xerostomia-related dental caries in irradiated cancer patients, *J Dent Res* 56:99, 1977.

12. Dury, DC et al: Dental root agenesis secondary to irradiation therapy in a case of rhabdomyosarcoma of the middle ear, *Oral Surg Oral Med Oral Pathol* 57:595-599, 1984.

13. Editorial, *Lancet* 2:1177-1178, 1983.

14. Evans JC, Ackerman LV: Submaxillary irradiated and obstructed salivary glands simulating cervical lymph node metastases, *Radiology* 62:550-555, 1954.

15. Fowler JF: The linear-quadratic formula and progress in fractionated radiotherapy, *Br J Radiol* 62:679-684, 1989.

16. Fromm M et al: Late effects after treatment of twenty children with soft tissue sarcomas of the head and neck, *Cancer* 57:2070-2076, 1986.

17. Goldwein JW: *Ototoxicity of radiotherapy and chemotherapy in children,* Second Annual International Symposium on Pediatric Neuro-Oncology, Philadelphia, 1990.

18. Helpin ML, Krejmas NL, Krolls SO: Complications following radiation therapy to the head, *Oral Surg Oral Med Oral Pathol* 61:209-212, 1986.

19. Jaffe W et al: Dental and maxillofacial abnormalities in long-term survivors of childhood cancer: effects of treatment with chemotherapy and radiation to the head and neck, *Pediatrics* 73:816-823, 1984.

20. Leach W: Irradiation of the ear, *J Laryngol Otol* 74:870-880, 1965.

21. Lockhart PB, Sonis ST: Alterations in the oral mucosa caused by chemotherapeutic agents—a histologic study, *J Dermatol Surg Oncol* 7:1019-1025, 1981.

22. Maguire A et al: The long-term effects of treatment on the dental condition of children surviving malignant disease, *Cancer* 60:2570-2575, 1987.

23. Mansson-Rahemtulla B et al: Analysis of salivary components in leukemia patients receiving chemotherapy, *Oral Surg Oral Med Oral Pathol* 73:35-46, 1992.

24. Marcial V: *The oral cavity and oropharynx.* In Moss WT, Cox JD, editors: *Radiation oncology,* St Louis, 1989, Mosby–Year Book.

25. Martin M, Remy J, Daubaron F: In vitro growth potential of fibroblasts isolated from pigs with radiation-induced fibrosis, *Int J Radiat Biol Relat Stud Phys Chem Med* 49:821-828, 1986.

26. McHaney V et al: *Effects of radiation therapy and chemotherapy on hearing.* In Green DM, D'Angio GL, editors: *Late effects of treatment for childhood cancer,* New York, 1992, Wiley-Liss.

27. Moore KL: *The developing human,* ed 2, Philadelphia, 1977, WB Saunders.

28. Nakai Y, Konishi K, Chang KC: Ototoxicity of the anticancer drug cisplatinum, *Acta Otolaryngol* 93:227-232, 1982.

29. Neuhauser EB et al: Irradiation effects of Roentgen therapy on the growing spine, *Radiology* 59:637-650, 1952.

30. Nguyen TD et al: Analysis of late complications after rapid hyperfractionated radiotherapy in advanced head and neck cancers, *Int J Radiat Oncol Biol Phys* 14:23-25, 1988.

31. Nunn JH et al: Dental caries and dental anomalies in children treated by chemotherapy for malignant disease: a study in the North of England, *Int J Ped Dent* 1:131-135, 1991.

32. Pajari U, Larmas M, Lanning M: Caries incidence and prevalence in children receiving antineoplastic therapy, *Caries Res* 22:318-320, 1988.

33. Pajari U, Lanning M, Larmas M: Prevalence and location of enamel opacities in children after anti-neoplastic therapy, *Community Dent Oral Epidemiol* 16:222-226, 1988.

34. Pietrokovski J, Menczel J: Tooth dwarfism and root underdevelopment following irradiation, *Oral Surg Oral Med Oral Pathol* 22:95-99, 1966.

35. Purdell-Lewis DJ et al: Long-term results of chemotherapy on the developing dentition: caries risk and developmental aspects, *Community Dent Oral Epidemiol* 16:68-71, 1988.

36. Rosenberg SW et al: Altered dental root development in long-term survivors of pediatric acute lymphoblastic leukemia, *Cancer* 59:1640-1648, 1987.

37. Rubin R: *Radiation biology and radiation pathology syllabus,* Chicago, 1975, *American College of Radiology.*

38. Shrieve DC et al: *Hyperfractionated radiation therapy for brain stem gliomas in children and adults,* Paper presented at the thirty-third annual ASTRO meeting, *Int Radiat Oncol Biol Phys* 21, Suppl 1:120, Washington, DC, 1991.

39. Sonis A et al: Dentofacial development in long-term survivors of acute lymphoblastic leukemia, *Cancer* 66:2645-2652, 1990.

40. Stevens KR: *The bone.* In Moss WJ, Cox JD, editors: *Radiation oncology,* St Louis, 1989, Mosby–Year Book.

41. Tange RA: Differences in the cochlear degeneration pattern in the guinea pig as a result of gentamicin and cis-platinum intoxication, *Clin Otolaryngol* 9:323-327, 1984.

42. Van der Brenk HAS et al: Serum amylase as a measure of salivary gland radiation damage, *Br J Radiol* 42:688-700, 1969.

43. Van der Hulst RJ, Dreschler WA, Urbanus NA: High frequency audiometry in prospective clinical research of ototoxicity due to platinum derivatives, *Ann Otol Rhinol Laryngol* 97:133-137, 1988.

44. Wei S: Clinical uses of fluoride: a state-of-the-art conference on the uses of fluoride in clinical dentistry (conference summary), *J Am Dent Assoc* 109:472, 1984.

45. Welburg RR et al: Dental health of survivors of malignant disease, *Arch Dis Child* 59:1186-1187, 1984.

7

The Thyroid Gland

Louis S. Constine
Cindy L. Schwartz

Thyroid dysfunction or deregulation may result from irradiation of the thyroid gland or hypothalamic-pituitary axis. Children irradiated to the cervical region for malignancies such as Hodgkin's disease and head and neck rhabdomyosarcoma, or to the spinal axis for central nervous system (CNS) tumors, may develop primary hypothyroidism manifested by an elevated serum thyroid-stimulating hormone (TSH) concentration with or without a concomitant decreased serum thyroxine concentration.[5,9,25] The development of benign thyroid nodules and malignancy after thyroid radiation therapy (RT) is also well documented.*

PATHOPHYSIOLOGY

The hypothyroidism that occurs in these patients could result from direct radiation damage to the thyroid follicular cells, the thyroid vasculature, or the supporting stroma. Less likely mechanisms that could be contributory include radiation-induced immunologic reactions or damage from the iodine load administered during lymphangiography (LAG). Support for the latter theory is based on the observation that iodine will induce hypothyroidism in patients with autoimmune thyroiditis after treatment with radioiodine.[2] Histopathologic changes in an irradiated thyroid gland include progressive obliteration of the fine vasculature, degeneration of follicular cells and follicles, and atrophy of the stroma.[24] Since radiation damage is dependent on the degree of mitotic activity and because the thyroid of a developing child grows in parallel with body growth,[12] this gland might be expected to show an age-related degree of injury and repair.

CLINICAL MANIFESTATIONS

The common clinical manifestations of hypothyroidism include cold intolerance, constipation, inordinate weight gain, dry skin, and slowed mentation. Specific signs include a round puffy face, slow speech, hoarseness, hypokinesia, generalized muscle weakness, delayed relaxation of deep tendon reflexes, cold and dry skin, brittle hair, and periorbital edema. The incidence of hypothyroidism following therapeutic irradiation for Hodgkin's disease varies in different reports. If an

---

*References 10, 11, 13, 14, 19, 33.

elevated serum TSH concentration is the determinant, then 4% to 79% of patients become affected. This large range exists because parameters relevant to the occurrence of hypothyroidism, such as radiation dose, technique, and the frequency and types of follow-up testing, differ in these reports. A recent study by Hancock and colleagues of 1677 children and adults with Hodgkin's disease in whom the thyroid was irradiated showed that the actuarial risk at 26 years for overt or subclinical hypothyroidism was 47%[13] (Table 7-1), with the peak incidence occurring 2 to 3 years after treatment. There are few reports specifically addressing the incidence of hypothyroidism in children as a function of radiation dose. Constine and colleagues noted thyroid abnormalities in 4 of 24 children (17%) who received mantle irradiation of 26 Gy or less and in 74 of 95 children (78%) who received greater than 26 Gy (Fig. 7-1).[5] The abnormality in all but three children (one with hyperthyroidism and two with thyroid nodules) included an elevated serum TSH concentration with or without a low serum T4 concentration. Spontaneous return of TSH to normal limits was observed in 20 of 75 (27%) patients.

Table 7-1
Thyroid Disease after Treatment of Hodgkin's Disease

Disease	No. of Patients/ Total No.*	Actuarial Risk (%)		Time to Occurrence (years)	
		20 yr	26 yr	Median	Range
At least one thyroid disease	573/1787	50	63	4.6	0.2-25.6
	570/1677	52	67	4.6	0.2-25.6
Hypothyroidism	513/1787	41	44	4.0	0.2-23.7
	512/1677	43	47	4.0	0.2-23.7
Graves' disease †	34/1787	3.1	3.1	4.8	0.1-17.6
	32/1677	3.3	3.3	4.9	0.1-17.6
Graves' ophthalmopathy †	21/1677	—	—	—	—
Silent thyroiditis	6/1677	0.6	0.6	3.7	0.8-15.3
Hashimoto's thyroiditis	4/1677	0.7	0.7	7.9	3.5-15.2
Thyroidectomy	26/1677	6.6	26.6	14.0	1.5-25.6
Thyroid cancer	6/1677	1.7	1.7	13.3	9.0-18.9
Benign adenoma	10/1677	—	—	12.0	1.5-25.6
Adenomatous nodule	6/1677	—	—	17.4	12.7-24.4
Multinodular goiter	4/1677	—	—	14.8	10.8-19.4
Clinically benign nodule	12/1677	3.3	5.1	12.6	2.4-22.6
Clinically benign cyst	4/1677	0.7	0.7	8.1	1.6-16.7
Multinodular goiter ‡	2/1677	0.5	0.5	13.8	10.5-17

*The total refers either to all 1787 patients at risk or to the 1677 patients who underwent irradiation of the thyroid region.
† Thirty of the 34 patients who had been given a diagnosis of Graves' disease had hyperthyroidism; ophthalmopathy developed in 3 during a period of hypothyroidism and in 1 during a period of euthyroidism.
‡ Identified by clinical examination.
From Hancock S, Cox R, McDougall I: Thyroid diseases after treatment of Hodgkin's disease, *N Engl J Med* 325:599-605, 1991.

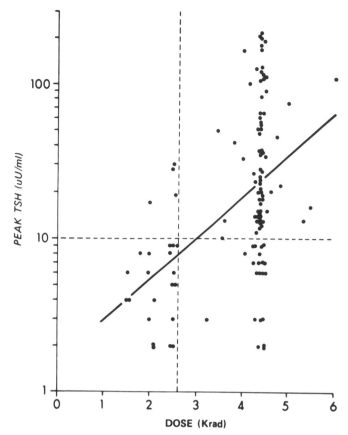

Fig. 7-1.   TSH value versus radiation dose in 116 patients treated for Hodgkin's disease in childhood. The horizontal dashed line denotes the upper limit of a normal serum TSH concentration, and the vertical dashed line denotes a radiation dose of 26 Gy (Krad), the level used to separate the low radiation dose from the high radiation dose group.

Although patients may become abnormal within 6 months of RT, most patients become abnormal after 3 to 5 years. Uncompensated hypothyroidism (decreased serum T4 and elevated serum TSH concentration) occurs in 6% to 27% of children receiving radiation to the thyroid. In Constine's study age did not affect the incidence of hypothyroidism but was weakly correlated with the degree of abnormality, as suggested by higher serum TSH concentrations in adolescents compared with younger children.[5] This may reflect the greater sensitivity of the thyroid gland in rapidly growing pubertal children compared with preadolescents. The iodine load from LAG may be a causal factor in the hypothyroidism observed in patients who are irradiated for Hodgkin's disease. There is a low but greater than expected incidence of hypothyroidism in patients having LAG without neck irradiation. Some recent reviews found that thyroid function was more likely to be abnormal in patients irradiated soon after LAG and mantle irradiation. However, no influence of LAG on thyroid dysfunction was noted in other studies.[25,28,32] The influence of chemotherapy on the development of thyroid dysfunction among Hodgkin's disease patients appears to be negligible in most reports,[5,9,31] although data from England suggest that chemotherapy may add to the frequency of compensated hypothyroidism.[21]

Primary hypothyroidism following irradiation of the spinal axis in the course of treating children with CNS tumors is also well documented. Ogilvy-Stuart evaluated 85 such children and found a 32% incidence of compensated hypothyroidism.[21] Constine evaluated eight children treated with 4 to 10 MV photon radiation to the spinal axis (mean dose 30 Gy). Three demonstrated primary thyroid injury with low serum-free T4 concentration and an exaggerated TSH response to provocative testing with thyrotropin releasing hormone (TRH).[4] Other reports indicate an incidence for compensated hypothyroidism of 20% to 68%, with overt hypothyroidism being rare.[15,20]

Patients undergoing a bone marrow transplant who receive total body irradiation (TBI) are also at risk for thyroid injury. Sklar found that a single dose of 7.5 Gy caused a decrease in serum T4 concentration in 9% of patients and an elevated serum TSH concentration in 35%.[27]

Thyroid abnormalities have been observed among long-term survivors of acute lymphoblastic leukemia (ALL). Robison collected data on 175 survivors first evaluated 7 years after diagnosis. Seventeen (10%) had thyroid function abnormalities including 5 with uncompensated primary hypothyroidism and 11 with compensated hypothyroidism. Eight in the latter group later reverted to normal without replacement therapy. No significant association was observed between hypothyroidism and the radiation dose (18 Gy versus 24 Gy), duration of chemotherapy (3 years versus 5 years), or age at the time of irradiation.[23]

The risk of Graves' disease also appears to be increased after RT for Hodgkin's disease, with a risk that is 7.2 to 20.4 times the expected risk.[13] Extensive data exist on the development of benign thyroid nodules and malignancy after thyroid RT. Representative incidences for thyroid nodules are 6% for malignant and 8% to 12% for benign lesions following lower dose (less than 15 Gy) external beam RT.[26] In a recent report from the Late Effects Study Group, of 9170 patients who had survived 2 or more years after the diagnosis of a cancer in childhood, the risk for thyroid cancer was increased fifty-threefold.[33] This risk was associated with both increasing radiation dose and time from treatment. Sixty-eight percent of the cancers occurred in areas directly within the radiation field, and all of the thyroid glands had received at least 1 Gy (via scatter for some patients). Patients treated for neuroblastoma and Wilms' tumor were affected more commonly than those treated for Hodgkin's disease; however, patients with the former two cancers were generally younger in age, which may be associated with an increase in the risk for thyroid cancer as a second malignancy when data from children are compared with those from adults. Finally, actinomycin D, but not alkylating agent therapy, may increase the risk of radiation-induced thyroid cancers. In Hancock's data, the risk for developing thyroid cancer was 15.6%, occurring 9 to 18 years after RT.[13] In a study by Schneider and colleagues, 318 of 5379 patients who had received RT for benign conditions of the head and neck developed thyroid cancer 3 to 42 years later.[26] Overall, in this setting (low dose RT, generally 2 to 5 Gy, for benign conditions) new nodules develop at a rate of about 2% per year, with a peak incidence at 15 to 25 years.[8] It is crucial to review the pathology of any biopsied nodule carefully, because adenomatous nodules with cytologic atypia can be difficult to distinguish from thyroid carcinoma.[3] The course of the cancer in these patients was the same as that of thyroid cancer found in other settings.[26] It is important to note that thyroid nodules have been found in as many as 35% to 50% of autopsies or during surgery in a nonirradiated population, and clinically palpable nodules are found in 4% to 7% of normal adults.[18,22,29,30]

DETECTION AND SCREENING

It is clearly important to obtain a comprehensive history and perform a thorough physical examination in all patients who received direct or scattered RT to the neck. Laboratory screening evaluations for asymptomatic patients should include serum concentrations of TSH and thyroxine (usually free T4) tests. The measurement of free T4 rather than other tests (usually total T4 by radioimmunoassay) is recommended because the former is not affected by changes in binding proteins.[34] Although some patients with normal serum-free T4 and TSH concentrations might show an exaggerated TSH response to provocative testing with TRH, the clinical significance of this finding is unclear. Screening for immunologic abnormalities can be performed by obtaining serum concentrations of antimicrosomal and antithyroglobulin antibodies, but abnormalities in asymptomatic patients are, again, of uncertain clinical significance. Patients with palpable abnormalities of the thyroid gland should undergo ultrasonography (US) (evaluating number, location, and density of nodules) and ^{99m}Tc scanning (functional status of nodules). Whether all patients who have received radiation to the thyroid gland should undergo periodic screening with one or the other of these techniques is controversial. Stewart and colleagues performed US on 30 patients treated with mantle radiation for Hodgkin's disease who did not have palpable abnormalities and found unilateral or bilateral atrophy in 8 patients, multiple hypoechoic lesions smaller than 0.75 cm in 18, and dominant cystic solid or complex lesions larger than 0.75 cm in 7 patients.[29] Biopsies were not performed. Soberman performed US on 18 long-term survivors of Hodgkin's disease who had received a mean dose of 34 Gy to the neck 1 to 16 years (mean 6.4) previously; 16 patients (89%) had abnormalities, including diffuse atrophy,[9] solitary nodules,[5] multiple nodules,[6] and gland heterogeneity[1]; only 2 patients had palpable nodules. Biopsies in four patients revealed multifocal papillary carcinoma in 1 patient, and adenomas in 3 patients. We have performed ^{99m}Tc scanning in 22 patients irradiated for Hodgkin's disease who are euthyroid and without palpable thyroid abnormalities and have diagnosed thyroid cancer in one patient. Patient numbers are currently too small to make firm recommendations. Although ^{99m}Tc scanning is less sensitive than US, its specificity for detecting clinically significant nodules is greater.

MANAGEMENT

Patients with uncompensated hypothyroidism (low serum concentration of thyroxine) clearly require thyroid replacement therapy. Patients with elevated serum concentrations of TSH but normal thyroxine are treated with thyroid replacement therapy in most institutions. The rationale for this approach is based on animal studies that have demonstrated that elevated levels of TSH in the presence of irradiated thyroid tissue can lead to the development of thyroid carcinoma. The observation of thyroid cancer following neck irradiation in humans and the high frequency of elevated serum TSH concentrations in children who have received radiation for Hodgkin's disease have prompted us to institute thyroid replacement therapy in this population. Approaches to decrease the risk of thyroid injury in the setting of RT for Hodgkin's disease have included shielding the gland from irradiation[16] and administering thyroxine during irradiation.[1] The former approach places patients at risk for shielding of involved cervical lymph nodes and the latter did not prevent subsequent hypothyroidism. Therefore, these approaches are not recommended. Patients with palpable thyroid abnormalities should undergo US or ^{99m}Tc scanning and be evaluated by an endocrinologist and surgeon. If nodules are discovered, then biopsy is necessary. Depending on the results, further therapy may be necessary, with treatment approaches varying in different centers, as recently reviewed by Mazzaferri.[17] For papillary thyroid carcinoma, treatment will generally involve near total thyroidectomy, radioactive iodine, and TSH suppression with thyroxine.[7] The optimal approach for patients who are not receiving replacement hormone and have clinically normal thyroid glands but nodules detected by US or ^{99m}Tc scanning is less clear. Multiple small 2- to 3-mm carcinomas have been found in irradiated thyroid glands.[14] Because autopsies have shown a high incidence of occult (less than 1 mm) papillary carcinomas, the significance of cancer found in clinically occult lesions is arguable. However, it would seem appropriate to biopsy nodules that are detectable until additional information is available for more definite guidelines.

REFERENCES

1. Bantle J, Lee C, Levitt S: Thyroxine administration during radiation therapy to the neck does not prevent subsequent thyroid dysfunction, *Int J Radiat Oncol Biol Phys* 11:1999-2002, 1985.
2. Braverman LE et al: Enhanced susceptibility to iodide myxedema in patients with Hashimoto's disease, *J Clin Endocrinol Metab* 32:515-521, 1971.
3. Carr R, Livolsi V: Morphologic changes in the thyroid after irradiation for Hodgkin's and non-Hodgkin's lymphoma, *Cancer* 64:825-829, 1989.
4. Constine L et al: Hypothalamic-pituitary dysfunction after radiation for brain tumors, *N Engl J Med* 328:87-94, 1993.

5. Constine LS, Donaldson SS, McDougall IR: Thyroid dysfunction after radiotherapy in children with Hodgkin's disease, *Cancer* 53:878-883, 1984.
6. Constine LS et al: Hyperprolactinemia and hypothyroidism following cytotoxic therapy for central nervous system malignancies, *J Clin Oncol* 5:1841-1851, 1987.
7. DeGroot L et al: Natural history, treatment, and course of papillary thyroid carcinoma, *J Clin Endocrinol Metab* 71:414-424, 1990.
8. DeGroot L: Clinical review 2: diagnostic approach and management of patients exposed to irradiation to the thyroid, *J Clin Endocrinol Metab* 69:925-928, 1989.
9. Devney RB et al: Serial thyroid function measurements in children with Hodgkin's disease, *J Pediatr* 105:223-229, 1984.
10. Donaldson SS, Kaplan HS: Complications of treatment of Hodgkin's disease in children, *Cancer Treat Rep* 66:977-989, 1982.
11. Doniach I: *Pathology of irradiation thyroid damage.* In DeGrott LJ et al, editors: *Radiation-associated thyroid carcinoma,* New York, 1977, Grune & Stratton.
12. Fisher DA, Dussault JH: *Development of the mammalian thyroid gland.* In Greep RO et al, editors: *Handbook of physiology,* sec 7, Endocrinology, vol 3, Thyroid, Bethesda, 1974, American Physiological Society.
13. Hancock S, Cox R, McDougall I: Thyroid diseases after treatment of Hodgkin's disease, *N Engl J Med* 325:599-605, 1991.
14. Hawkins M, Kingston J: Malignant thyroid tumours following childhood cancer, *Lancet* 2:455, 1988.
15. Livesey E, Brook C: Thyroid dysfunction after radiotherapy and chemotherapy of brain tumours, *Arch Dis Child* 64:593-595, 1989.
16. Marcial-Vega V et al: Prevention of hypothyroidism related to mantle irradiation for Hodgkin's disease: preparative phantom study, *Int J Radiat Oncol Biol Phys* 18:613-618, 1990.
17. Mazzaferri EL: Management of a solitary thyroid nodule, *N Engl J Med* 328:553-559, 1993.
18. Mazzaferri E, de los Santos E, Rofagha-Keyhani S: Solitary thyroid nodule: diagnosis and management, *Med Clin North Am* 72:1177-1211, 1988.
19. McDougall IR et al: Thyroid carcinoma after high-dose external radiotherapy for Hodgkin's disease, *Cancer* 45:2056-2060, 1980.
20. Oberfield S, Allen J, Pollack J et al: Long-term endocrine sequelae after treatment of medulloblastoma: prospective study of growth and thyroid function, *J Pediatr* 108:219-223, 1986.
21. Ogilvy-Stuart A, Shalet S, Gattamameni H: Thyroid function after treatment of brain tumors in children, *J Pediatr* 119:733-737, 1991.
22. Pelizzo M, Piotto A, Rubello D et al: High prevalence of occult papillary thyroid carcinoma in a surgical series for benign thyroid disease, *Tumori* 76:255-257, 1990.
23. Robinson LL, Nesbit ME, Sathes HN et al: Thyroid abnormalities in long-term survivors of childhood acute lymphoblastic leukemia, *Pediatr Res* 19:266A, 1985.
24. Rubin P, Cassarett GW: *Clinical radiation pathology, vols I and II,* Philadelphia, 1968, WB Saunders.
25. Schimpff SC, Diggs CH, Wiswell JD: Radiation-related thyroid dysfunction: implications for the treatment of Hodgkin's disease, *JAMA* 245:46-49, 1980.
26. Schneider A et al: Radiation-induced thyroid carcinoma: clinical course and results of therapy in 296 patients, *Ann Intern Med* 105:405-412, 1986.
27. Sklar CA, Kim TH, Ramsay NKC: Thyroid dysfunction among long-term survivors of bone marrow transplantation, *Am J Med* 73:688-694, 1982.

28. Smith RE et al: Thyroid function after mantle irradiation in Hodgkin's disease, *JAMA* 245:46-49, 1981.

29. Stewart R et al: Thyroid gland: US in patients with Hodgkin's disease treated with radiation therapy in childhood, *Radiology* 172:159, 1989.

30. Soberman N et al: Sonographic abnormalities of the thyroid gland in longterm survivors of Hodgkin's disease, *Pediatr Radiol* 21:250-253, 1991.

31. Sutcliffe S, Chapman R, Wrigley P: Cyclical combination chemotherapy and thyroid function in patients with advanced Hodgkin's disease, *Med Pediatr Oncol* 9:439-448, 1981.

32. Tamura L, Shimaoka K, Friedman M: Thyroid abnormalities associated with treatment of malignant lymphoma, *Cancer* 47:2704-2711, 1981.

33. Tucker M, Jones P, Boice J et al: Therapeutic radiation at a young age is linked to secondary thyroid cancer, *Cancer Res* 51:2885-2888, 1991.

34. Woolf P, Lee L, Hamill R et al: Thyroid test abnormalities in traumatic brain injury correlated with neurologic impairment and sympathetic-nervous system activities, *Am J Med* 84:201-208, 1988.

8

Cardiovascular Effects of Cancer Therapy

Susie Truesdell
Cindy L. Schwartz
Edward Clark
Louis S. Constine

During the last 20 years, advances in the treatment of cancer in children have enabled many to survive both the disease and the treatment. The cardiac sequelae that may affect these children are clearly a central concern in considering their chances for a normal adult life.

Late cardiac effects may occur within months or as long as 20 years after treatment with known cardiotoxic agents such as anthracyclines or radiation. For the newer regimens, results must be speculative and based on present knowledge.

Radiation therapy (RT) and chemotherapeutic agents may cause irreversible injury to the heart. Although many patients appear well and active, they may be compensating for some degree of heart damage. Although it is not known how many will eventually be debilitated by cardiac damage, it is clear that early recognition and treatment of problems will allow patients with cardiac damage to have a longer and more symptom-free life.

PATHOPHYSIOLOGY

Normal Organ Development

Cardiac development begins in the third week of gestation and primary morphogenesis is complete by the end of the eighth week. Myocardial cell replication rates are highest in the earlier weeks and decrease with septation of the embryonic heart.[10] Cell size remains constant during the period of rapid cardiac growth. With embryonic development and an increased workload, the embryonic heart increases its mass by cell proliferation (hyperplasia) rather than cell enlargement (hypertrophy).[12] In the late prenatal and early postnatal period, heart growth is achieved through both hypertrophy and hyperplasia.[25] By 6 months of postnatal age, however, the adult number of myocytes are present, and subsequent growth occurs by means of increasing size of existing myocytes. Beyond 6 months of age, myocytes that die are replaced through fibrosis. Such a loss is compensated by hypertrophy of existing cells.

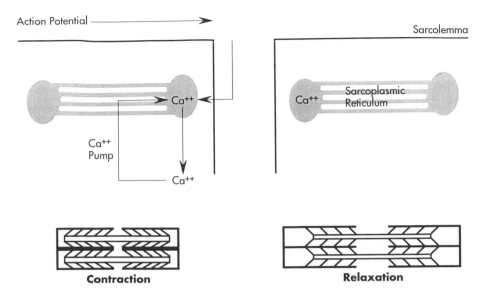

Fig. 8-1.   Cardiac myocyte. As the action potential is propagated down the length of the muscle, calcium leaves the sarcoplasmic reticulum through fast calcium channels and enters the sarcoplasm. In the sarcoplasm calcium activates the actin-myosin bridging, allowing the muscle to contract.

The pumping action of the heart occurs by synchronized contraction of the myocytes. This contraction is initiated by an electrical stimulus (action potential) that originates in the sinus node and is propagated through the atrioventricular (AV) node and His-Purkinje system to the ventricular myocytes. In order for the action potential to cause effective contraction of the myocyte, several factors must work optimally (Fig. 8-1). First, the actin and myosin filaments must be in their normal, relaxed state. If the myocytes are already stretched (as in doxorubicin-induced dilated cardiomyopathy), cross-bridging cannot occur effectively. Second, calcium must be available in the sarcoplasmic reticulum (SR) for release by the action potential into the sarcoplasm. Calcium catalyzes the cross-bridging, producing contraction of the myocyte. Third, the myocytes must return to their resting state in order for the next action potential to generate another contraction. Some types of cardiac damage, including doxorubicin or radiation-induced cardiomyopathy, impede the return to resting state, thus decreasing the diastolic compliance.

Natural History and Effects of Aging

The adult number of myocytes are present in the heart by the age of 6 months. Further growth of the heart is accomplished through hypertrophy of existing cells. Because both anthracyclines and cyclophosphamide cause myocyte death, children treated with these agents will enter adulthood with fewer myocytes than untreated children. The remaining myocytes will exhibit nonlethal changes described in later sections. Despite a normal clinical evaluation, each patient's heart has been injured by therapy.

The normal aging process within the heart consists of valvular degeneration (calcification and dysfunction) and coronary artery disease (ischemia and decreased ventricular function). Some children treated with mantle radiation incur valvular injury and are at high risk for early valvular degeneration as adults. These children may have a coronary and aortic vasculitis. Vascular damage may serve as a nidus for the development of plaque in the coronary arteries and aorta. Since atherosclerosis may be evident as early as age 18, young adults who require mantle radiation face the synergism of the valvular degeneration and vasculitis.

Changes Induced by Cytotoxic Therapy

Anthracyclines. The earliest changes seen in cardiac myocytes after exposure to doxorubicin include swelling of the SR and mitochondria with occasional nucleolar changes.[36,49] Large vacuoles that are probably distended SR displace mitochondria and contractile elements. Injuries to the mitochondria, SR, and sarcolemma affect both the calcium transport mechanisms and the intracellular calcium concentrations. These injuries, in concert with or due to the actions of other potential mediators of anthracycline-induced cardiac damage (e.g., free radicals, prostaglandins, histamines, and metabolites), result in the morphologic changes noted by Billingham and colleagues in endomyocardial biopsies taken from patients undergoing anthracycline therapy.[4]

The major types of myocyte damage described by Billingham and colleagues are myofibrillar loss and vacuolar degeneration. These changes are graded as follows:

1. Occasional myocytes show myofibrillar loss or sarcoplasmic swelling;
2. More widespread changes with clusters of myocytes showing myofibrillar dropout or definite cytoplasmic vacuolization; and
3. Diffuse injury with marked cellular damage and necrosis.

Electron micrographs show reduction in myofibrillar bundles, myofibrillar lysis, swollen mitochondria, and distortion of the Z-line substance. The severity of these changes correlates directly with the total anthracycline dosage.[21]

Since myocytes do not proliferate after age 6 months, all myocardial growth in childhood is a result of increased myocyte size. Anthracycline-induced myocyte death will, therefore, stimulate hypertrophy of other myocytes in order to generate (or maintain) a normal adult cardiac output.[40] Lipshultz and colleagues have noted such hypertrophy in association with reduced wall thickness and interstitial fibrosis in myocardial biopsy specimens from children treated with anthracyclines. Late-onset anthracycline-induced cardiac failure may be precipitated by the myocytes' inability to compensate adequately in accordance with the demand of growth, pregnancy, or other cardiac stress.

Cyclophosphamide. Cardiac effects of cyclophosphamide on the myocardium are described primarily in the setting of high-dose preparatory regimens for bone marrow transplant. Left ventricular wall mass and thickness increase as a result of intramyocardial edema or hemorrhage, often in association with a serosanguineous pericardial effusion with fibrinous pericarditis.[6] Multiple areas of myocardial hemorrhage are seen, with extravasation of blood, interstitial edema, and multifocal myocardial necrosis.[43] Myocardial edema has been attributed to endothelial damage by cyclophosphamide.[29,33,46] Myocardial fibrosis has also been thought to result from cyclophosphamide.[19] Chronic changes after cyclophosphamide administration have not been described, although cyclophosphamide may exacerbate anthracycline-induced cardiotoxicity.[58] Because the median lethal dose (LD_{50}) for cyclophosphamide-induced cardiotoxicity is decreased by glutathione depletion (which is induced by cyclophosphamide itself), sequential doses may result in an increase in myocardial sensitivity to the drug.[26]

Radiation. The chronic adverse cardiac effects of RT have been the subject of study since the 1940s.[37] Manifestations include pericarditis with chronic effusion and pancarditis that includes myocardial fibrosis with or without endocardial fibroelastosis, cardiomyopathy, coronary artery disease (CAD), valvular injury, and conduction defects. The histologic hallmark of these injuries is fibrosis in the interstitium with normal-appearing myocytes and capillary and arterial narrowing. The frequency of RT-related injuries varies considerably in patient reports, owing to the variability in radiation dosage and technique employed. Relevant radiation parameters include total and fractional doses, volume and specific region of the heart treated, and relative weighting of the radiation portals, which may determine the amount of radiation delivered to different depths of the heart. Other influential factors are the presence of other risk factors (e.g., tobacco use, hypertension) for cardiac disease and the use of specific chemotherapeutic agents.

Although clinically evident radiation-induced heart disease (RIHD) has a characteristic morphology, its pathophysiology remains a topic of active investigation. The most common manifestation is pericardial disease, and therefore the most common morphologic alterations from RIHD occur in the pericardium.[24] Pericardial fluid is almost invariably found in patients with pericardial disease. The fluid is protein rich and generally accumulates slowly so clinically significant tamponade occurs only rarely.[14,56] The parietal pericardium develops variable degrees of fibrosis that replaces the outer adipose tissue. There is always fibrinous exudate both on the surface of the pericardium facing the heart and in the stroma of the fibrotic pericardium. Although the pericardial fibrosis may progress to constriction, fibrous adhesions between epicardium and pericardium are practically never seen. Injury to the myocardium is characterized by patches of diffuse fibrosis. These fibrotic patches vary in size but never occupy the entire myocardium.[23,24] The fibrosis is made of a network of collagen fibers that separate individual myocytes or groups of myocytes.

The morphology of CAD, along with the resultant myocardial infarctions that can follow RT, is no different from that of spontaneous atherosclerosis; therefore, such lesions cannot be diagnosed specifically.[17,22,55] Because the endothelial cells are the most sensitive element in arteries of this size, it is presumed that the lesion in the coronary artery results from intimal injury and the eventual replacement of the damaged intima by myofibroblasts, deposition of platelets, and all of the other events that usually occur in atherosclerosis.

CLINICAL MANIFESTATIONS

Chemotherapy

Anthracyclines. Clinical abnormalities resulting from doxorubicin therapy are usually dose related and range from minor electrocardiogram (ECG) abnormalities to lethal congestive heart failure. During an infusion of doxorubicin, changes in the ECG can include an increase in the corrected QTc interval.[11] Rare patients will have ventricular arrhythmias. Echocardiographic evaluation may reveal minor, transient changes in left ventricular function. Some of these effects may be related to changes in calcium homeostasis. As the cumulative dose of anthracyclines increases, permanent changes occur.

Patients undergoing anthracycline therapy are generally asymptomatic in spite of subclinical changes. Although myocyte damage increases linearly with increasing cumulative dose, the incidence of congestive heart failure begins to increase logarithmically at a cumulative doxorubicin dose of approximately 550 mg/m^2. Young children may be more sensitive to anthracycline than are adults.[49] Mediastinal radiation and other chemotherapeutic agents, including cyclophosphamide and ifosfamide, may enhance the cardiotoxic effects of anthracyclines and potentially lower the critical cumulative anthracycline dose to approximately 350 to 400 mg/m^2.[3,44,45] Abnormalities noted that may indicate impending cardiac failure (and therefore suggest a need to limit further drug exposure) include prolongation of the corrected QT$_c$ interval; decreased fractional shortening by echocardiogram (ECHO); and decreased ejection fraction by radionuclear angiography (RNA).[2,38,44,50]

Clinically evident acute anthracycline-induced cardiotoxicity can be seen during or within approximately 6 months of completing therapy. Symptoms include fatigue, exercise intolerance, and dyspnea. Tachycardia, tachypnea, hepatomegaly, rales, and a new S3 or S4 may be noted on physical examination (Fig. 8-2). Some patients will succumb to the cardiomyopathy, and others will initially improve. (Therefore, it was once thought that the cardiac effects of anthracyclines were stable or reversible with time).[28] More recent information suggests that late cardiac decompensation may occur 10 to 14 years after treatment. The risk for late cardiac decompensation is greatest for those diagnosed (by ECHO) with abnormal cardiac function immediately after completing therapy (12% risk of late abnormalities if ECHO is normal at end of therapy, versus 70% risk of remaining abnormal or worsening if ECHO is abnormal at end of therapy.)[24]

Late-onset anthracycline-induced cardiomyopathy may manifest with congestive heart failure or ventricular arrhythmia. Steinherz and colleagues reported sudden and rapid cardiac decompensation in nine anthracycline-treated survivors of childhood cancer; the presenting symptoms were late cardiac failure, conduction abnormalities, and dysrhythmia.[37] Five survivors had cardiac symptoms within a year of treatment; four of whom initially improved. However, deterioration

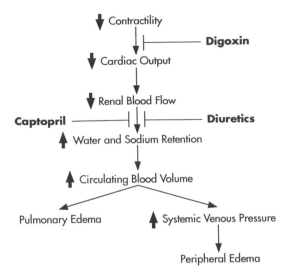

Fig. 8-2.   Mechanisms of congestive heart failure—signs and symptoms. As ventricular contractility decreases, cardiac output decreases, resulting in decreased renal blood flow and activation of the renin-angiotensin system with water and sodium retention. This results in an increase in circulating blood volume, which contributes to pulmonary and peripheral edema. Digoxin acts primarily to increase ventricular contractility. Diuretics and Captopril act, through different mechanisms, to decrease water and sodium retention, thus alleviating pulmonary and peripheral edema.

occurred 6 to 8 years later. Sudden death occurred in three of these patients, presumably due to dysrhythmia (documented in two patients). Two of the other four patients had mildly abnormal ECHOs during long-term follow-up and developed cardiac failure 12 to 18 years after completion of chemotherapy. Endomyocardial biopsies performed in five patients showed myocardial fibrosis with myocyte hypertrophy. Such observations prompted cohort studies of long-term, anthracycline-treated survivors of childhood cancer. Evaluation of 201 such patients by ECHO revealed the following proportions with decreased cardiac function: 11% after a cumulative dose of less than 400 mg/m², 23% after 400 to 599 mg/m², 47% after 500 to 799 mg/m², and 100% after more than 800 mg/m² of doxorubicin.[54]

Lipshultz and colleagues found abnormalities of left ventricular wall stress (afterload) or contractility in 57% of 115 children with acute lymphoblastic leukemia (ALL) who had received doxorubicin 1 to 15 years earlier.[40] Increased afterload was correlated with reduced ventricular wall thickness and progressed serially over time. Significant predictive factors included a high cumulative doxorubicin dose (predictive of decreased contractility) and age at diagnosis of less than 4 years (predictive of increased afterload). Symptoms of fatigue, shortness of breath, palpitations, and syncope correlated poorly with measures of ventricular function or exercise tolerance. Four percent of the patients had ventricular tachycardia on 24-hour ECG monitoring, always in association with severe left ventricular dysfunction and congestive heart failure. One third of patients had abnormal measures of exercise tolerance. Five of 11 patients with congestive failure at completion of therapy experienced recurrence of cardiac symptoms after initial improvement; 2 of the 5 required cardiac transplantation. Late cardiac failure as a new event was not noted.

Schwartz and colleagues have reported an increased frequency of QTc prolongation in patients who have received higher cumulative doses of anthracyclines.[51] This measure was more sensitive for cardiac injury than was the fractional shortening measured by ECHO. Those patients with a prolonged QTc (greater than 0.45) who underwent exercise testing were noted to have further prolongation with exercise, a finding reported in patients with congenital QTc prolongation who are at risk for sudden death. Since QTc prolongation has been associated both with impending cardiomyopathy in patients receiving anthracycline therapy[2] and with a potential for sudden death due to dysrhythmia,[48] it may be an excellent tool for screening this population of long-term survivors of childhood cancer. Jakacki and colleagues have recently confirmed the usefulness of this measure.[34] It has the benefit of being readily accessible to and interpretable by primary caretakers.

Life-style changes may allow a patient with progressive cardiac deterioration to compensate transiently, but the long-term effects of anthracyclines are usually irreversible. As ventricular contractility diminishes, the ventricle dilates to maintain cardiac output. A heart with ventricular dilatation is unable to compensate further when metabolic demands increase. Clinical congestive heart failure with tachycardia, tachypnea, and hepatomegaly ensues. Studies have shown an increased risk of cardiac decompensation when additional stress is imposed by growth hormone-induced growth spurts in children with ALL,[41] pregnancy-induced hypervolemic weight gain, or the increase in cardiac afterload associated with vaginal delivery or weight lifting.[18,54] Although the use of diuretics and agents that reduce afterload can enhance adaption to cardiac decompensation, its appearance during late follow-up is an ominous sign. Ventricular arrhythmia occurs as well, predisposing patients to sudden death. Death is likely within months to years after the onset of congestive heart failure. Cardiac transplant may improve the patient's immediate prognosis, but transplant currently remains a palliative treatment.

Radiation

The functional and structural complexity of the heart is reflected by the variety of irradiation injuries that can occur. A classification system modified from Fajardo and Stewart includes: (a) acute pericarditis during irradiation (rare and associated with juxtapericardial cancer); (b) delayed pericarditis that can present abruptly or as chronic effusion; (c) pancarditis that includes myocardial fibrosis with or without endocardial fibroelastosis (only after large doses); (d) cardiomyopathy in the absence of significant pericardial disease; (e) CAD (uncommon), usually involving the left anterior descending artery; (f) functional valvular injury; and (g) cardiac conduction defects. The histologic hallmark of these injuries is fibrosis in the interstitium with normal-appearing myocytes and capillary and arterial narrowing.[56]

Several parameters influence the degree of irradiation injury including (a) total and fractional doses; (b) volume and specific region of the heart treated; (c) relative weighting of the radiation portals, which determines the amount of radiation delivered to different depths of the heart; (d) the presence of juxtapericardial tumor; (e) the presence of other risk factors such as age, weight, blood pressure, family history, lipoprotein levels, and habits such as smoking; and (f) the use of specific chemotherapeutic agents.

Pericarditis. Delayed acute pericarditis can be clinically occult or associated with fever, dyspnea, pleuric chest pain, friction rub, and, on evaluation, ST and T wave changes, and decreased QRS voltage.[1,56] Up to 30% of patients treated for Hodgkin's disease irradiated with a mean midplane heart dose of 46 Gy (now rarely used) will develop delayed acute pericarditis.[42] With equally weighted anterior and posterior fields and the use of subcarinal blocking, the frequency decreases to 2.5%.[9] The onset of delayed acute pericarditis occurs on an average of 6 months of treatment, and 92% of effusions occur within 12 months of treatment. Up to 50% of patients (again, after treatment with older RT techniques) develop some degree of tamponade (paradoxical pulse, Kussmaul's sign), occasionally necessitating a pericardiocentesis.[57] The effusion usually resolves in 1 to 10 months but may persist for years. Chronic effusive-constrictive pericarditis develops in 10% to 15% of these patients and may necessitate pericardectomy. Constrictive pericarditis may develop 5 to 10 years after irradiation in patients without antecedent disease.[1,9,56]

Cardiomypathy. Reports that provide information regarding radiosensitivity of the myocardium are currently of limited clinical applicability, because the patients studied were treated with RT techniques that are considered suboptimal by current standards and certainly greater than most children would currently receive.[57] For example, Gottdiener and colleagues documented decreased LV function in 25 patients who were treated through a single anteroposterior port without the use of subcarinal cardiac blocking. The estimated doses to the anterior heart averaged 59.5 Gy, to the mid heart 50.7 Gy, and to the posterior heart 42.5 Gy.[30] Burns and colleagues found abnormal LV ejection fractions (LVEF) in 57% of 21 patients studied but irradiation doses ranged from 20 to 76 Gy and specific dose-response data were not provided.[8] Gomez and colleagues found lower LVEFs in patients irradiated for Hodgkin's disease but 44% and 32% of patients with low LVEFs were treated to 75% to 100% and 50% to 75% or more of the heart, respectively.[27]

Constine and colleagues used equilibrium radionuclide angiocardiography (ERNA), quantitative thallium scintigraphy, and ECG treadmill testing to evaluate 30 asymptomatic patients, aged 10 to 46 (mean 26.7) years at time of RT, who were tested 1.1 to 25.5 (mean 9.6) years after RT.[16] Radiation doses to the central cardiac volume ranged from 23.8 to 47.5 Gy (mean 38.4 Gy) in 1.5 to 2.0 daily fractions. The range of LVEFs was 48% to 73% (mean 60.0% ± 6.1%; normal ≥ 50%), and pulmonary flow rate (PFR) ranged from 1.9 to 4.7 end diastolic volume (EDV) per second (mean 3.41 ± 0.83 per second: normal ≥ 2.54) with 1 and 5 patients below normal, respectively. Thallium scintigraphy revealed areas of mild ischemia in two patients and borderline normal perfusion in three. ECG treadmill testing revealed mild abnormalities in three patients. One patient was abnormal at rest and had nondiagnostic changes with stress. In the nine patients who had repeat tests, the LVEF increased in six, decreased in two, and did not change in one. The PFR increased in seven patients and decreased in two. All changes were mild. Patients treated for Hodgkin's disease with modern techniques for mantle radiation generally had normal measures of cardiac function, and no significant deterioration occurred over time.

Valvular disease. Fibrous valvular endocardial thickening occurs in 80% of autopsied patients treated with high radiation doses. The mitral, aortic, and tricuspid valves were most frequently affected.[7] The frequency of this injury as a clinical problem in children after standard radiation doses is unknown.

Arrhythmia. High-degree atrioventricular conduction abnormalities are rarely seen but may be attributed to fibrosis of the AV node conduction branches.[13]

Coronary artery disease. Radiation delivered in therapeutic doses (35 to 45 Gy) for Hodgkin's disease using older techniques appears to produce clinically significant CAD or cardiomyopathy. Boivin's report on 4665 patients who were treated for Hodgkin's disease with various RT techniques at several medical centers documented a relative risk of death from CAD of 1.87, and in the subcategory of myocardial infarction of 2.56.[51] Hancock reviewed the records of 2232 patients treated at Stanford and found the relative risk of death from heart disease to be 3.5 after greater than 30 Gy to the mediastinum. The risk of death from acute myocardial infarction decreased from 3.7 to 3.2 after pericardial and subcarinal blocking techniques were instituted.[32]

Cardiac irradiation in children. There are few data specific to the clinical effects of cardiac irradiation in children. Among 120 children treated at Stanford with greater than 40 Gy for Hodgkin's disease, 13% developed cardiac damage. Six patients were asymptomatic, five had valvular or myocardial abnormalities, three required pericardectomy, and two had premature CAD. Among 35 children treated with 15 to 26 Gy, none developed cardiac damage.[20] Another series of 28 children treated with 30 Gy (average dose) showed pericardial thickening in 43% but no functional abnormalities.[31] Exercise testing with a variety of measurements may detect and quantitate important cardiopulmonary abnormalities. Among 12 patients treated at the Mayo Clinic with 19.5 to 55 Gy (median dose 35 Gy) for Hodgkin's disease, 33% had abnormal ECHOs and 50% had abnormal exercise studies.[35] In summary, it appears that cardiac doses of up to 25 Gy are generally safe, and 40 Gy may be administered to small cardiac regions. However, longer follow-up of patients treated with cardiac irradiation may reveal an unexpected frequency of cardiac-related difficulties.

DETECTION AND SCREENING

Long-term survivors of childhood cancer who have received therapies that are potentially cardiotoxic should undergo annual or biannual evaluations of cardiac status, even if the patient is asymptomatic. Patients at risk include (but may not be limited to) those who have received anthracyclines, high-dose cyclophosphamide (e.g., after bone marrow transplantation), and cardiac irradiation (mediastinal, mantle, and possibly spinal; whole lung; and left renal bed). The minimal baseline evaluation for all high-risk patients includes a thorough history, physical examination, chest radiograph, 12-lead ECG, and ECHO. The necessity for subsequent studies and the frequency of studies should be determined by individual risk factors.

The Anthracycline-Treated Patient

Lipshultz could not find a correlation between patient- or parent-reported symptoms and measures of LV function or exercise tolerance.[40] This may be due in part to patient expectation and interpretation of health status, rather than to the true incidence of symptomatology. It is essential that information is determined by specific, quantitative parameters (e.g., "Can you walk up two flights of stairs without becoming short of breath?"). Changes in exercise tolerance, dyspnea on exertion, palpitations, and syncope should be evaluated, because the manifestations of late anthracycline-related cardiotoxicity are congestive heart failure and dysrhythmias. Worrisome findings on physical examination include tachypnea, tachycardia, a new S3 or S4, rales, hepatomegaly, peripheral edema, diminished peripheral pulse volume, and perfusion, any of which is suggestive of congestive failure.

Steinherz and colleagues have recommended that all patients treated with anthracycline have an ECG and ECHO every 2 to 3 years.[53] We agree with this, particularly for those who have received greater than 200 mg/m^2 of doxorubicin or any doxorubicin with mediastinal radiation. Those patients who have had an abnormal study either at the end of therapy or at the time of initial long-term follow-up (5 years after diagnosis) should have more frequent cardiac screening. Pertinent ECG findings include low voltage, prolonged QTc ($\geq$ 0.45 or longer), second-degree AV block, complete heart block, ventricular ectopy, ST elevation or depression, and T wave changes. In some patients, serially determining the QTc by ECG may prove to be a simple method of screening on an annual basis, with ECHOs every 2 to 3 years. Others will need annual ECHOs as well.

Fractional shortening (FS) and the velocity of circumferential fiber shortening (VCF) are reliable echocardiographic measures of left ventricular contractility. FS is the percentage of change in left ventricular dimension between systole and diastole. VCF incorporates ejection time into the equation. Both measurements, however, are sensitive to preload. Interpretation is therefore most valid in normovolemic nonsedated patients. For the long-term patient who is usually in a normal physiologic state at clinic visits, serial measures of FS and VCF are reliable, easily performed indexes of myocardial systolic function. The evaluation of LV wall stress (used as a measure of afterload) requires simultaneous measurements of the left ventricle by ECHO, external carotid pulse tracings, phonocardiographic recordings, and blood pressure readings.[15] This evaluation is less dependent on preload and is normalized for heart rate. It is especially useful in the case of altered hemodynamic states and may be used to detect small changes in FS or VCF. ERNA determines an ejection fraction that is more accurate than that derived from ECHO by calculating the change in radioactivity at end diastole to that at end systole. Although it has been recommended as a baseline study to be repeated every 5 years in anthracycline-treated children,[53] further studies are necessary to determine whether ERNA is of clinical value for the entire cohort of asymptomatic patients. It is useful for those in whom a good ECHO cannot be obtained.

Steinherz and colleagues have recommended that 24-hour continuous ECG monitoring be performed at baseline and every 5 years thereafter to detect a risk for dysrhythmia.[53] It is not clear that the risk is sufficiently high to justify continuous ECG monitoring in patients with normal ECGs and ECHOs who have received low cumulative doses of doxorubicin. We are performing such studies in patients with prolongation of the QTc, ventricular dysfunction, or high cumulative doses of anthracyclines.

ECHO and ECG exercise testing have been shown to reveal cardiac injury that is not discernible on resting studies.[51,59] Further studies are necessary to determine the appropriate use of such studies in the clinical setting. Because anthracycline-treated patients appear to decompensate at times of cardiac stress, it is likely that such tests will be of good predictive value.

Asymptomatic patients who will be subjected to increased cardiac stress should undergo careful baseline evaluations and systematic follow-up monitoring. Examples of such patients include those anticipating pregnancy or general anesthesia, those beginning a growth hormone regimen, or those starting a new exercise regimen.

The Cyclophosphamide-treated Patient

Because long-term cardiovascular effects of standard-dose cyclophosphamide have not been described, routine evaluation of the cyclophosphamide-treated patient should include only a full history and physical examination unless cardiovascular instability was noted during treatment. For children with such instability and those who received high-dose cyclophosphamide for bone marrow transplantation, a baseline follow-up (5 years after diagnosis) ECG and ECHO are warranted. Pertinent findings that would precipitate a more in-depth evaluation include ST and T wave changes on ECG or diminished contractility or abnormal wall motion by ECHO.

The Radiation-treated Patient

Children who have received mediastinal or spinal irradiation should undergo a history and physical examination with attention given to the signs and symptoms of pericarditis (fever, dyspnea, pleuritic chest pain, friction rub, ST and T wave changes, decreased QRS voltage); cardiomyopathy; valvular disease (new murmur); arrhythmia (palpitations, syncope); and CAD (left arm and chest pain, diaphoresis, dyspnea). In young patients, chest pain is most commonly due to costochondritis (Tietze's syndrome), characterized by point tenderness, discomfort with inspiration, and response to nonsteroidal analgesics. However, crushing pain (especially with exercise), diaphoresis, dyspnea, and nausea suggest the possibility of myocardial ischemia. These complaints must be considered seriously and require additional evaluation.

A baseline ECHO and ECG are recommended and should be repeated every 3 to 5 years in asymptomatic patients. Pertinent positive ECG findings include: complete heart block, ST wave changes, decreased QRS voltage, and abnormalities of the P wave axis. ECHO should include evaluation of left ventricular function, valve function, and pericardial status. Consultation with a cardiologist is recommended if any abnormalities are seen.

There are no definitive recommendations for ECG stress testing or quantitative thallium scintigraphy in patients who have received mediastinal irradiation, but the probable increased risk for CAD necessitates such testing if any symptoms are present.

MANAGEMENT OF ESTABLISHED PROBLEMS

Cardiomyopathy and Ventricular Arrhythmia

Late anthracycline-induced cardiomyopathy is a progressive disorder, the course of which extends over months to years. At the onset, the patient may be asymptomatic while his or her life-style unconsciously adjusts to match the decreasing cardiac function. It is essential that the physician informs the patient and reminds other physicians that rapid progression of symptoms may occur with pregnancy, anesthesia, isometric exercise, and the use of illicit (e.g., cocaine) and prescription (e.g., beta-blockers) drugs or alcohol.

As signs and symptoms such as exercise intolerance, dyspnea, peripheral edema, pulmonary rales, S3 and S4, and hepatomegaly are noted, therapy becomes necessary. Many patients experience a major reduction in symptoms for months to years if treated with diuretics alone. Owing to its ability to increase cardiac contractility, digoxin is another mainstay in the treatment of congestive heart failure. Increased cardiac contractility results in increased renal blood flow, increased diuresis, and decreased venous pressure. Angiotensin converting enzyme–inhibiting agents can decrease afterload and natriuresis. Enalapril has been used in survivors of childhood cancer who have poor contractility or increased afterload, with promising results.[39]

Patients with cardiomyopathy are at risk for ventricular arrhythmias. All such patients should undergo 24-hour ECG monitoring on a regular basis. If arrhythmias are occurring, antiarrhythmic agents may be necessary. Unfortunately, many of the drugs used to treat arrhythmias also depress myocardial function. Referral to a cardiologist is recommended.

The poor prognosis of late-onset congestive heart failure necessitates that physicians consider cardiac transplantation. Starnes[52] reported the results of cardiac transplantation in 37 children with cardiomyopathy. Actuarial survival rates at 1, 2, and 5 years were 84%, 80%, and 77% respectively. Deaths resulted from infection (three patients), rejection (two), pulmonary hypertension (two), and late CAD (one). CAD is a major concern, occurring in 5 of the 37 children. At the present time, heart transplantation cannot be considered curative therapy owing to the limited follow-up of patients so treated.

Coronary Artery Disease

Patients with CAD should be followed by a cardiologist. Clinical evaluation includes ECG and ECHO to evaluate overall function and to look for segmental regions of ischemia-induced dyskinesis. An ECG stress test is helpful in the evaluation of ischemic changes and exercise-induced arrhythmias. However, ECG changes seen on a stress test may not correlate well with the presence of CAD in an already damaged myocardium. Depending on the results of the above studies, an ERNA with exercise to evaluate the myocardial response to stress and a thallium scan with exercise or dipyridamole to look for areas of ischemic myocardium may be warranted. Stress echocardiography is another noninvasive method of evaluating for segmental areas of abnormal wall motion that may indicate clinically significant CAD. Cardiac catheterization may be necessary.

Those treated with mantle radiation are at risk for CAD; the condition may be exacerbated by treatment with anthracyclines and cyclophosphamide. Patients should be evaluated for other risk factors such as hypertension, smoking, hyperlipidemia, obesity, diabetes mellitus, and a sedentary life-style. Counseling to reduce such risk factors is appropriate.

Valvulitis

The clinical significance of valvulitis is highly variable. Mild to moderate insufficiency of the tricuspid or pulmonary valves is often well tolerated. Degeneration of mitral or aortic valves, however, may lead to sudden death, congestive heart failure, or the need for valve replacement. All patients with evidence of valvular insufficiency need antibiotic prophylaxis prior to dental or surgical procedures to decrease the risk of bacterial endocarditis. Frequent follow-up by a cardiologist is necessary to evaluate the type and timing of interventions.

Pericarditis

Pericardial disease can result in constrictive pericarditis as the thickened pericardium restricts diastolic relaxation. The treatment consists of surgical stripping of the pericardium. In spite of initial symptomatic improvement, many patients continue to have compromised cardiovascular function.

Preventive Measures

Prevention is the best treatment for cardiovascular sequelae. Many new treatment regimens now address the issues of dose and method of delivery of cardiotoxic therapy for a particular patient group, but the treating clinician must monitor the individual's cardiac studies closely for early evidence of enhanced sensitivity. Once late cardiac injury is present, it appears to be irreversible.

Long-term follow-up must include education regarding the effects of life-style choices on a previously damaged heart. In particular, smoking and drinking alcohol are extremely risky and should be discouraged emphatically. Obesity, a sedentary life-style, hyperlipidemia, and diabetes mellitus are interrelated risk factors. Since the life-style choices that lead to these problems occur early in life, a major focus of annual visits should be to encourage aerobic exercise and a low-fat diet. Exercise need not be exhaustive; the American Heart Association (AHA) recommends 20 to 30 minutes of aerobic exercise 3 to 5 times a week. The best types of exercise are those that can be performed any time of the year, by individuals of any age; thus walking, bike riding, tennis, and swimming are highly recommended. As previously noted, isometric exercise increases cardiac wall stress and should be avoided. Weight lifting also should be avoided, as should competitive football (the training for which includes weight lifting). Rigid dietary restrictions are not necessary, but the following AHA recommendations are appropriate for all adults: two or fewer eggs weekly, no organ meats, and low-fat forms of or substitutes for dairy products (frozen yogurt, skim milk, liquid margarine). In general, less than 30% of the total calories should be derived from fat, and cholesterol intake should be less than 100 mg/day. A dietician may be helpful in teaching families to incorporate such changes into their diets.

Induction of general anesthesia in anthracycline-treated patients has been associated with ventricular arrhythmias. Anesthesiologists should be made aware of a patient's prior history and the associated risks. Similarly, ideal care of a woman of reproductive age may include the involvement and education of her obstetrician. Although many cancer patients have tolerated pregnancy and childbirth well, cardiac consultation should be sought prior to pregnancy. Close monitoring throughout pregnancy may be necessary.

All of our patients are pioneers. The cytostatic therapies that cured their cancers may have caused cardiac damage. Careful long-term surveillance, early diagnosis, and prompt treatment will allow each patient the maximum opportunity to lead a productive and healthy life.

REFERENCES

1. Applefield M: The late appearance of chronic pericardial disease in patients treated by radiotherapy for Hodgkin's disease, *Ann Intern Med* 94:338-341, 1981.
2. Bender KS et al: QT interval prolongation associated with anthracycline cardiotoxicity, *J Pediatr* 105:442-444, 1984.
3. Billingham ME et al: Adriamycin cardiotoxicity: endomyocardial biopsy evidence of enhancement by irradiation, *Am J Surg Pathol* 1:17-23, 1977.
4. Billingham ME et al: Anthracycline cardiomyopathy monitored by morphologic changes, *Cancer Treat Rep* 62:865, 1978.
5. Boivin J et al: Coronary artery disease mortality in patients treated for Hodgkin's disease, *Cancer* 69:1241-1247, 1992.
6. Braverman AC et al: Cyclophosphamide cardiotoxicity in bone marrow transplantation: a prospective evaluation of new dosing regimens, *J Clin Oncol* 9:1215-1223, 1991.
7. Brosius FC III, Waller BF, Roberts WC: Radiation heart disease. Analysis of 16 young (aged 15-33 years) necropsy patients who received over 3,500 rads to the heart, *Am J Med* 70:519-530, 1981.

8. Burns R et al: Detection of radiation cardiomyopathy by gated radionuclide angiography, *Am J Med* 74:297-302, 1983.

9. Byhardt R, Brace K, Ruckdeschel J: Dose and treatment factors in radiation-related pericardial effusion associated with the mantle technique for Hodgkin's disease, *Cancer* 35:795, 1975.

10. Clark EB: *Growth, morphogenesis, and function: the dynamics of heart development.* In Moller JH, Neal WA, Lock JE, editors: *Fetal, neonatal, and infant heart disease,* New York, 1990, Appleton-Century-Crofts.

11. Clark EB: Unpublished data, 1989.

12. Clark EB et al: Effect of increased ventricular pressure on ventricular growth in stage 21 chick embryo, *Am J Physiol* 257:1455-1461, 1989.

13. Cohen SI et al: Radiotherapy as a cause of complete atrioventricular block in Hodgkin's disease: an electrophysiological-pathological correlation, *Arch Intern Med* 141:676-679, 1981.

14. Cohn K et al: Heart disease following irradiation, *Medicine* 46:281-298, 1967.

15. Colan SD, Borow KM, Neumann A: Left ventricular end-systolic wall stress-velocity of fiber shortening relation: a load-independent index of myocardial contractility, *J Am Coll Cardiol* 4:715-724, 1984.

16. Constine LS: Left ventricular function and myocardial perfusion in patients irradiated for Hodgkin's disease, *Int J Radiat Oncol Biol Phys* 24:126, 1992.

17. Corn B, Trock B, Goodman R: Irradiation-related ischemic heart disease, *J Clin Oncol* 8:741-750, 1990.

18. Davis LE, Brown CE: Peripartum heart failure in a patient treated previously with doxorubicin, *Obstet Gynecol* 71:506-508, 1988.

19. Dickout WJ et al: Prevention of acute pulmonary edema after bone marrow transplantation, *Chest* 92:303-309, 1987.

20. Donaldson SS, Kaplan HS: Complications of treatment of Hodgkin's disease in children, *Cancer Treat Rep* 66:977-989, 1982.

21. Ewer MS et al: A comparison of cardiac biopsy grades and ejection fraction estimations in patients receiving Adriamycin, *J Clin Oncol* 2:112, 1984.

22. Fajardo L: Radiation-induced coronary artery disease, *Chest* 71:563-564, 1977.

23. Fajardo L, Stewart J: *Radiation-induced heart disease. Human and experimental observations.* In Bistow MR, editor: *Drug-induced heart disease.* Amsterdam, 1980, Elsevier, North-Holland Biomedical Press.

24. Fajardo L, Stewart J, Cohn K: Morphology of radiation-induced heart disease, *Arch Pathol* 86:512-519, 1968.

25. Fishman NH et al: Models of congenital heart disease in fetal lambs, *Circulation* 58:354-364, 1978.

26. Friedman HS et al: Glutathione protects cardiac and skeletal muscle from cyclophosphamide-induced toxicity, *Cancer Res* 50:2455-2462, 1990.

27. Gomez G et al: Heart size and function after radiation therapy to the mediastinum in patients with Hodgkin's disease, *Cancer Treat Rep* 67:1099-1103, 1983.

28. Goorin AM et al: Congestive heart failure due to Adriamycin cardiotoxicity: its natural history in children, *Cancer* 47:2810-2816, 1981.

29. Gottdiener JS et al: Cardiotoxicity associated with high dose cyclophosphamide therapy, *Arch Intern Med* 141:753-763, 1981.

30. Gottdiener JS et al: Late cardiac effects of mediastinal irradiation, *N Engl J Med* 308:569-572, 1983.
31. Green D et al: The effect of mediastinal irradiation on cardiac function of patients treated during childhood and adolescence for Hodgkin's disease, *J Clin Oncol* 5:239-245, 1987.
32. Hancock S et al: Intercurrent death after Hodgkin's disease in radiotherapy and adjuvant MOPP trials, *Ann Intern Med* 109:183-189, 1988.
33. Hopkins HA et al: Cyclophosphamide-induced cardiomyopathy in the rat, *Cancer Treat Rep* 66:1521-1527, 1982.
34. Jakacki R et al: *Cardiac function in survivors of childhood cancer: effects of anthracyclines, mediastinal and spinal irradiation,* Proceedings of the Second International Conference on Long-Term Complications of Treatment of Children and Adolescents for Cancer, Buffalo, NY, 1992.
35. Kadota R et al: Cardiopulmonary function in long-term survivors of childhood Hodgkin's lymphoma: a pilot study, *Mayo Clin Proc* 63:362-367, 1988.
36. Kim DH et al: Doxorubicin-induced calcium release from cardiac sarcoplasmic reticulum vesicles, *J Mol Cell Cardiol* 21:433-436, 1989.
37. Leach J: Effect of roentgen therapy on the heart, *Arch Intern Med* 72:715-745, 1943.
38. Lewis AB et al: Echocardiographic assessment of anthracycline cardiotoxcity in children, *Med Pediatr Oncol* 5:167, 1978.
39. Lipshultz SE, Colan SD: *The use of echocardiography and holter monitoring in the assessment of anthracycline-treated patients,* Proceedings of the Second International Conference on Long-Term Complications of Treatment of Children and Adolescents for Cancer, Buffalo, NY, 1992.
40. Lipshultz SE et al: Late cardiac effects of doxorubicin therapy for acute lymphoblastic leukemia in childhood, *N Engl J Med* 324:808-814, 1991.
41. Lipshultz S et al: Cardiac mechanics after growth hormone therapy in pediatric Adriamycin recipients, *Proc Am Soc Clin Oncol* 8:296, 1989 (abstract).
42. Martin RG et al: Radiation-related pericarditis, *Am J Cardiol* 35:216-220, 1975.
43. Mills BA, Roberts RW: Cyclophosphamide-induced cardiomyopathy, *Cancer* 43:223-226, 1979.
44. Minow RA et al: Adriamycin cardiomyopathy-risk factors, *Cancer* 39:1397-1402, 1977.
45. Oberlin O et al: No benefit of ifosfamide in Ewing's sarcoma: a nonrandomized study of the French Society of Pediatric Oncology, *J Clin Oncol* 10:1407-1412, 1992.
46. O'Connell TX, Berenbaum MC: Cardiac and pulmonary effects of high doses of cyclophosphamide and isophosphamide, *Cancer Res* 34:1586-1691, 1974.
47. Olson RD, Mushlin PS: Doxorubicin cardiotoxicity: analysis of prevailing hypotheses, *FASEB J* 4:3076-3086, 1990.
48. Phillips J, Ichinose H: Clinical and pathologic studies in the hereditary syndrome of a long QT interval, syncopal spells and sudden death, *Chest* 58:236-243, 1970.
49. Pratt CB, Ransom JL, Evans WE: Age-related Adriamycin cardiotoxicity in children, *Cancer Treat Rep* 62:1381-1385, 1978.
50. Ritchie JL et al: Anthracycline cardiotoxicity: clinical and pathologic outcomes assessed by radionuclide ejection fraction, *Cancer* 46:1109-1116, 1980.
51. Schwartz CL et al: QTc prolongation in anthracycline treated survivors of childhood cancer, *Proc Am Soc Clin Oncol* 9:292, 1990.
52. Starnes V: Heart transplantation in children with cardiomyopathies, *J Heart Lung Transplant* 10:815-819, 1991.

53. Steinherz LJ et al: Guidelines for cardiac monitoring of children during and after anthracycline therapy: report of the Cardiology committee of the children's cancer study group, *Pediatrics* 89:942-949, 1992.

54. Steinherz LJ et al: Cardiac toxicity 4 to 20 years after completing anthracycline therapy, *JAMA* 266:1672, 1991.

55. Stewart J, Fajardo L: Cancer and coronary artery disease, *Int J Radiat Oncol Biol Phys* 4:915-916, 1978.

56. Stewart J, Fajardo L: Radiation-induced heart disease: an update, *Prog Cardivasc Dis* 27:173-194, 1984.

57. Stewart J et al: Radiation-induced heart disease: a study of twenty-five patients, *Radiology* 89:302-310, 1967.

58. Watts RG: Severe and fatal anthracycline cardiotoxicity at cumulative doses below 400 mg/m^2: evidence for enhanced toxicity with multiagent chemotherapy, *Am J Hematol* 36:217-218, 1991.

59. Weesner KM: Exercise echocardiography in the detection of anthracycline cardiotoxicity, *Cancer* 68:435-438, 1991.

9

Pulmonary Effects of Antineoplastic Therapy

Sandra McDonald
Philip Rubin
Cindy L. Schwartz

Anticancer therapy can cause significant toxicity in the respiratory system, ranging in effect from acute lethal events to degrees of chronic pulmonary compromise, which can manifest years after the initial cancer therapy. Additionally, lung and thoracic development can be impaired in young children, augmenting the direct pulmonary sequelae of therapy. Although pulmonary side effects could be prevented by avoiding offending drugs and irradiation of the lung, this is often not feasible in the pursuit of tumor control. Thus, an understanding of the pathophysiology of radiation or chemotherapy lung injury and its quantification are essential in planning new directions of treatment and in evaluating survivors of childhood cancer for chronic pulmonary effects.

PATHOPHYSIOLOGY
Development of the Lung

The development of the lung includes periods of proliferation, hypertrophy, and maturation. During the first 4 months of fetal life the primary lung bud develops into the bronchial tree, which continues to divide further with increased number of blood vessels entering the lung. By 28 weeks gestation, a total of three generations of respiratory bronchioli and one generation of transitional duct has arisen. The latter gives rise to two primitive saccules. By birth, three generations of saccules are found, all ending in terminal saccules. No true alveoli exist, although indentations representing future alveoli are present. Inflation of the saccules occurs at birth, and within a few months the infant's alveoli resemble those of the adult. After birth, minor structural changes continue to occur, the alveolar surfaces becoming more complex and the alveoli more numerous with the increase in body size. However, the exact amount of time necessary for multiplication and proliferation is not certain. The most rapid phase of pulmonary growth probably occurs within the first years of life, followed at 4 to 6 years by a slow growth phase. The number of alveoli that will be present in adulthood is reached at approximately 8 years of age, after which alveolar surface enlarges by increases in volume or size.[29,75] Radiographic measurement of lung diameters demonstrates linear growth during childhood and a spurt at puberty.[71]

Both radiation therapy (RT) and chemotherapy can acutely and chronically affect lung function. Thoracic irradiation in children can cause developmental abnormalities including inhibition of growth of the thoracic cage—a condition that can result in impaired pulmonary function. Effects of direct radiation on the lungs include developmental abnormalities, pneumonitis, and fibrosis. Pulmonary effects of cytotoxic drugs can also cause clinical problems, usually as acute effects and less frequently as long-term effects.

Pathophysiologic Changes Induced by Cytotoxic Therapy

Relatively similar histopathologic changes and resultant physiologic abnormalities are found in the lung following RT and chemotherapy.

Radiation. Histologically, lesions in the lung due to irradiation are most likely present in all patients, even after very small doses of radiation. A large spectrum of histologic changes have been documented in animals; however, data for humans are incomplete. The effects of lethal radiation doses on the lung parenchyma become evident within weeks to months after exposure. There is exudation of proteinaceous material into the alveoli, leading to impairment of gas exchange. An infiltration of inflammatory cells and desquamation of epithelial cells from the alveolar walls occur.[47] In a few weeks the interstitial edema organizes into collagen fibrils, which eventually leads to thickening of the alveolar septa. These exudative changes may resolve in a few weeks to a few months. However, depending on the volume of lung parenchyma irradiated, the total dose, and the dose per fraction, these changes can result in an acute radiation pneumonitis. Although no specific lesion is entirely characteristic of pneumonitis, current evidence[49,76,77,85] suggests that damage to the type II pneumocyte and to the endothelial cell are closely linked to the pneumonitic process. The type II pneumocyte, which produces surfactant and maintains patent alveoli, has been well studied. After radiation exposure a rapid decrease in the content of cytoplasmic surfactant–containing lamellar bodies occurs followed by ultimate sloughing of some of the cells into the alveolar lumen.[46,48] Changes in the surfactant system that lead to alterations in alveolar surface tension and low compliance are most likely a direct result of the radiation,[49,63,64] although it has been postulated that the changes indirectly result from exudation of plasma proteins.[24]

Endothelial cell damage results in changes in perfusion and permeability of the vessel wall. In the first few days to weeks after irradiation, ultrastructural alterations in the capillary endothelial lining become evident. The cells become pleomorphic and vacuolated and may slough, thereby producing areas of denuded basement membrane and occlusion of the capillary lumen by debris and thrombi.[23,33,38,52] It must be noted that these phenomena are dose dependent; scattered changes can be seen at 5.0 Gy, but lesions become widespread at lethal doses of irradiation.

The late lung injury is characterized by progressive fibrosis of alveolar septa, which become thickened by bundles of elastic fibers. The alveoli collapse and are obliterated by connective tissue. Studies in animals have confirmed the protective effect of fractionation, indicating a significant degree of recovery of lung tissue between fractions.[70,84] The mechanisms of chronic injury may be related to the effects of radiation on the pulmonary vasculature (endothelial cells) or somatic cells. The nature of the triggering event in the pathogenesis of radiation-related lung fibrosis is unknown. The classic hypothesis that fibrosis is a connective tissue replacement process following parenchymal cell death is currently being challenged. New evidence[62] suggests that cytokine-mediated multicellular interactions that initiate and sustain the fibrogenic process take place within hours to days after radiation.

Chemotherapy. As increasing numbers of patients are cured with chemotherapy, reports of agents responsible for acute pulmonary toxicity are expanding. Drug-related pulmonary disease may be the result of toxicity, allergy, or idiosyncrasy.[32] Toxicity, with a dose response, has been shown for bleomycin, chlorambucil, and the nitrosoureas. Pulmonary damage, likely mediated through allergic mechanisms, is caused by cyclophosphamide, methotrexate, procarbazine, and bleomycin. Lung injury following low-dose bleomycin has been explained by idiosyncrasy, possibly due to genetically impaired drug metabolism. Pulmonary disease has also been associated with mitomycin, cytosine arabinoside, the vinca alkaloids, and alkylating agents. The pathogenesis of bleomycin injury has been studied extensively.[11,28,31] Its mechanism of cell toxicity appears to include formation of free radicals and lipid peroxidation of phospholipid membranes. This may also be the mechanism by which cyclophosphamide and mitomycin damage the capillary endothelium.[12] Permeability increases, resulting in interstitial edema. Thereafter, swelling and necrosis of type I pneumocytes occur. Hyaline membranes are produced by plasma proteins and fluid entering the alveoli through the denuded epithelium. Type I pneumocytes are replaced by cuboidal cells and then proliferation of fibroblasts occurs, with resulting fibrosis. Interstitial pneumonitis (either the desquamative type that appears to be an earlier stage or the usual type with fibrinous exudation, hyaline membranes, and interstitial fibrosis) is also seen with alkylating agents and nitrosoureas. This pneumonitis may lead to the development of chronic pulmonary fibrosis that is characterized by the enhanced production and deposition of collagen and other matrix components. Pulmonary venoocclusive disease, with vasculitis and intimal fibrosis resulting in pulmonary hypertension, has been reported with bleomycin and mitomycin.[15]

Developmental Effects

The mechanism for respiratory damage in young children is different from that in the adult or adolescent. In the child, impairment by cytotoxic therapy of proliferation and maturation of alveoli can lead to chronic respiratory insufficiency. Inhibition of growth of the thoracic cage (i.e., muscle, cartilage, and bone) can limit chest-wall compliance, with resultant restrictive problems. Therefore, younger children are more at risk than adults or adolescents for developing chronic toxicity, as will be discussed in the clinical manifestations section of this chapter.

CLINICAL MANIFESTATIONS

Clinical Presentation

There is little reaction noted within the first month following radiotherapy. There may be irritation of the larger bronchioles and bronchi resulting in cough during treatment. With high doses exceeding clinical thresholds (8.0 to 12 Gy single dose), pulmonary reactions clinically express themselves as a pneumonitic process 1 to 3 months after the completion of thoracic irradiation. Lethality can occur if both lungs are irradiated to high doses (8.0 to 10 Gy single dose) or if threshold doses of drugs are exceeded. However, recovery from pneumonitis usually occurs, and the second phase of fibrosis follows almost immediately and progresses with time. The clinical syndromes of pneumonitis and fibrosis are associated with RT and several cytotoxic drugs, including bleomycin, methotrexate, mitomycin (with vinca alkaloids), nitrosoureas, and alkylating agents.

The clinical pathologic course is biphasic and is dependent upon the dose and volume of lung exposed. Lower doses of lung irradiation (less than 7.0 Gy single dose) produce subclinical pathologic effects that can be expressed by added insult such as infection or drugs.

Acute Pneumonitis

Acute pneumonitis may be more accurately called pneumonopathy because it is not an infective process. The clinical syndrome usually occurs 1 to 3 months after the completion of radiation or drug therapy, but occasionally an accelerated phase develops within a period of days after chemotherapy. Five to 15 percent of irradiated patients develop acute injury that is more likely to be evident radiologically (particularly on computed tomography [CT] studies[37]) than symptomatically, or on pulmonary function studies. During the period when clinical pneumonitis would occur, some radiologic abnormalities can be found in about 50% of all irradiated patients. The severity of symptoms of the acute pneumonitis syndrome is both dose and volume dependent. There may be low-grade fever and nonspecific respiratory symptoms such as congestion, cough, and fullness in the chest. In more severe cases, dyspnea, pleuritic chest pain, and nonproductive cough may be present. Later, small amounts of sputum, sometimes bloodstained, may be produced. Physical signs in the chest are usually absent, although evidence of consolidation is sometimes found in the region corresponding to pneumonitis. Pleural friction rub or pleural fluid may be detected. When radiation tolerance doses are exceeded, pneumonitis can be very severe and produce acute respiratory distress with the patient experiencing spiking temperatures and acute cor pulmonale that can lead to death.[61] Patients who survive this phase experience protracted pneumonitis — possibly lasting several months — that will generally resolve unless death occurs. No gross abnormalities in lung function occur before 4 to 8 weeks after completion of a course of RT. Restrictive changes gradually develop and progress with time.[23] Gas exchange abnormalities occur approximately at the same time as the changes in lung volumes. These abnormalities consist of a fall in diffusion capacity, mild arterial hypoxemia that may be manifest only with exercise, and a normal or low $Paco_2$ level. These changes appear to be consistent with a parenchymal lung defect and ventilation-perfusion inequality that results in a component of effective shunt.[24] Radionuclide evaluations have demonstrated that under perfusion, rather than under ventilation, is the cause of these inequalities, reflecting radiation injury to the microvasculature.[55,56,82] Larger doses of irradiation cause reductions in lung compliance that start at the time of acute pneumonitis and persist thereafter.[54] The compliance of the chest wall is usually much less affected in adults and adolescents than in young children, in whom interference with growth of both lung and chest wall leads to marked reductions in mean total lung volumes and DLCO.[90] Whole-lung irradiation in doses of 11 to 14 Gy has resulted in restrictive changes in lungs of children treated for various malignancies.[5,35,41] Consequently, RT in younger children, particularly those younger than 3 years old, results in increased chronic toxicity.[41]

The radiation injury seen on chest radiograph (1 to 3 months after the radiation) is usually a diffuse infiltrate corresponding to the radiation field.[25] This results from an acute exudative edema that is initially faint but may progress to homogenous or patchy air-space consolidation. There is frequently an associated volume loss in the affected portion of the lung. CT studies of the lung have been used to evaluate lung density in this situation, and increases are correlated with radiation effects.[34,80] Because of its sensitivity to slight changes in lung density, CT is presently favored for radiographic detection of pulmonary damage in humans.[34,37] CT findings demonstrate a well defined dose-response relationship.[36] Libshitz and Shuman[34] identified four patterns of radiation-induced changes in lung on CT: homogenous (slight increase in radiodensity); patchy consolidation; discrete consolidation; and solid consolidation. These patterns have varying timetables and may appear weeks to years after radiotherapy corresponding to both pneumonitic and fibrotic phases.

Fibrosis

In contrast to the acute reaction, chronic effects of cytotoxic therapy may be observed from months to years following treatment, even though histologic and biochemical changes are evident sooner. Pulmonary fibrosis develops insidiously in the previously irradiated field and stabilizes after 1 or 2 years.

The clinical symptomatology related to radiographic changes is proportional to the extent of the lung parenchyma involved and preexisting pulmonary reserve. Most patients with radiation fibrosis are asymptomatic. In a few patients, particularly those who have had severe pneumonitis, chronic respiratory failure may be present and may be characterized by dyspnea on effort, reduced exercise tolerance, orthopnea, cyanosis, chronic cor pulmonale (sometimes), and finger clubbing. Symptoms are minimal if fibrosis is limited to less than 50% of one lung.[86] If the volume increases above this limit, dyspnea may manifest clinically and progressive chronic cor pulmonale leading to right heart failure may occur.

A mild deterioration in pulmonary function may be demonstrated as fibrosis develops. There is a reduction in maximum breathing capacity that is particularly evident in patients with bilateral radiation fibrosis. Tidal volume usually decreases, and breathing frequency tends to increase, resulting in an overall moderate increase in minute ventilation.[68] Most studies have found these changes to persist indefinitely, with little recovery. Conversely, improvements in pulmonary function can occur as the lung tumor responds to therapy, compensating for losses due to radiation fibrosis.[17,20,25] Owing to functional compensation by adjacent lung regions,[46] pulmonary function tests do not demonstrate significant changes when small volumes of lung are irradiated. These tests are therefore not an ideal endpoint for measurement of radiation-induced lung injury.

Radiologic changes consistent with fibrosis are seen in most patients who have received lung irradiation even if they do not develop acute pneumonitis. Chest radiographs have linear streaking, radiating from the area of previous pneumonitis and sometimes extending outside the irradiated region, with concomitant regional contraction, pleural thickening, and tenting of the diaphragm. The hilum or mediastinum may be retracted with a densely contracted lung segment, resulting in compensatory hyperinflation of adjacent or contralateral lung tissue. This is usually seen 12 months to 2 years after radiation. When chronic fibrosis occurs in the absence of an earlier clinically evident pneumonitic phase.[49,60,69] chest radiography generally reveals scarring that corresponds to the shape of the radiation portal. Eventually, dense fibrotic nodules can develop, especially in the area of previous tumor.[59] CT is currently favored to image regions subjected to RT.[34,37,80] Magnetic resonance imaging (MRI) is being explored and may have promise in accurately distinguishing radiation fibrosis from recurrent tumor.[22] Although radiation tolerance doses may be exceeded, not all patients will develop complications because sensitivity to radiation varies from patient to patient.

Radiation: Tolerance Doses and Tolerance Volumes

Single dose, whole lung volume. Since the introduction of total-body irradiation (TBI) in the setting of bone marrow transplantation and half-body irradiation (HBI) for the treatment of metastatic cancer, substantial human data on lung tolerance have been accumulated.[19,31] When first used, these radiation techniques generally entailed doses of 8.0 to 10 Gy without lung correction factors (for lung density). With TBI, bone marrow transplantation resulted in long-term survival for leukemia patients, and death resulting from interstitial pneumonitis was often attributed to secondary opportunistic infection. With HBI for metastatic patients, the onset of pulmonary failure 1 to 3 months later was mistaken for lymphangitic carcinomatosis. At autopsy, the presence of radiation pneumonopathy became evident when recurrent tumor or infection was not found. Studies of fatal pneumonitis following TBI and HBI, conducted by Keane et al[31] and Fryer et al,[19] provided precise dose-response curves for injury both with and without lung inhomogeneity correction. The threshold dose for fatal pneumonitis was 7.0 Gy with the TD_5 (tolerance dose for 5% probability of death) at 8.2 Gy, the TD_{50} at 9.3 Gy, and the TD_{90} at 11 Gy, corrected for pulmonary transmission. The dose response is so sharp that a difference of 2.0 Gy could change zero mortality to 50% lethality. Decreasing the dose rate from 0.5 to 0.1 Gy per minute decreases the incidence of injury from 90% to 50%.[19,31]

Fractionated dose, whole lung volume. The tolerance of the whole lung to fractionated doses of radiation is well described, particularly in Wilms' tumor patients.[5,35,41,51,90] In the absence of chemotherapy and with daily doses of 1.3 to 1.5 Gy, the TD_5 is 26.5 Gy and the TD_{50} is 30.5 Gy. Young children experience more chronic toxicity at lower doses than older children and adults because of interference with lung and chest-wall development in addition to fibrosis and volume loss. After 20 Gy, mean total lung volumes and DLCO are reduced to 60% of predicted values[90] and 11 to 14 Gy causes restrictive changes.[5,35,41]

Fractionated dose, partial lung volume. Clinical tolerance of partial lung volumes to fractionated radiation is not well quantified. Some relevant data come from Mah and colleagues.[37] Using an increase in lung density within the irradiated volume on CT in the posttreatment period as an endpoint, each 5% increase in effective dose was associated with a 12% increase in incidence of pneumonitis. Doses above 30 Gy in 10 to 15 days and 45 to 50 Gy in 25 to 30 days caused radiographic changes in 30% to 90% of patients.

Chemotherapy: Clinical Manifestations

Drug-related lung injury is most commonly an acute phenomenon, occurring during or shortly after the chemotherapeutic agent(s) are administered.[12] Three typical patterns of pulmonary toxicity have been described: pneumonitis or fibrosis, acute hypersensitivity, and noncardiogenic pulmonary edema. Hypersensitivity reactions (induced by methotrexate, procarbazine, and bleomycin) or noncardiogenic pulmonary edema (induced by methotrexate, cytosine arabinoside, ifosfamide, and cyclophosphamide) usually arise within days of the beginning of treatment[12,32,73] and are unlikely to result in late-onset pulmonary toxicity. Drug-induced pneumonitis or fibrosis has a similar clinical presentation to that described after RT. Bleomycin, the nitrosoureas, and cyclophosphamide are most commonly the etiologic agents, although methotrexate and vinca alkaloids have also been implicated.[12] This syndrome is particularly worrisome because symptoms may not be detectable until months after a critical cumulative dose has been reached or exceeded. In addition, persistent subclinical findings may indicate a potential for late decompensation.

Bleomycin. Patients with acute bleomycin toxicity most commonly present with dyspnea and a dry cough. Fine bibasilar rales may progress to coarse rales involving the entire lung. Radiographs reveal an interstitial pneumonitis with a bibasilar reticular pattern or fine nodular infiltrates. In advanced cases, widespread infiltrates are seen, occasionally with lobar consolidation.[65] Large nodules may mimic metastatic cancer.[40] Loss of lung volume may occur. Pulmonary function testing reveals a restrictive ventilatory defect with hypoxia, hypocapnia, and chronic respiratory alkalosis due to impaired diffusion and hyperventilation.[79]

A major risk factor for bleomycin-induced pulmonary toxicity is the cumulative dose (10% of adults after 400 IU).[7,65] The elderly[7] and children or adolescents[18] may be more sensitive, especially when bleomycin is administered in conjunction with RT.[9] Renal insufficiency[50] and chemotherapeutic agents such as cisplatin or cyclophosphamide[3,57] also increase the risk. Exposure to high levels of oxygen or to pulmonary infection, especially within a year of treatment, is associated with a risk for immediate progressive respiratory failure.[21] These risks may persist for longer periods of time.

The DLCO is thought by some to be the most sensitive screening tool for bleomycin toxicity.[78] Of children treated for Hodgkin's disease with 800 IU/m^2 of bleomycin, 9% had grade 3 or grade 4 pulmonary toxicity according to DLCO. Five percent had clinical symptomatology, and 1.6% died. In patients who develop mild toxicity, discontinuation of bleomycin leads to reversal of abnormalities in some,[13] but others will have persistent radiographic or pulmonary-function abnormalities.[4,45,88]

Nitrosoureas. Patients who have received high cumulative doses of nitrosoureas (e.g., greater than 1500 mg/m^2 in adults and 750 mg/m^2 in children) may present with an interstitial pneumonitis that is identical to that seen after bleomycin therapy. Bibasilar rales with a bibasilar reticular pattern by chest radiograph and a restrictive ventilatory defect are seen. A decreased diffusion capacity may precede all other signs.[66]

Discontinuation of therapy may alter the course of BCNU-induced pulmonary disease. However, once pulmonary infiltrates are noted, the disease may be irreversible.[87] In a documented study, 35% of survivors of childhood brain tumors treated with BCNU and radiation died of lung fibrosis, 12% within 3 years of treatment. However, 24% experienced progressive lung fibrosis resulting in death after a symptom-free interval of 7 to 12 years. The surviving patients were also noted to have evidence of restrictive disease with small lung volume and may remain at risk for late decompensation.[44]

Although pulmonary fibrosis has been most commonly associated with BCNU, it has been described after other nitrosoureas as well.[6,14]

Cyclophosphamide. Makipernaa and colleagues[39] found that 4 of 15 children treated with high-dose cyclophosphamide (no mediastinal RT) had significantly decreased forced vital capacities; two of these children also had a decreased FEV_1. One of these children also had pulmonary fibrosis and a chest deformity. Two children who received more than 50 g/m^2 of cyclophosphamide have been reported to have delayed (greater than 7 years) fatal pulmonary fibrosis with severe restrictive lung disease. Severely decreased anteroposterior chest dimensions in these patients were attributed to inability of the lung to grow in accordance with body growth.[1]

Other agents. Acute pulmonary effects have occurred with cytosine arabinoside (noncardiogenic pulmonary edema)[2,27] and vinca alkaloids in association with mitomycin (bronchospasm or interstitial pneumonitis),[11,26] but delayed pulmonary toxicity has not been described. Hypersensitivity reactions to the antimetabolites (methotrexate, mercaptopurine, and azathioprine) may cause either a desquamative interstitial pneumonitis or an eosinophilic pneumonitis.[32,80,83] Recovery usually occurs within 10 to 45 days after methotrexate-induced pulmonary toxicity.[72]

However, long-term follow-up of 26 childhood-leukemia survivors revealed that 17 (65%) patients had one or more abnormalities of vital capacity, total lung capacity, reserve volume, or diffusion capacity.[67] All children with these deficiencies were diagnosed and treated before age 8. These findings have also been attributed to an impairment of lung growth, which normally proceeds exponentially by cell division in the first 8 years of life.

Radiation and Chemotherapy Combinations: Interaction and Tolerance

Many antineoplastic agents potentiate the damaging effects of radiation on the lung. Phillips[52] and Wara[84] demonstrated that dactinomycin administration lowered the radiation-dose threshold for pneumonitis. Testing the effects of commonly used chemotherapeutic agents, Phillips and colleagues[53] reported that the administration of dactinomycin, cyclophosphamide, and, to a lesser extent, vincristine enhanced the lethal potential of thoracic irradiation. The effect of dactinomycin was seen when given as long as 30 days before the irradiation but was not seen when given 30 days after the irradiation. The administration of bleomycin and lung irradiation together produces a lung toxicity that is more common and severe than when either agent is given alone. Catane[9] found pulmonary toxicity in 19% of patients; it was fatal in 10%. This toxicity appears to be maximal when bleomycin is given concurrently with radiation.[16] Although 500 IU of bleomycin without RT can be lethal in 1% to 2% of patients, as little as 30 IU can be fatal when given with RT. The effects of RT are potentiated by doxorubicin. In addition to the enhanced toxicity observed in skin, intestines, and heart, the lung also appears to be very sensitive to this combination.[8,10] Of 24 patients treated with low-dose doxorubicin and RT, 13 developed pneumonitis.[81]

Chemotherapy-Chemotherapy Interactions

Toxicity is seen at much lower doses than expected with drug combinations such as: nitrosoureas and cyclophosphamide,[74] bleomycin, and cisplatin; or vincristine, doxorubicin, and cyclophosphamide.[3,32,57] Vinca alkaloids appear to cause pulmonary toxicity only in the presence of mitomycin.[11,32]

DETECTION AND SCREENING

Pulmonary disease occurring in patients treated for cancer can present a diagnostic problem because of the multiplicity of possible etiologies. Progressive cancer, infections, emboli, allergy, irradiation, or drugs (and their interaction) can be causative. Clinical findings, radiologic studies, and pulmonary function tests can be nonspecific; however, these factors represent measurable endpoints to quantify toxicity.

Measurable Endpoints

Symptoms. Fever, cough, and shortness of breath are the most common symptoms of radiation-induced pneumonopathy. Temperature, respiratory rate,

Table 9-1
Shortness-of-Breath Scoring System

Grade	Description
0	No shortness of breath with normal activity. Shortness of breath with exertion, comparable to a well person of the same age, height, and sex.
1	More shortness of breath than a person of the same age while walking quietly on the level or on climbing an incline or two flights of stairs.
2	More shortness of breath and unable to keep up with persons of the same age and sex while walking on the level.
3	Shortness of breath while walking on the level and while performing everyday tasks at work.
4	Shortness of breath while carrying out personal activities, e.g., dressing, talking, walking from one room to another.

From: Morgan W, Seaton A: *Occupational lung diseases,* Philadelphia, 1989, WB Saunders.

frequency of cough, and the nature of sputum produced should all be recorded. Varying degrees of dyspnea, as well as orthopnea, can be present depending on the severity of pulmonary damage. A grading system has been suggested by Morgan and Seaton[42] to correlate the degree of shortness of breath with the amount of disability caused by pulmonary injury (Table 9-1).

Signs. The principal signs of both acute and delayed radiation-induced pneumonopathy are increase in respiratory rate, percussion of a pleural effusion, auscultation of rales or rhonchi, and, in severe cases, cyanosis.

Analytic: pulmonary function tests (PFTs). The various PFTs that are available can be divided primarily into those performed in a pulmonary function laboratory and those performed in a nuclear medicine unit. Classic PFTs include measurement of static lung volumes, static and dynamic mechanical properties, airway reactivity, small airway function, and gas exchange functions. A wide range of abnormalities in PFTs has been reported during both the acute and chronic phases of radiation-induced pneumonopathy. The abnormalities will, of course, relate to the volume of lung irradiated as well as the dose. Decreases have been noted in the vital capacity, the inspiratory capacity, the total lung capacity, the residual volume, and the FEV_1. Decreases in lung compliance have also been measured.

The goal of classic PFTs is to determine what pattern of pulmonary disease affects the patient (see Table 9-2 for definitions of restrictive, obstructive, and interstitial disease). Restrictive patterns are generally found after RT or chemotherapy injury with reductions in the vital capacity, lung volumes, and total lung capacity. Combined obstructive restrictive patterns may be seen in which lung volumes are reduced, but the fibrotic injury also reduces airway patency. Finally, there is abnormal gas transfer because of the change in the alveolar capillary barrier. This can be measured by the carbon monoxide lung-diffusion test and, in more severe cases, will also be reflected in the arterial oxygen and carbon dioxide levels, which can be elevated.

Table 9-2
Grading System for Impaired Pulmonary Function

Test	Mild	Moderate	Severe
Obstructive impairment			
MVV, % predicted	65-80	45-60	Less than 45
VC, % predicted	Normal	Usually normal	Slight to moderate reduction
FEV_1, % predicted	65-80	45-60	Less than 45
$FEV_1/FVC_\%$*	55-75	45-55	Less than 45
Blood gases,† % sat	Normal	Usually normal	Hypoxemia
DL_{CO}, % predicted	Normal	Normal or slight reduction	Slight to moderate reduction
Restrictive impairment			
MVV, % predicted	Normal	Normal	50-80
VC, % predicted	60-80	50-60	Less than 50
FEV_1, % predicted	60-80	50-60	Less than 50
$FEV_1/FVC_\%$*	Normal	Normal	Normal
Blood gases, % sat	Normal	Normal	Usually normal
DL_{CO}, % predicted	Normal	50-75	Below 50
Interstitial lung disease			
MVV, % predicted	Normal	Normal	60 or above
VC, % predicted	70 or greater	50-70	Less than 50
FEV_1, % predicted	70 or greater	50-70	Less than 50
$FEV_1/FVC_\%$*	Normal	Normal	Normal
Blood gases, % sat	94-96	90-94	90 or less
$(A-a)P_{O_2}$, mm*	15-30	30-40	Above 40
DL_{CO}, % predicted	Normal	40-75	Less than 40

*Age-related.
†Unreliable in obstructive impairment.
From: Morgan W, Seaton A: *Occupational lung diseases,* Philadelphia, 1989, WB Saunders.

The basic evaluation that is most valuable in studying patients who have had lung injury consists of the measurement of maximum inspiratory and expiratory pressures, forced vital capacity and the FEV_1, as well as the $FEV_1/FVC\%$. The findings usually indicate whether there is an obstructive or restrictive pattern and to what degree pulmonary function is impaired. The evaluation consists of a screening spirometry panel followed by an examination of static lung volume such as total lung capacity, functional residual capacity, and residual volume. Finally, it is essential to perform a carbon monoxide diffusing test to measure the degree of alveolar-capillary block.

All these tests are quantitative but must be related to the expected level of function in a person of the same age and size, or preferably to measurements performed before the anticancer therapy is begun.

Table 9-3
Summary of Clinical, Radiologic, and Quantitative Assessments of Pulmonary Function

Symptoms	Signs	PFTs	Nuclear medicine tests	Radiography	Blood tests
Cough	Fever	Vital capacity	Perfusion scan	Quantitative CT	Surfactant apoprotein
Dyspnea	Dullness to percussion	FEV_1	Ventilation scan	Total aerated lung volume	Procollagen type 3
Pain	Sputum	$FEV_1/$ FVC%	Gallium scan	Total opacified volume	Angiotensin converting enzyme
		Carbon monoxide diffusing capacity (DLCO%)	Quantitative V-Q scan	Percentage of opacified	Plasminogen-activating factor
			Ventilation per unit volume Blood flow to ventilated alveoli Blood flow per unit ventilated lung volume		Prostacyclin

Combining these various measurements into a grading system of pulmonary function is difficult. One attempt has been made by Morgan and Seaton and is shown in Table 9-3.[42]

Nuclear medicine tests. Extremely important in evaluating radiation-induced pneumonopathy in particular are the qualitative and quantitative radionuclide studies. These consist of perfusion studies, ventilation studies, gallium scans, and quantitative ventilation-perfusion scintigraphy.

A perfusion scan is usually obtained with microaggregated albumin labeled with ^{99m}Tc or similarly labeled microspheres, which are injected intravenously and imaged in eight views to ensure that the entire lung is viewed. Ventilation studies can be carried out either with ^{133}Xe or ^{127}Xe by inhalation. The wash-in, equilibration, and wash-out phases can be observed, generally through posterior and oblique views. Because of energy and half-life, the ^{133}Xe test is done before the perfusion study and the ^{127}Xe test after the perfusion scan. Generally, both should be employed and, if possible, quantified. The advantage over classic PFTs is that scans will show regional function, which can be correlated with irradiated volumes.

In some situations the ventilation study with xenon may be done with krypton, although krypton is more expensive. Finally, aerosols of ^{99m}Tc diethylenetriamine-pentaacetic acid (DTPA) can be substituted for an inspiration gas study. The pair of studies (i.e., perfusion and ventilation), is often termed a *V-Q scan;* the letter *V* stands for ventilation, and the letter *Q* stands for perfusion.

Gallium scans of the lungs can be useful in assessing and quantifying bleomycin, cyclophosphamide, and busulfan chemotherapy injury to the lung and can also be used to separate radiation-induced pneumonopathy from *Pneumocystis carinii* pneumonopathy because the latter will label heavily with gallium.[30,58]

Quantitative ventilation-perfusion scintigraphy consists of three different studies. The first is ventilation per unit volume; the second is blood flow to ventilated alveoli; and the third is blood flow per unit ventilated lung volume. The second, that is, blood flow to ventilated alveoli, has proven most useful in quantifying RT injury.

Radiography. Plain anteroposterior (AP) and lateral chest films are useful when disease involves a large volume of lung. The acute pneumonitic phase manifests as a fluffy infiltrate, and the late fibrotic phase can follow the intermediate phase of contraction. However, routine chest radiography has a low level of reliability in detecting small volumes of pneumonopathy, particularly if they are located close to the chest wall. Chest radiography also lacks the ability to quantify the volume of affected lung versus the total lung volume.

CT scans have the capability of presenting three-dimensional images and calculating three-dimensional volumes of functional lung with a defined range of Hounsfield units. One can also detect small infiltrates that may be adjacent to the chest wall, for example, in the case of tangential field RT, where infiltrates are calculated as a percentage of the total lung volume. Mah[36,37] has shown a quantitative relationship between the volume of abnormality on CT and RT dose (converted to a single-dose equivalent).

Laboratory tests of serum or blood. Although the usefulness of serum or blood laboratory tests is as yet undefined, there is a need for early biochemical markers of normal-tissue damage that would predict late effects and that would allow the radiation oncologist and medical oncologist to determine if their treatment is exceeding normal tissue tolerance.[60] If biochemical markers of tissue damage could be detected in the subclinical phase, prior to the accumulation of significant injury, one could terminate therapy or institute treatment to prevent or attenuate later lesions. An ideal marker would be a simple, reproducible positive or negative biochemical test. There are many substances the release of which could reflect or predict the degree of RT and chemotherapy injury to the lung. Besides the surfactant apoprotein, procollagen type 3 can be measured in the blood. It is possible that angiotensin-converting enzyme, blood plasminogen-activating factor, and prostacyclin can be measured as well. These various substances have been correlated with either acute or delayed radiation-induced pneumonopathy. Significant additional work is required to evaluate the usefulness of such blood level measurements.

MANAGEMENT OF ESTABLISHED PULMONARY TOXICITY INDUCED BY CYTOTOXIC THERAPY

Optimally, pulmonary toxicity will be prevented rather than managed. Strict attention should be paid to drug doses and cumulative drug-dose restrictions. When RT is given, volumes and doses should be minimized and given in accordance to accepted tolerance. During drug (e.g. bleomycin) therapy, monitoring of symptoms and signs, PFTs, and chest radiographs can aid in detecting problems early, and the causative agent can be withdrawn. After withdrawal of bleomycin, early stages of bleomycin-induced pneumonitis have reversed clinically and radiographically.[40]

Therapy for Established Toxicity

Corticosteroids play a useful role in the relief of symptoms from pneumonitis caused by a variety of drugs and RT. Severe symptoms necessitating treatment can be relieved markedly and rapidly by corticosteroids in half of affected patients;[43,88,89] however, prevention or reversal of the fibrotic phase does not occur. Supportive care with bronchodilators, expectorants, antibiotics, bed rest, and oxygen can be beneficial for relief of symptoms in pneumonitis and fibrosis.

Precautions for Minimizing Potential Complications

When following survivors of cancer, vigilant evaluation of symptoms of respiratory compromise is necessary and should be anticipated when thoracic RT or drugs with known pulmonary toxicity have been used. Chronic cough or dyspnea should be further evaluated with PFTs and chest radiography. This is imperative in patients scheduled for general anesthesia. In the absence of symptoms, chest radiographs and lung function testing are recommended every 2 to 5 years. Depending on the circumstances, lung biopsy should be considered to confirm fibrosis or exclude recurrence of cancer. In cases of radiation-induced pneumonitis in which corticosteroids have been used, it is important to withdraw steroids very slowly to avoid reactivation. Prophylactic administration of steroids before therapy has no proven use and may do more harm than good.

Counseling to Prevent Further Compromise

Strenuous counseling on the risks of smoking is imperative in these patients, as is awareness of the risks of general anesthesia.

Future Studies

An understanding of the new molecular mechanisms (involving immediate cytokine release[62]) in the initiation of the fibrosis process allows for timely intervention and proper protection. Substances, such as certain interferons that oppose or inhibit fibrosis-promoting growth factors, could be used during therapy, resulting in the desired enhanced therapeutic ratio.

REFERENCES

1. Alvarado CS, Boat TF, Newman AJ: Late-onset pulmonary fibrosis and chest deformity in two children treated with cyclophosphamide, *J Pediatr* 92:443-446, 1978.
2. Anderson BS, Cogan BM, Keating MJ et al: Subacute pulmonary failure complicating therapy with high dose ara-C in acute leukemia, *Cancer* 56:2181-2184, 1984.
3. Bauer KA, Skarin AT, Balikian JP et al: Pulmonary complications associated with combination chemotherapy programs containing bleomycin, *Am J Med* 74:557-563, 1983.
4. Bellamy EZ, Husband JE, Blaquiere RM et al: Bleomycin related lung damage: CT evidence, *Radiology* 156:155-158, 1985.
5. Benoist MR et al: Effects on pulmonary function of whole lung irradiation for Wilms' tumor in children, *Thorax* 37:175-180, 1982.
6. Block M, Lachowiez RM, Rios C et al: Pulmonary fibrosis associated with low-dose adjuvant methyl-CCNU, *Med Pediatr Oncol* 18:256-260, 1990.
7. Blum RH, Carter SK, Agre K: A clinical review of bleomycin—a new antineoplastic agent, *Cancer* 31:903-914, 1973.
8. Cassady JR, Richter MP, Piro AJ et al: Radiation-adriamycin interactions: preliminary clinical observations, *Cancer* 36:946-949, 1975.
9. Catane R, Schwade JG, Turrisi AT et al: Pulmonary toxicity after radiation and bleomycin: a review, *Int J Radiat Oncol Biol Phys* 5:1513-1518, 1979.
10. Chan PYM, Kagan AR, Byfield JE et al: Pulmonary complications of combined chemotherapy and radiotherapy in lung cancer, *Front Radiat Ther Oncol* 13:136-144, 1979.
11. Cooper JA, Zitnik R, Matthay RA: Mechanisms of drug-induced pulmonary disease, *Ann Rev Med* 39:395-404, 1988.
12. Cooper JAD, White DA, Matthay RA: Drug induced pulmonary disease. Part I. Cytotoxic drugs, *Am Rev Respir Dis* 133:321-340, 1986.
13. DeLana M, Guzzon A, Monfardini S et al: Clinical radiologic and histopathologic studies on pulmonary toxicity induced by treatment with bleomycin, *Cancer Chemother Rep* 343-355, 1972.
14. Dent RG: Fatal pulmonary toxic effects of lomustine, *Thorax* 37:627-629, 1982.
15. Doll DC, Ringenberg Q, Yarbo JW: Vascular toxicity associated with antineoplastic agents, *J Clin Oncol* 4:1405-1417, 1986.
16. Einhorn L, Krause M, Hornback N et al: Enhanced pulmonary toxicity with bleomycin and radiotherapy in oat cell lung cancer, *Cancer* 37:2414-2416, 1976.
17. Evans RF, Sagerman RH, Ringrose TL: Pulmonary function following mantle field irradiation for Hodgkin's disease, *Radiology* 111:729, 1974.
18. Fryer CJ, Hutchinson RJ, Krailo M et al: Efficacy and toxicity of 12 courses of ABVD chemotherapy followed by low-dose regional radiation in advanced Hodgkin's disease in children: a report from the children cancer study group, *J Clin Oncol* 8:1971-1980, 1990.
19. Fryer CJH, Fitzpatrick PJ, Rider WD et al: Radiation pneumonitis: experience following a large single dose of radiation, *Int J Radiat Oncol Biol Phys* 4:931-936, 1978.
20. Germon PA, Brady LW: Physiologic changes before and after radiation treatment for carcinoma of the lung, *JAMA* 206:808, 1968.

21. Gilson AJ, Sahn SA: Reactivation of bleomycin lung toxicity following oxygen administration, *Chest* 88:304-306, 1985.

22. Glazer HS, Lee JKT, Levitt RG et al: Radiation fibrosis: differentiation from recurrent tumor by MR imaging, *Radiology* 156:721-726, 1985.

23. Gross NJ: Experimental radiation pneumonitis IV. Leakage of circulatory proteins onto the alveolar surface, *J Lab Clin Med* 95:19-31, 1980.

24. Gross NJ: The pathogenesis of radiation-induced lung damage, *Lung* 159:115-125, 1981.

25. Gross NJ: Pulmonary effects of radiation therapy, *Ann Intern Med* 86:81-92, 1977.

26. Gunstream SR, Seidenfeld JJ, Sobonya RE et al: Mitomycin associated lung disease, *Cancer Treat Rep* 67:301-304, 1983.

27. Haupt HM, Hutchins GM, Moore GW: Ara-C lung: non-cardiogenic pulmonary edema complicating cytosine-arabinoside therapy of leukemia, *Am J Med* 70:256-261, 1981.

28. Hay J, Shahriar S, Laurent G: Mechanisms of bleomycin-induced lung damage, *Arch Toxicol* 65:81-94, 1991.

29. Hodson WA: *Development of the lung,* New York, 1977, Marcel Dekker.

30. Kataoka M, Kawamura M, Itoh H et al: Ga-67 citrate scintigraphy for the early detection of radiation pneumonitis, *Clin Nucl Med* 17(1):27-31, 1992.

31. Keane TJ, Van Dyk J, Rider WD: Idiopathic interstitial pneumonia following bone marrow transplantation: the relationship with total body irradiation, *Int J Radiat Oncol Biol Phys* 7:1365-1370, 1981.

32. Lehne G, Lote K: Pulmonary toxicity of cytotoxic and immunosuppressive agents. A review, *Acta Oncol* 29(2):113-124, 1990.

33. Leroy EP, Liebner EJ, Jensick RJ: The ultrastructure of canine alveoli after supervoltage irradiation of the thorax, *Lab Invest* 15:1544-1558, 1966.

34. Libshitz HI, Shuman LS: Radiation induced pulmonary change: CT findings, *J Comput Assist Tomogr* 8:15-19, 1984.

35. Littman P, Meadows AT, Polgar G et al: Pulmonary function in survivors of Wilms' tumor: patterns of impairment, *Cancer* 37:2773-2776, 1976.

36. Mah K, Poon PY, Van Dyk J et al: Assessment of acute radiation-induced pulmonary changes using computed tomography, *J Comput Assist Tomogr* 10:736-743, 1986.

37. Mah K, Van Dyk J, Keane T et al: Acute radiation-induced pulmonary damage: a clinical study on the response to fractionated radiation therapy, *Int J Radiat Oncol Biol Phys* 13:179-188, 1987.

38. Maisin JR: The influence of radiation on blood vessels and circulation. III. Ultrastructure of the vessel wall, *Curr Top Radiat Res Q* 10:29-57, 1974.

39. Makipernaa A, Heino M, Laitnen L et al: Lung function following treatment of malignant tumors with surgery, radiotherapy, or cyclophosphamide in childhood, *Cancer* 63:625-630, 1989.

40. McCrea ES, Diaconis JJN, Wade C et al: Bleomycin toxicity simulating metastatic nodules to the lungs, *Cancer* 48:1096-1100, 1981.

41. Miller RW, Fusner JE, Fink R et al: Pulmonary function abnormalities in long term survivors of childhood cancer, *Med Pediatr Oncol* 14:202-207, 1986.

42. Morgan W, Seaton A: *Occupational lung diseases,* Philadelphia, 1989, WB Saunders.

43. Moss WT, Haddy FJ, Sweany SK: Some factors altering the severity of acute radiation pneumonitis: variation with cortisone, heparin and antibiotics, *Radiology* 75:50-54, 1960.

44. O'Driscoll BR, Hasleton PS, Taylor PM et al: Active lung fibrosis up to 17 years after chemotherapy with carmustine (BCNU) in childhood, *N Engl J Med* 323:378-382, 1990.

45. Osanto S, Bukman A, Van Hoek F et al: Long term effects of chemotherapy in patients with testicular cancer, *J Clin Oncol* 10:574-579, 1992.

46. Penney DP, Rubin P: Specific early fine structural changes in the lung following irradiation, *Int J Radiat Oncol Biol Phys* 2:1123-1132, 1977.

47. Penney DP: *Ultrastructural organization of the distal lung and potential target cells of ionizing radiation.* International Conference on New Biology of Lung and Lung Injury and Their Implications for Oncology, Porvoo, Finland, June 1987.

48. Penney DP, Shapiro DL, Rubin P et al: Effects of radiation on the mouse lung and potential induction of radiation pneumonitis, *Virchows Arch B Cell Pathol* 37:327-336, 1981.

49. Penney DP, Siemann DW, Rubin P et al: Morphologic changes reflecting early and late effects of irradiation of the distal lung of the mouse review, *Scanning Microsc* I:413-425, 1982.

50. Perry DJ, Weiss RB, Taylor HG: Enhanced bleomycin toxicity during acute renal failure, *Cancer Treat Rep* 66:592-593, 1982.

51. Philips T: Pulmonary section—cardiorespiratory workshops, *Cancer Clin Trial* 4(suppl):45-52, 1981.

52. Phillips TL, Margolis L: Radiation pathology and the clinical response of lung and esophagus, *Front Radiat Ther Oncol* 6:254-273, 1972.

53. Phillips TL, Wharam MD, Margolis LW: Modification of radiation injury to normal tissues by chemotherapeutic agents, *Cancer* 35:1678-1684, 1975.

54. Phillips TL, Wyatt JP: *Radiation fibrosis.* In Fishman AP: Pulmonary diseases and disorders, *vol I,* New York, 1980, McGraw-Hill.

55. Prato FS, Kurdyak R, Saibil EA et al: Regional and total lung function in patients following pulmonary irradiation, *Invest Radiol* 12:224-237, 1977.

56. Prato FS, Kurdyak R, Saibil EA et al: Physiological and radiographic assessment during the development of pulmonary radiation fibrosis, *Radiology* 122:389-397, 1977.

57. Rabinowitz M, Souhami L, Gil RA et al: Increased pulmonary toxicity with bleomycin and cisplatin chemotherapy combinations, *Am J Clin Oncol* (CCT) 13(2):132-138, 1990.

58. Richman S, Levenson SM, Bunn PA et al: Ga-67 accumulation in pulmonary lesions associated with bleomycin toxicity, *Cancer* 36:1966, 1975.

59. Rubin P: The Franz Busche lecture: late effects of chemotherapy and radiation therapy: a new hypothesis, *Int J Radiat Oncol Biol Phys* 10:5-34, 1984.

60. Rubin P: Radiation toxicity: quantitative radiation pathology for predicting effects, *Cancer* 39(suppl 2):729-736, 1977.

61. Rubin P, Casarett GW: *Clinical radiation pathology,* Philadelphia, 1968, WB Saunders.

62. Rubin P, Finkelstein J, McDonald S et al: The identification of new early molecular mechanisms in the pathogenesis of radiation induced pulmonary fibrosis, *Int J Radiat Oncol Biol Phys* 21(suppl 1):163, 1991.

63. Rubin P, Siemann DW, Shapiro DL et al: Surfactant release as an early measure of radiation pneumonitis, *Int J Radiat Oncol Biol Phys* 9:1669-1673, 1983.

64. Rubin P, Shapiro DL, Finklestein JN et al: The early release of surfactant following lung irradiation of alveolar type II cells, *Int J Radiat Oncol Biol Phys* 6:75-77, 1980.

65. Samuels ML, Douglas EJ, Holoye PV et al: Large dose bleomycin therapy and pulmonary toxicity, *JAMA* 235:1117-1120, 1976.

66. Selker RG, Jacobs SA, Moore PB et al: 1,3-Bis (2-chloroethyl)-1-nitrosourea (BCNU)-induced pulmonary fibrosis, *Neurosurgery* 7:560-565, 1980.

67. Shaw NJ, Tweeddale PM, Eden OB: Pulmonary function in childhood leukemia survivors, *Med Pediatr Oncol* 17:149-154, 1989.

68. Shrivastava PN, Hans L, Concannon JP: Changes in pulmonary compliance and production of fibrosis in x-irradiated lungs of rats, *Radiology* 112:439-440, 1974.

69. Siemann DW, Hill RP, Penney DP: Early and late pulmonary toxicity in mice evaluated 180 and 420 days following localized lung irradiation, *Radiat Res* 89:396-407, 1982.

70. Siemann DW, Rubin P, Penney DP: Pulmonary toxicity following multi-fraction radiotherapy, *Br J Cancer* 53:365-367, 1986.

71. Simon G, Reiol L, Tanner SM et al: Growth of radiobiologically determined heart diameter, lung width and lung lengths from 5-19 years with standard for clinical use, *Arch Dis Child* 47:373-382, 1972.

72. Sostman HD, Matthay RA, Putnam CE et al: Methotrexate induced pneumonitis, *Medicine* 55:371-89, 1976.

73. Spector I, Zimbler H, Ross S: Early-onset cyclophosphamide induced interstitial pneumonitis, *JAMA* 242:2852-2854, 1979.

74. Stewart P, Buckner CD, Thomas ED et al: Intensive chemotherapy with autologous marrow transplantation for small cell carcinoma of the lung, *Cancer Treat Rep* 7:1055-1059, 1983.

75. Thurlbeck WM: Postnatal growth and development of the lung, *Am Rev Respir Dis* 111:803-843, 1975.

76. Travis EL, Hanley RA, Fenn JO et al: Pathologic changes in the lung following single and multi-fraction irradiation, *Int J Radiat Oncol Biol Phys* 2:475-490, 1977.

77. Travis EL: Early indicators of radiation injury on the lung: are they useful predictors for late changes? *Int J Radiat Oncol Biol Phys* 6:1267-1269, 1980.

78. Umezawa H, Crooke ST, editors: *Bleomycin status and new developments,* New York, 1978, Academic Press.

79. van Barneveld PWC, Veenstra G, Sleifer DT et al: Changes in pulmonary function during and after bleomycin treatment in patients with testicular carcinoma, *Cancer Chemother Pharmacol* 14:168-171, 1985.

80. Van Dyk J, Hill RP: Postirradiation lung density changes measured by computerized tomography, *Int J Radiat Oncol Biol Phys* 9:847-852, 1983.

81. Verschoore J, Lagrange JL, Boublil JL et al: Pulmonary toxicity of a combination of low-dose doxorubicin and irradiation for inoperable lung cancer, *Radiother Oncol* 9:281-288, 1987.

82. Vieras F, Bradley EW, Alderson PO et al: Regional pulmonary function after irradiation of the canine lung: radionuclide evaluation, *Radiology* 147:839-844, 1983.

83. Wall MA, Wohl MEB, Jaffe N: Lung function in adolescents receiving high dose methotrexate, *Pediatrics* 63:741-746, 1979.

84. Wara WM, Phillips TL, Margolis LW et al: Radiation pneumonitis: a new approach to the derivation of time-dose factors, *Cancer* 32:547-552, 1973.

85. Ward WF, Molteni A, Solliday SH et al: The relationship between endothelial dysfunction and collagen accumulation in irradiated rat lung, *Int J Radiat Oncol Biol Phys* 11: 1985-1990, 1985.

86. Weichselbaum RR, Awan AM: *Principles of radiation oncology.* In JD Bitran et al, editors: *Lung cancer—a comprehensive treatise,* Orlando, 1987, Grune and Stratton.

87. Weinstein AS, Diener-West M, Nelson DF et al: Pulmonary toxicity of carmustine in patients treated for malignant glioma, *Cancer Treat Rep* 70:943-946, 1986.
88. White DA, Stover DE: Severe bleomycin induced pneumonitis. Clinical features and response to corticosteroids, *Chest* 86:723-728, 1984.
89. Whitfield AGW, Bond WH, Kunkler PB: Radiation damage to thoracic tissues, *Thorax* 18:371-380, 1963.
90. Wohl ME, Griscom NT, Traggis DG et al: Effects of therapeutic irradiation delivered in early childhood upon subsequent lung function, *Pediatrics* 55:507-514, 1975.

10

Late Gastrointestinal and Hepatic Effects

J. Blatt
D. Neigut
J.M. Robertson
T. S. Lawrence

Treatment-related gastrointestinal (GI) toxicities in long-term survivors of childhood cancer have received relatively little attention. This may be for one of several reasons. GI toxicity may truly be uncommon among survivors of the common pediatric malignancies. The Late Effects Study Group, reporting on follow-up of 110 5-year survivors of childhood leukemia (the single most common pediatric cancer), identified only one patient with liver disease and another who required a bowel resection.[19] Also, GI toxicity may be underdetected. Hepatic fibrosis, for example, which has been reported in surveillance liver biopsies of patients treated with methotrexate, may be asymptomatic and unassociated with abnormal liver function tests. Finally, the latency for other GI toxicities may not yet have been reached in a large enough number of patients to be noticeable.

In this chapter, we will summarize abnormalities of the upper and lower GI tracts and hepatobiliary tree that are seen in survivors of childhood cancer. These abnormalities will be related to therapeutic modalities (radiation, chemotherapy, surgery, bone marrow transplant) and to supportive therapies such as tranfusions. Toxicities that first develop during treatment and persist, as well as those that are delayed in onset, will be discussed. An attempt will be made to place these abnormalities in the context of normal organ pathophysiology and to provide guidelines for surveillance and management.

Upper and Lower Gastrointestinal Tract
PATHOPHYSIOLOGY
Normal Anatomy and Physiology

The upper GI tract extends from the oropharynx to the ileocecal valve and is composed of the esophagus, the stomach, and the small intestine. The esophagus is a distensible tube that consists of an inner mucosa lined by stratified squamous epithelium, a submucosa, muscularis externa that contains both striated and smooth muscle, and an outermost connective tissue layer. The neurovascular supply and mucous glands (which open into the lumen of the esophagus) are located primarily in the submucosa. The esophagus is at risk for injury from reflux of gastric contents, and the lower esophageal sphincter acts to prevent gastroesophageal reflux. The epithelium and mucous glands help protect the esophagus from peptic injury. Other protective factors include salivation and esophageal peristalsis, which aid in acid clearance.

The stomach, which lies inferior to the left hemidiaphragm, is anatomically divided into the cardia, the fundus, the body, and the antrum. The distal aperture of the stomach—the pylorus—has a thick muscular wall that forms the sphincter connecting the antrum to the duodenum. The stomach wall includes a mucosal layer lined by columnar epithelium, a submucosa, and an outer muscularis that consists of longitudinal and circular smooth muscle. The gastric mucosa contains many glands that, depending on location, secrete mucus, hydrochloric acid, or hormones that participate in regulation of gastric secretion and motility. The mucosa of the gastric fundus secretes an intrinsic factor that is necessary for absorption of vitamin B_{12} from the small intestine.

The layers of the small intestine have a configuration similar to that of the stomach. However, unlike other tubular organs, the small intestine is lined with villi that increase the absorptive and digestive surface area. The epithelium is rapidly proliferating, and mitoses are commonly seen. Microvilli form the brush border of the luminal surface of the columnar cells that form the villi. Disaccharidases and peptidases are located on the microvillous surface. The duodenum is located primarily in the retroperitoneum. It is fixed by several ligaments and forms a shape like the letter C with the head of the pancreas in the concavity. In contrast to the duodenum, the jejunum and most of the ileum are normally freely mobile within the abdominal cavity and are suspended by the mesentery. The ileocecal valve acts as a sphincter, preventing bacterial contamination of the small bowel.

The colon originates in the right lower quadrant, ascends to the hepatic flexure, traverses the abdomen to the splenic flexure, and descends to the anus in a somewhat tortuous fashion. The splenic flexure and rectosigmoid are two "watershed" areas in the arterial supply to the colon and are, therefore, predisposed to ischemia. The colon is lined with columnar epithelium, and there are no villi. Microvilli are located on the luminal surface of the epithelial cells, where active transport of electrolytes and water takes place. Copious goblet cells secrete mucus onto the luminal surface of the colon.

Changes Induced by Cytotoxic Therapy

Several interacting causes of enteritis and fibrosis after cancer therapy are shown in the box on the next page. Fibrosis is among the most common change to affect the GI tract in survivors of childhood cancer. It may involve any site from the esophagus to the rectum. Pathologically, fibrosis may develop within the wall of the upper GI tract with thickening of the serosa, muscularis, and especially (because of its rapid cell turnover) the submucosa (Fig. 10-1, *A*) leading ultimately to stricture formation. In addition, the fibrosis may be extraintestinal with formation of

---

Etiology of GI Fibrosis and Enteritis following Cancer Therapy

Radiation
Intraabdominal surgery
Chemotherapy
Chronic GVHD
Postinfection
Other (unrelated to therapy)

GVHD = graft-versus-host disease.

---

adhesions.[8,9] Enteritis, or inflammation of the mucosa or lamina propria; ulceration; and villous atrophy are associated, but sometimes independent, findings (Fig. 10-1, B). Focal vascular changes with chronic ischemia in the submucosa and mesentery may be responsible for these lesions. Other pathologic changes in survivors of cancer include those of chronic graft-versus-host disease (GVHD) (mononuclear infiltration of the lamina propria, mucosal ulceration, and reepithelialization) in survivors of bone marrow transplant[26]; the anatomic revisions that follow intraabdominal exenteration and bowel resections; rare dysmotility from neuronal toxicity[13]; and esophageal varices from portal hypertension. Second malignancies may develop and will be discussed elsewhere (see Chapter 16).

CLINICAL MANIFESTATIONS

Presenting clinical signs depend on the degree of injury in the GI tract. If injury is mild, patients may remain asymptomatic indefinitely, and the abnormalities may be detected incidentally, for example at the time of a radiographic procedure, surgery, or autopsy. If the injury is more severe, fibrosis may lead to partial or complete obstruction. Enteritis, ulceration, and bowel resection may lead to malabsorption, perforation, or fistulization. Manifestations of GI toxicity also vary with the location of the damage but may include dysphagia; odynophagia; vomiting; abdominal pain (which may be local or generalized); colic; obstipation; diarrhea; bleeding with or without anemia; anorexia; fatigue; wasting; and the central nervous system manifestations of the rare chronic hyperchloremic metabolic acidosis. In a young child, upper GI obstruction with reflux may lead to aspiration and symptoms of pneumonia.

Radiation

Radiation has been the best-studied cause of fibrosis and enteritis. Data from large series of adults with intraabdominal or pelvic tumors[25] suggest that most patients with late-occurring symptoms of radiation change will have experienced GI toxicity during therapy and will present with delayed symptoms within 5 years. However, there have been reports of patients first presenting with strictures or inflammatory

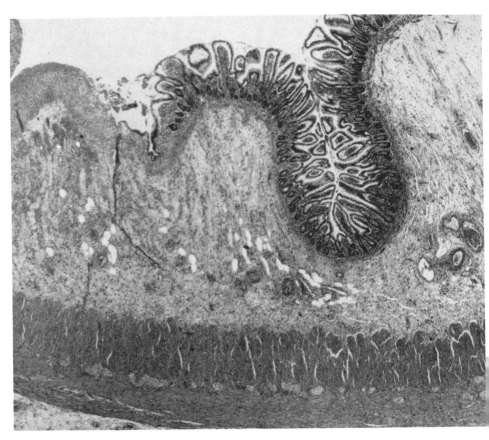

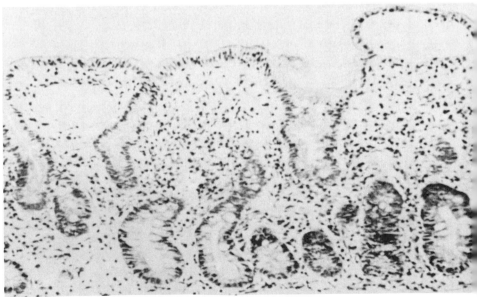

Fig. 10-1. See opposite page for legend.

lesions more than 20 years after therapy.[2,15,25] The effects of radiation are dependent on the total dose, volume, and site of radiation. Fixed loops of the duodenum and terminal ileum are more sensitive than the esophagus or other intestinal sites.[2,22] After 40 to 50 Gy, a 5% incidence of small bowel fibrosis has been reported, rising to 40% after more than 60 Gy.[9]

The chronic effects of GI radiation therapy (RT) have been less well studied in children than in adults. In a comprehensive review of 44 children who received whole-abdominal radiation for various malignancies, 11 developed severe small bowel obstruction that occurred within 2 months of radiation therapy (10 to 40 Gy whole abdomen with 25 to 40 Gy to involved fields) and was uniformly preceded by small bowel toxicity during treatment.[8] Of patients surviving 19 months to 7 years, five (36%) developed a late small bowel obstruction. Infants and children less than 2 years old appeared to have a higher rate of acute and chronic toxicity. Data from smaller series of patients with pelvic or intraabdominal rhabdomyosarcoma[10,29] and central axis Ewing's sarcoma[29] are consistent with these observations. However, one report of patients with Hodgkin's disease who were treated with RT (35 to 44 Gy) reported only one late-bowel obstruction in 79 patients treated.[7] As with adults, a dose-response relationship appears to exist, because patients irradiated with lower doses for Wilms' tumor only rarely develop chronic gastrointestinal toxicity.[28] It may be anticipated that multiple laparotomies (occasionally used for neuroblastoma and rhabdomyosarcoma) would be associated with a higher incidence of adhesions and obstruction than the 2% reported following single laparotomy,[11,24] and that abdominal radiation therapy would increase the risk further. In older children and young adults, definitive RT for Hodgkin's disease has been associated with an approximately 1% incidence of nonspecific abdominal pain a decade later[5] that can be attributed to retroperitoneal fibrosis involving the genitourinary tract rather than the intestine.

Fig. 10-1, cont'd.   **Top,** Delayed radiation injury in wall of ileum. Notice chronic ulceration (left third), extensive fibrosis of submucosa, and subserosa. Villous atrophy is slight in this case. Approximately 10 years after exposure to an undetermined (kilorad) dose of external radiation for adjacent intraabdominal neoplasm. (Hematoxylin-eosin stain; ×21.) **Bottom,** Histologic picture of the small bowel at the time of obstruction, demonstrating severe villus blunting, distended lymphatics, and an abnormally dense mucosal round cell infiltrate. The normal columnar epithelium is lost, with only low cuboidal cells present. Villi are shortened. (Hematoxylin-eosin stain; ×10.) **Top** from Fajardo LF: *Radiation-induced pathology of the alimentary tract.* In Whitehead R, editor: *Gastrointestinal and oesophageal pathology,* Edinburgh, 1989, Churchill Livingstone. **Bottom** from Donaldson SS et al: Radiation enteritis in children, *Cancer* 35:1167-1178, 1975.

Chemotherapy

The role of chemotherapy in the development of chronic enteropathy is less prominent. Although a number of commonly used chemotherapeutic agents cause acute mucositis, most of these changes resolve with discontinuation of therapy. Similarly, the radiomimetic effects of dactinomycin and the anthracyclines wane with time. Nonetheless, it seems likely that these drugs potentiate the long-term GI toxicities of radiation.[8,10,29] Rapid lysis of tumors induced by chemotherapy has been associated with local intestinal necrosis and subsequent fistulization.[20]

Surgery

Beyond the side effects caused by radiation and chemotherapy, surgery alone may cause GI complications. For example, although radiation enteropathy frequently occurs in segments of bowel with surgically induced adhesions,[2] surgery alone may cause fibrosis. In a series of 234 children with nonabdominal Hodgkins' disease who had undergone staging laparotomy a mean of 3.8 years earlier, 1.8% required surgical intervention for intestinal obstruction occurring 11 to 19 months after completion of therapy (abdominal RT in one patient).[11] Although small bowel obstruction is seen in approximately 7% of patients treated for Wilms' tumor, late obstruction (more than 1 year after diagnosis and resulting from adhesions, intussusception, or unknown causes) occurs in fewer than 2% of patients, with events rarely occurring more than 5 years postoperatively. Partial bowel resection is also necessary in approximately 2% of all Wilms' tumor patients.[24] It is anticipated that these and other patients who undergo multiple laparotomies (as in treatment for neuroblastoma and rhabdomyosarcoma) will have a higher rate of bowel obstruction than the 2% reported following single laparotomy.[10,29] Other late effects caused by surgery include the problems of stoma care and hyperchloremic metabolic acidosis associated with ureterosigmoidostomies.[33]

Bone Marrow Transplant

Since the advent of GVH prophylaxis and therapy, chronic GVHD following allogeneic bone marrow transplant rarely affects the upper GI tract.[26] When GVHD does occur, the esophagus is most commonly affected with characteristic weblike intraluminal membranes that form strictures. Some patients have developed perimuscular fibrosis similar to that seen in scleroderma.[17] The unusual occurrence of chronic GVHD in the stomach and small bowel is due to persistence of damage from acute GVHD or by flares of GVHD that result during tapering of prophylactic therapy. Case reports indicate that GVHD may terminate in segmental stenosis with obstruction. Bacterial overgrowth with stasis syndrome (steatorrhea, diarrhea) may be a complication of both chronic GVHD and partial bowel obstruction.

Other Factors

Infections that occur during cancer therapy may have chronic sequelae. Notably, strictures may result from subacute or chronic candidal esophagitis.[21,27] These strictures usually involve the upper third of the esophagus and have been associated

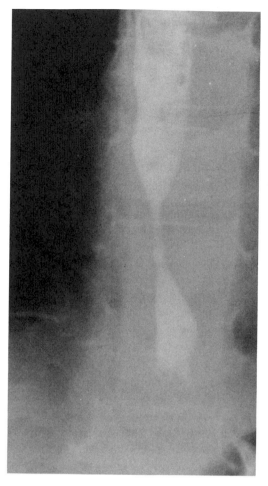

Fig. 10-2.   Barium study of 5-year-old girl with ALL showing distal esophageal stricture.
(Courtesy of Dr. S. Kocoshis.)

with intramucosal pseudodiverticulitis, an inflammatory disorder characterized by digitation of excretory ducts of submucosal glands. Mucosal bridges resulting in webs may also be seen.

Figure 10-2 shows an esophagogram of a 5-year-old girl who had completed treatment for acute lymphoblastic leukemia (ALL) several years previously. The above-noted risk factors were not present. The distal location of the stricture and its endoscopic appearance suggest that gastroesophageal reflux may have played a part in formation of the structure. Although this could be a result of chemotherapy-induced hyperemesis, it is also important to remember that GI fibrosis occurs in age-related normal controls not exposed to cancer therapy.

DETECTION AND SCREENING

Significant GI pathology may be clinically obvious in some patients. In others the signs and symptoms summarized above will need to be recognized and evaluated. Physical examination should include measurement of height and weight as a screen for significant malabsorption. Annual rectal examination with stool guaiac is recommended by the American College of Physicians (ACP) for any adult over 50 years of age. Although it may be worthwhile to perform this exam on younger patients who have received abdominal radiation as children, there are no data demonstrating that this is efficacious.

Some abnormalities may be detected only with laboratory tests. Complete blood counts, which likely will be followed yearly or every other year to monitor for a number of the long-term toxicities described in this text, may reveal anemia associated with macrocytosis, suggesting B_{12} or folate deficiency from malabsorption; anemia and microcytosis may be among the first clues to iron deficiency from GI blood loss. We think it is reasonable to check serum total protein and albumin levels every 3 to 5 years in patients at particular risk for enteritis, that is, those with a history of intraabdominal radiation or surgery and patients with chronic GVHD after a bone marrow transplant. The ACP recommends routine sigmoidoscopy every 3 years for all adults over the age of 50. Again, we think it is reasonable to be at least this conservative for long-term survivors of childhood cancer with the above-noted risk factors.

MANAGEMENT

Further evaluation of suspected late GI effects requires cooperation between primary physician and subspecialist. Symptoms of bowel obstruction should be evaluated with abdominal radiographs, decompression (if necessary), and the appropriate contrast studies based on the suspected location of the lesion. Suspected upper GI strictures should be evaluated by barium swallow and subsequent endoscopy. Long-term management of esophageal strictures may require repetitive endoscopy with dilations, during the course of which biopsy may be necessary to screen for peptic esophagitis. Antireflux surgical procedures, in conjunction with dilation, may be appropriate to minimize the chance of restricturing. Esophagitis can be managed pharmacologically using H_2 antagonists and a prokinetic agent such as metoclopramide, or with drugs such as omeprazole, which antagonize the parietal cell proton pump and eliminate acid production. Sucralfate (carafate), which appears to bind to proteins of denuded mucosa and act as a physical barrier to esophageal irritation, can be used in conjunction with other therapies. When dysmotility secondary to neuronal injury is identified by barium swallow and motility studies as a cause of dysphagia, calcium channel blockers may be beneficial.

Chronic intestinal obstruction secondary to strictures or adhesions may require surgical resection or balloon dilatation. Depending on the extent of malnutrition, a preoperative period of parenteral hyperalimentation may be necessary. Obstipation also may result from motility abnormalities that may be discerned by manometric studies. Abnormal motility is difficult to manage, and the efficacy of many medications is being evaluated currently. The most important first step is the removal of impacted stool with enemata followed by the initiation of therapy with stool softeners and peristaltic stimulants such as Senokot. When malabsorption is the primary problem, evaluation includes contrast studies to document the site of involvement, small bowel biopsies to document the histologic features, and individual tests of absorption to define the defects. Studies documenting malabsorption include the D-xylose absorption test, the lactose breath hydrogen test, 72-hour fecal fat determinations, measurement of serum B_{12} and folate levels, measurements of stool pH and reducing substances, and the Schilling test. Stool also should be examined for ova and parasites. Evidence from intubation and quantitative cultures of bacterial contamination of the small bowel may be important, particularly if the ileocecal valve is absent or small bowel stasis is present. Bacterial overgrowth may be treated with tetracycline or metronidazole, but consideration should be given to potentially correctable causes such as strictures. After ileal resection, diarrhea due to bowel salt malabsorption may improve with cholestyramine. If malabsorption is found to be secondary to villous atrophy without a treatable cause, enteral nutrition or parenteral hyperalimentation may be necessary.

When GI blood loss is identified by screening studies (as mentioned earlier), a more extensive evaluation should be undertaken to localize the site of bleeding. In addition to barium studies, endoscopy will be important to document inflammation or ulceration. Biopsy of mucosal lesions is helpful in determining their etiology. Rarely, enterolysis, a bleeding scan, or even exploratory laparotomy in conjunction with intraoperative endoscopy may be necessary to localize a bleeding site. The management of acute GI bleeding will be familiar to the generalist.

Hepatobiliary Tree
PATHOPHYSIOLOGY
Normal Anatomy and Physiology

The largest organ in the body, the liver consists of right and left lobes joined posteroinferiorly at the porta hepatis. Under the visceral surface of the liver lies the gallbladder. The hepatic lobule is the basic ultrastructural unit of the liver. Each contains a central vein that is a tributary of the hepatic vein, which drains into the inferior vena cava. From the center of each lobule radiate columns of hepatocytes separated by sinusoids that are lined with reticuloendothelial or Kupffer's cells. Functionally, the lobule is divided into three zones, each receiving blood of different nutrient and oxygen content. Zone 3 receives the least oxygen and nutrients and is, therefore, most susceptible to injury. In portal triads between the lobules are hepatic arterioles, portal vein radicles, and branches of the left and right hepatic ducts. These latter fuse at the porta hepatis to form the common hepatic duct. This joins the cystic duct, which drains the gallbladder, and together they form the common bile duct that drains into the duodenum.

Hepatic function is diverse. It includes synthesis of a variety of enzymes, albumin, coagulation proteins, urea, and steroids such as cholesterol and primary bile acids; bilirubin conjugation and drug detoxification; and storage of fat-soluble vitamins. Hepatocytes are also responsible for gluconeogenesis and glycolysis. The Kupffer's cells have an immunoregulatory function, engaging in phagocytosis as well as secretion of a number of biologic response modifiers such as tumor necrosis factor and interleukins.

Changes Induced by Cytotoxic Therapy

As in the GI tract, fibrosis is among the best-documented findings in the liver. Regardless of etiology (to be discussed), fibrosis is generally periportal and concentric (Fig. 10-3).[23] It may be associated with fatty infiltration, focal necrosis, nodular regeneration of cirrhosis, and portal hypertension. Fibrosis, piecemeal necrosis, and portal-periportal lymphoplasmacytic infiltrate are the cardinal features of chronic active hepatitis, a syndrome with multiple etiologies. The pathologic changes of chronic venoocclusive disease (VOD) and chronic GVHD have been extensively described.[23,26] Hepatocellular carcinoma has occurred in rare long-term survivors, notably patients with Wilms' tumor who have had abdominal radiation.[3]

CLINICAL MANIFESTATIONS

Radiation

Hepatic pathology is often subclinical and may develop without prior acute toxicity. In one series of 99 patients evaluated within 6 months of irradiation and then again an average of 47 months after irradiation, 36 who initially had normal physical examinations, liver function testing, and liver scans developed abnormalities.[30] Clinical findings, including ascites and pleural effusion, sometimes with death due to liver decompensation, have developed more than 2 years after RT.[32] Chronic fibrosis[14] leading to increased portal pressures, varices, and hematemesis, has been described in a child treated with partial liver irradiation and chemotherapy for Wilms' tumor.[1] We have seen asymptomatic atrophy in a lobe of the liver 6 months to 1 year after treatment with doses greater than or equal to 45 Gy, with compensating hypertrophy-hyperplasia in the untreated portions of the liver (Robertson, Lawrence, unpublished observation). Liver functions may improve after localized treatment with chemoradiotherapy as a result of compensatory changes in the liver.

There has been a single report of cholelithiasis in 16 of about 6000 patients (without a history of hemolytic anemia or gallstones at presentation) 3 months to 17 years following diagnosis of cancer; this incidence is higher than the risk in the general population.[16]

Chemotherapy and Surgery

The role of other modalities in the development of chronic hepatopathy is somewhat limited. Methotrexate, given in daily oral low doses for $2\frac{1}{2}$ to 5 years to children with ALL (a schedule no longer used), has been found to cause

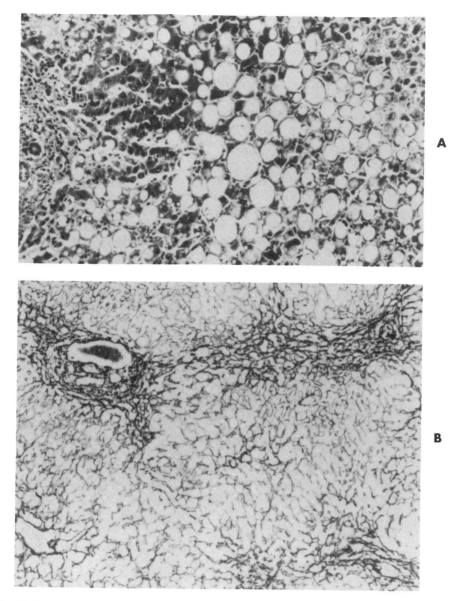

Fig. 10-3.   Chronic methotrexate liver damage. There is fatty change together with chronic portal inflammation and fibrosis. **A,** Hematoxylin-eosin stain; ×180. **B,** Reticulin stain ×72. (From reference 23; reprinted with the kind permission of Dr. R.S. Patrick and Chapman Hall, Ltd.)

biopsy-proven hepatic fibrosis in as many as 80% of children.[12] When intermediate doses of intravenous methotrexate have been administered, the incidence of fibrosis has been below 5%.[18] In contrast to what is seen after RT, methotrexate-related hepatic fibrosis stabilizes or resolves after discontinuation of the drug.[6] Neither the contribution of other acute hepatotoxins (e.g., 6-mercaptopurine [6-MP] or actino-mycin) to chronic liver disease nor the long-term liver function of patients who have developed carmustine-related VOD in the setting of bone marrow transplant has been studied.

Other Factors

Several newer approaches to the treatment of gastrointestinal malignancy (includ-ing both administration of radiolabeled monoclonal antibodies for the therapy of hepatomas and intrahepatic arterial chemotherapy) have not yet been examined with respect to possible delayed effects. In patients who have undergone a bone marrow transplant, chronic GVHD[26] and chronic active hepatitis[31] are the most common causes of chronic liver disease. Following transplantation or conventional therapy, symptomatic or subclinical hepatitis may be related to transfusion-mediated infections (hepatitis A, B, C, CMV).[4] Human immunodeficiency virus (HIV) contracted in the course of treatment is at present only a theoretic cause of hepatitis in long-term survivors. Surgery, including partial hepatectomy, does not appear to have major long-term repercussions on liver function, although ileal conduits may enhance the risk of gallstones.[16] Long-term liver function in patients undergoing liver transplant as primary management for hepatic tumors has not been studied.

DETECTION AND SCREENING

Foolproof guidelines for long-term follow-up are unavailable because significant hepatitis or cirrhosis, with the attendant risks of liver failure or hepatic tumors, may be impossible to detect without liver biopsy. We suggest annual or biannual evaluations with attention to hepatomegaly, icterus, and malabsorption. For patients who experienced acute hepatotoxicity during therapy and for patients treated with hepatectomy, multiple blood transfusions, hepatotoxic chemotherapy (e.g., metho-trexate, 6-MP, actinomycin) or hepatic irradiation (or right-sided abdominal irra-diation, as used in some Wilms' tumor patients), we recommend a chemistry screen—including transaminase, alkaline phosphatase, and bilirubin levels—every 2 to 5 years. Liver transplant patients require closer monitoring, which is best done in collaboration with a gastroenterology or transplant service. Patients with elevated transaminases, and who have been transfused, should have serologic tests for hepatitis A, B, and C. Because lower doses of hepatic radiation and shorter courses of oral methotrexate are being prescribed, and in view of the relatively infrequent development of end-stage liver disease with current anticancer regimens, we do not advocate routine liver scans or biopsies. Although the possibility of additional risks from other hepatotoxins, such as alcohol, have not been studied in the long-term survivors of childhood cancer, it is reasonable to advise against the use (and especially, the abuse) of alcohol.

MANAGEMENT

There is no current therapy to reverse fibrosis, either in the presence or absence of cirrhosis. It is, therefore, imperative to preserve residual hepatocyte function. Consequently, radiation-induced liver disease is usually treated conservatively with diuretics. Most adult patients will respond to this therapy, with symptoms resolving over 1 to 2 months. Patients should be made aware of the danger of ethanol ingestion and exposure to other hepatotoxins.

Patients with cirrhosis may remain asymptomatic for many years. Decompensated cirrhosis, as manifested by jaundice, hepatic encephalopathy, hypoproteinemia, progressive ascites, and coagulopathies, is present when hepatocyte dysfunction exceeds the capability for regeneration. Portal hypertension and GI hemorrhage may precipitate decompensation. The management of decompensated cirrhosis depends on the patient's symptoms and is the same regardless of etiology. Unfortunately, a substantial portion of these patients will die of liver failure. An abdominal ultrasound should be performed to rule out potentially treatable factors, such as obstruction of the biliary tract. Hepatic encephalopathy is managed with a low-protein diet and with lactulose and neomycin therapy to minimize urea production. Hypoproteinemia and coagulopathy may require albumin and fresh frozen plasma infusions, respectively. Ascites and associated electrolyte derangements may be treated with salt restriction, diuretics, and, in refractory cases, paracentesis. Life-threatening bleeding due to esophageal varices requires sclerosis during endoscopy or, if bleeding persists, esophageal transection or a vascular shunting procedure to decrease portal pressure.

When persistent transaminase elevation leads to abnormal hepatitis serologies, liver biopsy is indicated, because chronic active hepatitis B and C may respond to alpha-interferon therapy. Although there is no specific therapy for end-stage liver disease from these and other causes, such as VOD, liver transplant has been effective. When this is a consideration, consultation with a transplant service should be undertaken promptly.

REFERENCES

1. Barnard JA et al: Noncirrhotic portal fibrosis after Wilms' tumor therapy, *Gastroenterology* 90:1054-1056, 1986.
2. Berthrong M, Fajardo LF: Radiation injury in surgical pathology, part II, alimentary tract, *Am J Surg Pathol* 5:153-178, 1981.
3. Blatt J et al: Second malignancies in very long term survivors of childhood cancer, *Am J Med* 93:57-60, 1992.
4. Buchanan GR: *Hematologic supportive care*. In Pizzo PA, Poplack DG, editors: *Principles and practice of pediatric oncology,* Philadelphia, 1989, JB Lippincott.
5. Chao N, Levine J, Hornig SJ: Retroperitoneal fibrosis post Hodgkin's Disease 9-13 years after definitive radiation therapy, *J Clin Oncol* 5:231-232, 1987.
6. Dahl MGC, Gregory MM, Schever PJ: Liver damage due to methotrexate in patients with psoriasis, *Br Med J* 1:625-630, 1971.
7. Donaldson SS et al: Pediatric Hodgkin's disease. II. results of therapy, *Cancer* 37:2436-2447, 1976.

8. Donaldson SS et al: Radiation enteritis in children, *Cancer* 35:1167-1178, 1975.

9. Fajardo LF: *Radiation-induced pathology of the alimentary tract.* In Whitehead R, editor: *Gastrointestinal and oesophageal pathology,* Edinburgh, 1989, Churchill Livingstone.

10. Flamant F et al: Long-term sequelae of conservative treatment by surgery, brachytherapy and chemotherapy for vulval and vaginal rhabdomyosarcoma in children, *J Clin Oncol* 8:1847-1853, 1990.

11. Hays DM et al: Complications related to 234 staging laparotomies performed in the Intergroup Hodgkin's Disease in Childhood Study, *Surgery* 96:471-478, 1984.

12. Hutter RVP et al: Hepatic fibrosis in children with acute leukemia: a complication of therapy, *Cancer* 13:288-307, 1960.

13. Kaplinsky C et al: Esophageal obstruction 14 years after treatment for Hodgkin's Disease, *Cancer* 68:903-905, 1991.

14. Lewin K, Millis RR: Human radiation hepatitis. A morphologic study with emphasis on the late change, *Arch Pathol* 96:21-26, 1973.

15. Localio SA, Stone A, Friedman M: Surgical aspects of radiation enteritis, *Surg Gynecol Obstet* 129:302-307, 1969.

16. Mahmoud H, Schell M, Pui C-H: Cholelithiasis after treatment for childhood cancer, *Cancer* 67:1439-1442, 1991.

17. McDonald GB et al: Esophageal abnormalities in chronic graft-versus-host disease in humans, *Gastroenterology* 80:914-921, 1981.

18. McIntosh S et al: Methotrexate hepatotoxicity in children with leukemia, *J Pediatr* 90:1019-1021, 1977.

19. Meadows AT, Krejmas NL, Belasco JB: *The medical cost of cure: sequelae in survivors of childhood cancer.* In Von Eys J, Sullivan MP, editors: *Status of the curability of childhood cancers,* New York, 1980, Raven Press.

20. Myers PA et al: Bowel perforation during initial treatment of childhood non-Hodgkin's lymphoma, *Cancer* 56:259-261, 1985.

21. Orringer MB, Sloan H: Monilial esophagitis: an increasingly frequent cause of esophageal stenosis? *Ann Thorac Surg* 26:364-374, 1978.

22. Papazian A et al: Mucosal bridges of the upper esophagus after radiotherapy for Hodgkin's disease, *Gastroenterology* 84:1028-1031, 1983.

23. Patrick RS, McGee JO'D: *Biopsy pathology of the liver,* London, 1980, Chapman Hall, Ltd.

24. Ritchey ML et al: Surgical complications following nephrectomy for Wilms' Tumor: a report of the National Wilms' Tumor Study-3, Manuscript submitted for publication.

25. Roswit B: Complications of radiation therapy: the alimentary tract, *Semin Roentgenol* 9:51-63, 1974.

26. Shulman HM: *Pathology of chronic graft-vs.-host disease.* In Burakoff SJ et al, editors: *Graft-vs-host disease immunology, pathophysiology and treatment,* New York, 1990, Marcel Dekker.

27. Simson JN et al: Mucosal bridges of the oesophagus in Candida oesophagitis, *Br J Surg* 72:209-210, 1985.

28. Tefft M: Radiation related toxicity in National Wilms' Tumor Study Number One, *Int J Radiat Oncol Biol Phys* 2:455-463, 1977.

29. Tefft M et al: Acute and late effects on normal tissues following combined chemo- and radiotherapy for childhood rhabdomyosarcoma and Ewing's sarcoma, *Cancer* 37:1201-1213, 1976.

30. Tefft M et al: Irradiation of the liver in children: review of experience in the acute and chronic phases, and in the intact normal and partially resected, *Am J Roentgenol* 108:365-385, 1970.
31. Vernant JP: Hepatitis B and non-A–non-B hepatitis after allogeneic bone marrow transplantation in leukemia, *Bone Marrow Transplant* 1:183-184, 1986.
32. Wharton JT et al: Radiation hepatitis induced by abdominal irradiation with the cobalt 60 moving strip technique, *Am J Roentgenol* 117:73-80, 1973.
33. Zincke H, Segura SW: Ureterosigmoidostomy: critical review of 173 cases, *J Urol* 113:324-327, 1975.

11

The Ovary

Angel E. Torano
Edward C. Halperin
Brigid G. Leventhal

In the course of the treatment of pediatric malignancies, the ovaries often sustain exposure to radiation (either directly or indirectly) as well as to chemotherapy. Understanding the possible adverse effects of these treatment modalities necessitate an understanding of normal ovarian function and of its role in growth, sexual development, and reproduction. In general, radiation to subdiaphragmatic regions in standard therapeutic doses will produce some diminution in fertility. Alkylating agents in high doses will also affect female fertility. In all of these cases, the effect is more marked in older than in younger women; in fact, there may be no substantial effect on fertility in those treated before the age of 20 years. In one large study, the relative fertility of female survivors of childhood cancer treatment was 0.93 when compared with controls.[6]

PATHOPHYSIOLOGY

Brief Overview of Normal Organ Development

The human ovary produces oocytes and secretes steroid hormones.[17] In human embryos, primordial germ cells are first recognized among endodermal cells in the wall of the yolk sac. They migrate to the primitive gonads in the fifth to sixth week of development. The gonads begin to acquire sexual characteristics at the seventh week of gestation. At that time the surface epithelium continues to proliferate in the female gonad and gives rise to the cortical cords, which split into irregular cell clusters, each surrounding one or more primitive germ cells at about the fourth month of gestation. It is these cells that develop into mature oocytes, while the surrounding epithelial cells form the follicle cells. Active mitosis of oogonia occurs during fetal life, producing thousands of primitive germ cells. Oocyte number in the human ovary is a function of age, reaching a peak of 6 million at 5 months after conception, dropping to 2 million at birth, with only 100,000 present at puberty. No oogonia form postnatally in full-term humans.

From late gestation to adulthood, steroidogeneis and follicular growth and maturation undergo a predictable sequence of changes with age.[11] The initiating event of puberty is an increasing secretion of gonadotropin releasing hormone

(GnRH) by the hypothalamus, which stimulates the pituitary to release its stores of the gonadotropins (GNs), follicle-stimulating hormone (FSH), and luteinizing hormone (LH). FSH stimulates follicular growth, and LH promotes luteinization of the ovary. The hallmark of sexual maturity is the development of positive feedback on the pituitary by estrogen to stimulate the mid-cycle surge of pituitary GNs. After the onset of puberty, follicular maturation and ovulation are dependent on the 28-day cyclic secretion of FSH and LH from the pituitary. After ovulation, the corpus luteum forms and produces progesterone, estradiol, and 17 hydroxyproges-terone. This stimulates secretory changes in the endometrium and an increase in blood supply. In the absence of increasing chorionic GN from a conceptus, the corpus luteum is exhausted and progesterone and estrogen levels fall. As FSH levels rise, the endometrium sloughs, giving rise to menstrual flow and the initiation of the next cycle.

Adrenal cortical androgens also play a role in pubertal maturation (adrenarche). Levels of dehydroepiandrosterone (DHEA) and its sulfate, DHEAS, begin to rise before the earliest physical changes of puberty are apparent.

Puberty is a complex growth and developmental process initiated by the central nervous system, but influenced by many physiologic factors. Pubertal stages have been described by Marshall and Tanner[24,28] (Tables 11-1 and 11-2). There is considerable normal variation in the timing and sequence of these events. Age of onset of puberty is more closely correlated with osseous maturation than with chronological age. In conjunction with the appearance of secondary sexual characteristics there is a second peak in growth velocity. Girls generally have a short period of moderately rapid growth prior to menarche. The epiphyses then close, preventing further growth. Normal growth is therefore closely tied to normal sexual development.

Table 11-1
Stages of Breast Development in Girls

	Mean Age	Range (95%)
1. Preadolescent. Only papilla is elevated.		
2. Breast Bud Stage. Breast and papilla are elevated as small mound. Areola diameter is enlarged.	11.2	9.0-13.3
3. There is further enlargement of breast and areola with no separation of their contours.	12.2	10.0-14.3
4. Areola and papilla project to form a secondary mound above the level of the breast.	13.1	10.8-15.3
5. Mature stage. There is projection only of papilla because of recession of the areola to the general contour of the breast.	15.3	11.9-18.8

From Marshall WA, Tanner JM: Variation in the pattern of pubertal changes in girls, *Arch Dis Child* 44:291-303, 1969, as cited in Odell WD: *Puberty.* In DeGroot LJ, editor: *Endocrinology,* ed 2, Philadelphia, 1989, WB Saunders.

With the depletion of oocytes by radiation, chemotherapy, or advancing age, menstruation will cease and, eventually, estrogen production will cease as well. This estrogen depletion can bring about hot flashes, decreased vaginal secretions, osteoporosis, and other menopausal symptoms.

Description of Organ Damage Induced by Cytotoxic Therapy

Cytotoxic effects of radiation. Many physical and environmental factors can influence the radiosensitivity of the ovary. There are marked differences reported in the radiosensitivity of the oocyte among species, which makes it difficult to define a good animal model. Oocytes, like lymphocytes, die in interphase within a few hours of irradiation exposure. Post mortem examinations of ovaries have established the histologic changes seen after radiotherapy. There is a decrease in the number of small follicles, impaired follicular maturation, cortical fibrosis, generalized hypoplasia, and hyalinization of the capsule. Vascular changes are also common with severe sclerosis, myointimal proliferation, and obliteration of the lumen. The most consistent and obvious change is atrophy of the cortex.[12]

Cytotoxic effects of chemotherapy. Alkylating agents may affect the ovary in an age-related fashion, with older women more susceptible to damage than prepubertal girls. Alkylating agents cause cytotoxicity in a direct, dose-dependent cell-cycle–independent manner that could explain the effects of these agents on the resting oocyte.[8] On histologic examination,[40] the ovaries of women treated with

Table 11-2
Stages of Pubic Hair Growth in Girls

	Mean Age	Range (95%)
1. Preadolescent vellus over pubis is no further developed than that over anterior abdominal wall (i.e., no pubic hair).		
2. There is sparse growth of long, slightly pigmented, downy hair, straight or only slightly curled, appearing chiefly along the labia.	11.7	9.3-14.1
3. Hair is considerably darker, coarser and more curled. Hair spreads sparsely over pubic junction.	12.4	10.2-14.6
4. Hair is now adult in type but area covered by it is still considerably smaller than in most adults. There is no spread to medial surface of the thighs.	13.0	10.8-15.1
5. Adult in quantity and type distributed as coarse triangle of classically feminine pattern. Spread to medial surface of thighs but not linea alba or elsewhere above base of triangle.	14.4	12.2-16.7

From Marshall WA, Tanner JM: Variation in the pattern of pubertal changes in girls, *Arch Dis Child* 44:291-303, 1969, as cited in Odell WD: *Puberty.* In DeGroot LJ, editor: *Endocrinology,* ed 2, Philadelphia, 1989, WB Saunders.

cyclophosphamide show an absence of thecal cells and ova, suggesting a direct action on the oocyte by the drug. Histologic examination of ovaries of patients treated with alkylating agents containing drug combinations for Hodgkin's disease showed destruction of resting oocytes and absent primordial follicles, with resultant arrest of follicular maturation and decrease in estrogen secretion.[8] Ovarian failure is relatively common after busulfan therapy. Histologic study of the ovaries of one patient at autopsy showed the presence of numerous primordial follicles but no maturation beyond the primary follicle stage.[37] Busulfan apparently has a toxic effect on developing germ cells, and one case report[10] describes a pregnant woman under treatment with busulfan who delivered a female baby born with hypoplastic ovaries consisting of ovarian stroma and only occasional primordial ova. Antimetabolites, which interfere with synthesis of deoxyribonucleic acid (DNA), in general do not affect ovarian function, because oocytes are not dividing cells.

Developmental effects. In general, because most therapies deplete ova rather than ablating them entirely, girls treated before puberty will progress normally through puberty. Even those with complete ovarian ablation may develop early adrenarchal changes with pubic hair as a result of adrenal cortical androgen (DHEA and DHEAS). Patients who have received whole-abdomen irradiation[39] or whole-body irradiation[35] may require estrogen replacement therapy to develop secondary sexual characteristics; the same has been true of some patients treated with busulfan.[23,37] Radiation can also affect growing breast buds, even to the extent of lack of development of an ipsilateral breast after 10 to 20 Gy to the chest in young girls (see Chapter 14). These changes are irreversible and do not respond to hormonal therapy.[31] The capacity for lactation is variable in breasts treated with surgery and radiotherapy for breast cancer (and, therefore, presumably after irradiation involving the breast in older girls). Breastfeeding is generally successful from the nonirradiated breast, but a previously existing disparity in size may be exaggerated by pregnancy and lactation.[38]

CLINICAL MANIFESTATIONS

Because the sum total of the effects of both radiation and chemotherapy is the depletion of ova, the age at which depletion occurs will be critical in regard to subsequent clinical manifestations. Prepubertal girls may suffer delay in pubertal development and delayed onset of menses. Those who have received cranial radiation, on the other hand, may be at risk of precocious puberty (see Chapter 4). Those who have already passed through puberty may develop oligomenorrhea, amenorrhea, and even menopausal symptoms. The degree to which these syndromes are to be expected from each type of treatment is described below.

Effects of Irradiation

Wallace and colleagues[39] followed 19 patients treated in childhood with whole abdominal radiotherapy (total dose 30 Gy). Using the assumption that the number of oocytes within the ovary declines exponentially by atresia from approximately

Table 11-3
Effect of Fractionated Ovarian X-irradiation on Ovarian Function in Women of Reproductive Age Irradiated for Malignant or Nonmalignant Disease*

Minimum Ovarian Dose in Gy	Effect
0.6	No deleterious effect.
1.5	No deleterious effect in most young women. Some risk of sterilization especially in women aged >40.
2.5-5.0	Variable. Aged 15-40 years: about 60% sterilized permanently, some with temporary amenorrhea. Aged >40: usually 100% permanently sterile.
5-8	Variable. Aged 15-40 years: about 70% sterilized permanently; of the remainder, some temporary amenorrhea.
>8	100% permanently sterilized.

*No attempt has been made to allow for variation in mode of fractionation.
Modified from Ash P: The influence of radiation on fertility in man, *Br J Radiol* 53:271-278, 1980.

2,000,000 at birth to approximately 2000 at menopause, they were able to estimate that the LD_{50} for the human oocyte does not exceed 4 Gy. Ash's summary of clinical information on radiation to the human ovary is shown in Table 11-3.[2] Artificial menopause was induced by a dose of 12 to 15 Gy in women under 40 years of age, whereas women over 40 years of age required only 4 to 7 Gy. Permanent sterility occurred in 60% of females 15 to 40 years of age receiving 5 to 6 Gy. This corresponds to Rubin and Casarett's TD 50/5 (i.e., 50% incidence at 5 years) of 6 to 12 Gy for induction of sterility.[33] Rubin reports a dose of 20 Gy for a 95% incidence of sterility in young females, whereas a dose of only 10 Gy is needed in older, premenopausal women.[34] Even a dose as low as 1.5 Gy has produced sterility in older women. In a study of 103 women aged 40 years or younger at the time of radiation treatment for Hodgkin's disease, only age at the time of treatment and radiation dose were significant variables in a multivariate analysis predicting normal menses.[17]

The cytotoxic effects of radiation on the ovary are related to the nonreplaceable population of cells that exist within the organ, so one would expect the prepubertal ovary to be less sensitive.[4] A significant delay in the onset of menses (or in some girls, failure to achieve menarche) has been shown, however, in prepubertal girls receiving total-body irradiation as part of bone marrow transplant preparative regimens[35] or ovarian radiation as part of combined modality therapy for acute lymphoblastic leukemia (ALL),[16] especially if treated before the age of 8. These patients also showed elevated FSH and LH and low estradiol levels.

Hamre and colleagues assessed FSH and LH levels in 163 long-term survivors of childhood ALL treated with the same induction chemotherapy and with one of the following radiation fields[15]: cranial-spinal (18 to 24 Gy) plus abdominal radiation therapy (RT) including ovaries (12 Gy); cranial-spinal RT (18 to 24 Gy) with the ovaries out of the field; or cranial RT alone (18 to 24 Gy). There was a statistical correlation between the radiotherapy port dose to the ovary and the elevated LH and FSH levels. The actuarial estimated median age at menarche was 14 years in patients treated with cranial RT only, although it has not been reached and is at least 16 years in patients receiving cranial-spinal and whole-abdomen RT. This correlated well with elevated FSH and LH levels. Clayton[7] described 21 girls who had received neuroaxis irradiation for brain tumors followed by adjuvant chemotherapy with carmustine (BCNU) or lomustine (CCNU) and procarbazine. Thirteen received chemotherapy before the age of 11 years. At last assessment 10 remained prepubertal, 9 of whom showed biochemical evidence of primary ovarian failure. The remaining three were pubertal or adult, although all had shown abnormalities of gonadotropin secretion previously. Eight girls received chemotherapy after 11 years of age. All girls entered or progressed through puberty spontaneously; although four had previously exhibited elevated basal FSH levels, these had returned to normal. Therefore, the majority of girls showed evidence of primary ovarian dysfunction, but there was some evidence of return to normal in the years after treatment. These chemotherapy agents have been shown to deplete stem cells in hematopoietic model systems, which may explain the marked effect in the younger girls in this study. These effects may be due both to radiation and chemotherapy exposure.

Effects of Chemotherapy

The prepubertal gonad may be more resistant than the postpubertal gonad to damage by alkylating agents. A factor in the resistance may be the larger number of primordial follicles in the prepubertal adolescents, compared with older patients. In one report 24 female survivors of Burkitt's lymphoma were treated at age 3 to 17 years (median 9). They had received a total of 2.8 to 9.0 g/m^2 of cyclophosphamide, and fertility seemed to be unimpaired with 16 of 17 (94%) bearing children, although the average age at menarche was significantly later than controls (age 13.5 versus 12.2 years, $p < 0.05$).[26] Nevertheless, primary ovarian failure has been reported in patients given cyclophosphamide therapy before puberty.[27] Alkylating-agent therapy is also used in some regimens for the treatment of Hodgkin's disease (nitrogen mustard, vincristine, procarbazine, prednisone [MOPP]; nitrogen mustard, vinblastine, procarbazine, prednisone [MVPP][17]; cyclophosphamide, vincristine, procarbazine, prednisone [COPP][20]). Here, too, the effect on the ovary seems proportional to the age at treatment, with women treated after the age of 30 having a high likelihood of amenorrhea after 5 to 6 cycles of alkylating-agent therapy whereas those treated as teenagers were most likely to retain regular menses.[17]

In bone marrow transplantation, an increasingly common treatment for cancer patients, conditioning regimens that include melphalan or busulfan may be used. Both of these agents in high doses can cause irreversible fibrosis of the ovary.[8,18] Mitoxantrone[36] and Velban[8] have also been associated with development of menopausal symptoms.

Female patients treated for acute leukemia generally receive antimetabolites, vincristine, and prednisone as the mainstays of therapy rather than alkylating agents. Most children, whether they are prepubertal or postpubertal at the time of therapy, will maintain normal ovarian function; however, in one early study, 30% of those who were pubertal when leukemia developed had abnormal function.[37] In one study of women with acute leukemia, aged 14 to 36 years (median 23), aggressive chemotherapy with combinations that included anthracyclines and cyclophosphamide had no effect on reproductive or endocrine function.[21]

Ovarian tumors. The vast majority of patients treated for malignant ovarian germ cell tumors who have an intact ovary and uterus are fertile.[13] This is true after vincristine, actinomycin, cyclophosphamide-type regimens, cisplatin-based regimens,[30] or etoposide.[1] Patients with ovarian germ cell tumors should have a unilateral salpingooophorectomy rather than more radical surgery, and radiotherapy to the gonads should be avoided. Methotrexate therapy for gestational malignancies has not affected fertility.[32]

DETECTION AND SCREENING

Delayed Puberty

If there is a concern that puberty is delayed, the concern should be addressed. It is not inappropriate to start an evaluation by age 12 or 13 years if there is no evidence of pubertal development (e.g., breast buds). A complete history and physical is required, including information about parental height and the age at onset of maternal menarche. Because hypothyroidism may present as developmental delay, check for symptoms such as sensitivity to cold, dry skin, or constipation. Height and weight should be measured carefully, comparing the two to determine proportionality. A hypogonadal individual may be overweight for age, whereas someone who has anorexia nervosa as a cause of delayed puberty will have a different body habitus. It is important to remember that having a history of childhood cancer does not rule out other causes of delayed development.

Tanner stage should be accurately assessed (see Tables 11-1 and 11-2). A careful examination of breast development with determination of whether glandular tissue actually appears can provide some indication of estrogen effect. The onset of breast development is one of the earliest manifestations of puberty and the first readily identifiable signs of puberty in 85% of females. Thelarche occurs at 11 years of age on the average (SD = 1 year).[19] Vaginal color and secretion should be assessed. Uterine size is often best appreciated on a rectal examination. Some androgenic manifestations (e.g., pubic hair) may reflect adrenal steroid secretion rather than gonadal function.

Amenorrhea is not a disease but a symptom and may be arbitrarily defined as the absence of menses for 6 months or longer.[42] Primary amenorrhea is defined as the failure of menses to appear initially, and secondary amenorrhea is defined as that in a woman who previously had menstrual periods. The evaluation of a patient with primary amenorrhea is indicated if she has reached age 16 years without menarche, if secondary sex development has not progressed to Tanner 2 or 3 by age 14 years, and if more than 3 years have elapsed since the first signs of development. In women with secondary amenorrhea, menopausal symptoms such as hot flashes, decreasing size of breasts, breast discharge, and headaches should be elicited in the review of systems. It is important to be sure that the patient is not taking birth control pills, because menstruation under these circumstances does not represent ovulation. Evaluation of fertility in such a patient requires discontinuation of the medication, probably for at least 6 months before a reasonable assessment of her intrinsic potential for ovulation can be made.

Laboratory workup of primary or secondary amenorrhea
Radiology   Bone age
              Ultrasound of ovaries may help define size, morphology, and presence of
                  cysts or follicles
Blood tests   Free T4, TSH
              DHEAS
              Testosterone, prolactin, FSH, LH, estradiol

Blood levels of FSH and LH should be repeated 2 to 3 times to be sure that any particular level is consistently abnormal.

Interpretation of hormonal studies
Differential diagnosis (modified from Wentz[42])

High gonadotropins (LH/FSH)	Patients with high gonadotropins invariably have physiologic or premature menopause secondary to ovarian failure.
High FSH with normal LH	This generally means impending menopause with ovarian failure. The FSH rises first, and, with repeat tests, the LH will rise as well.
Low LH and FSH	Pituitary or hypothalamic dysfunction is indictated. This may occur after cranial radiation. A syndrome of precocious puberty (described in Chapter 4) has also been reported in these children.
Very high LH with low FSH	Indicates pregnancy or trophoblastic disease.
Increased LH with normal to low FSH	Polycystic ovary syndrome is indicated.
Normal LH, very low FSH	Indicates an endogenous or exogenous source of estrogen (e.g., granulosa theca cell tumor, birth control pills, respectively).
Normal DHEAS with high FSH/LH	In patients with isolated hypogonadal hypogonadism, levels of adrenal sex steroids are in the normal range relative to chronologic age. In contrast, in individuals with constitutional delay of puberty, there is a lag in the maturation of both gonadal and adrenal function. This distinction appears most useful after 16 years.

Growth, secondary sexual characteristics, menstrual history, menopausal symptoms, and pregnancy history should be obtained at each visit in any girl over the age of 13 years.

MANAGEMENT OF ESTABLISHED PROBLEMS

Ovarian Failure

Once it appears that ovarian failure has ensued, a pediatric endocrinologist should be consulted. The endocrinologist will discuss the possibility of estrogen replacement in girls as young as 12 to 13 years. Growth hormone therapy may also be considered at this time, because prepubertal girls experiencing ovarian failure are at risk for both short stature and pubertal delay. The next challenge is to induce puberty. Premarin 0.3 to 0.625 mg daily for 3-6 months is usually effective in inducing puberty, although currently pediatric endocrinologists may prefer a more complex integrated regimen with growth hormone and gonadotropins as well. If spontaneous sexual maturation has not occurred with short term therapy, longer term oral therapy with the lowest possible estrogen dose that produces the desired effect should be given. In general, these patients should be cycled for some period of time and allowed to have withdrawal bleeding. A number of girls will not wish to continue this therapy indefinitely, because the bleeding is merely a pharmacologic response and does not indicate ovulation. However, estrogen plays an important physiologic role in females (e.g., feminization, prevention of osteoporosis). In a situation in which ova are depleted but not ablated, one author (BGL) believes it may be worth trying to suppress ovulation to conserve ova until the patient wants to try to get pregnant. There are no solid data to support this opinion. A return of normal menses and pregnancy has been reported following valuable lengths of time in patients with amenorrhea after chemotherapy and RT. Infertility in women who are not ovulating (i.e., having menstrual periods) spontaneously is a condition that may be treated with newer agents and techniques such as clomiphene and in vitro fertilization, but this discussion is beyond the scope of this text.

Pregnancy and delivery. As noted previously, the older the woman at the time of cytotoxic therapy, the greater the depletion of ova. Women treated with abdominal radiation or with alkylating agents may undergo menopause as early as age 30 and be unable to become pregnant. Once the cancer patient has managed to become pregnant, what are the chances of a normal delivery? With one exception—women who have received radiation to the abdomen—they appear to be good. Preliminary analysis of data from the National Cancer Institute series of offspring born to survivors of childhood and adolescent cancer showed that the rate of birth defects was 4%, similar to that in the general population and in sibling controls.[25] However, there appears to be a high relative risk for perinatal mortality and a fourfold excess risk for low birth weight in the offspring of women treated with abdominal RT for Wilms' tumor.[5] Damage to the vasculature and elastic properties of the uterus may impair adequate expansion and lead to positional deformities and early delivery. Women with known abdominal or pelvic RT for a childhood cancer should be identified before advanced pregnancy and enrolled in a high-risk clinic.

Cardiovascular and pulmonary late effects may complicate delivery. At least three case reports have appeared of primiparae who went into congestive heart failure, two with constrictive pericarditis after radiation[3,15] and a third with peripartum heart failure, which was shown on biopsy to be associated with vacuolar degeneration, fibrosis, and myofibrillar dropout consistent with doxorubicin toxicity.[9] As we follow these children farther into adulthood, other problems may present themselves.

Prevention. Because there is a dose-response relationship for induction of amenorrhea, it follows that decreasing the radiation dose to the ovaries will decrease the risk of ovarian failure. This has been confirmed in studies using various techniques of ovarian displacement and shielding, which have demonstrated intact fertility and ovarian function using the technique of oophoropexy (ovarian transposition) at the time of exploratory laparotomy in Hodgkin's disease patients undergoing definitive RT.[29] In a Stanford University study with oophoropexy and adequate shielding, the ovary was reported to receive a dose of 3.5 to 4.0 Gy. Two thirds of the women receiving pelvic RT retained normal menses, and nine have become pregnant. Noncomplicated deliveries have resulted from those pregnancies carried to term.[22]

Unfortunately it has not been so easy to control the sterilizing effects of chemotherapy. Attempts to "down regulate" the gonad to render it less vulnerable to the effects of cytotoxic chemotherapy have generally not met with success.[41]

Summary

Normal ovarian function is essential for normal growth, sexual development, and fertility. Because of the age-dependent number of limited nonreplaceable oocytes, the ovary is particularly sensitive to the cytotoxic effect of RT and alkylating-agent chemotherapy. This is reflected in the age-dependent response to dose, with younger females being more resistant than older females. Great care must be taken in planning appropriate treatment strategies to help minimize the potential adverse effects of therapy while maintaining or improving survival rates. In those patients who continue to menstruate, it is likely that there will be a normal outcome to the pregnancy. Return of normal menses and pregnancy has been reported following variable lengths of time in patients with amenorrhea after RT and chemotherapy. A periodic trial of replacement hormone therapy is therefore indicated in patients with normal menses prior to therapy.

REFERENCES

1. Adewole IF et al: Fertility in patients with gestational trophoblastic tumors, treated with etoposide, *Eur J Cancer Clin Oncol* 22:1479-1482, 1986.
2. Ash P: The influence of radiation on fertility in man, *Br J Radiol* 53:271-278, 1980.
3. Bakri YN et al: Pregnancy complicating irradiation-induced constrictive pericarditis, *Abstr Obstet Gynecol Scand* 71:143-144, 1992.

4. Bianchi M: *Germinal tissue: ovary.* In Potten CS, Hondry JH, editors: *Cytotoxic insult to tissue; effects on cell lineages,* New York, 1983, Longman Group.

5. Byrne J: Fertility and pregnancy after malignancy, *Semin Perinatol* 14:423-429, 1990.

6. Byrne J et al: Effects of treatment on fertility in long-term survivors of childhood or adolescent cancer, *N Engl J Med* 317:1315-1321, 1987.

7. Clayton PE et al: Ovarian function following chemotherapy for childhood brain tumours, *Med Pediatr Oncol* 17:92-96, 1989.

8. Damewood MD, Grochow LB: Prospects for fertility after chemotherapy or radiation for neoplastic disease, *Fertil Steril* 45:443-459, 1986.

9. Davis LE, Brown CEL: Peripartum heart failure in a patient treated previously with doxorubicin, *Obstet Gynecol* 71:506-508, 1988.

10. Diamond I, Anderson MM, McCreade SR: Transplacental transmission of busulfan (Myleran) in a mother with leukemia. Production of fetal malformation and cytomegaly, *Pediatrics* 25:85-90, 1960.

11. DiGeorge AM: *The endocrine system.* In Behrman RE, editor: *Nelson's textbook of pediatrics,* ed 14, Philadelphia, 1992, WB Saunders.

12. Fajardo LF: *Pathology of radiation injury,* New York, 1982, Masson.

13. Gershenson DM: Menstrual and reproductive function after treatment with combination chemotherapy for malignant ovarian germ cell tumors, *J Clin Oncol* 6:270-275, 1988.

14. Gray SF, Myers MF, Scott JS: Maternal death from constrictive pericarditis 15 years after radiotherapy, case report, *Brit J Obstet Gynaecol* 95:518-520, 1988.

15. Hamre MR et al: Effects of radiation on ovarian function in long-term survivors of childhood ALL: a report from the Childrens Cancer Study Group, *J Clin Oncol* 5:1759-1765, 1987.

16. Horning SJ: Female reproductive potential after treatment for Hodgkin's disease, *N Engl J Med* 304:1377-1382, 1981.

17. Jones HW III: *Cyclic histology and cytology of the genital tract.* In Jones HW III, Wentz AC, Burnett LS, editors: *Novak's textbook of gynecology,* ed 11, Baltimore, 1988, Williams & Wilkins.

18. Kellie SJ, Kingston JE: Ovarian failure after high-dose melphalan in adolescents, *Lancet* 1:1425, 1987.

19. Kreipe RF: *Normal somatic growth and development.* In McQuerrey ER et al, editors: *Textbook of adolescent medicine,* Philadelphia, 1992, WB Saunders.

20. Kreuser ED et al: Reproductive and endocrine gonadal capacity in patients treated with COPP chemotherapy for Hodgkin's disease, *J Cancer Res Clin Oncol* 113:260-266, 1987.

21. Kreuser ED et al: Reproductive and endocrine gonadal function in adults following multidrug chemotherapy for acute lymphoblastic or undifferentiated leukemia, *J Clin Oncol* 6:588-595, 1988.

22. LeFloch O, Donaldson SS, Kaplan HS: Pregnancy following oophoropexy and total nodal irradiation in women with Hodgkin's disease, *Cancer* 38:2263-2268, 1976.

23. Lopez-Ibor B, Schwartz AD: Gonadal failure following busulfan therapy in an adolescent girl, *Am J Pediatr Hematol Oncol* 8:85-87, 1986.

24. Marshall WA, Tanner JM: Variation in the pattern of pubertal changes in girls, *Arch Dis Child* 44:291-303, 1969.

25. Mulvihill J, Byrne J: Offspring of long-term survivors of childhood cancer, *Clin Oncol* 4:333-343, 1985.

26. Neequaye JE, Byrne J, Levine PH: Menarche and reproduction after treatment for African Burkitt's lymphoma, *BMJ* 303:1033, 1991.

27. Nicosia SV, Matus-Ridley M, Meadows AT: Gonadal effects of cancer therapy in girls, *Cancer* 55:2364-2372, 1985.

28. O'Dell WD: *Puberty.* In DeGroot LJ, editor: *Endocrinology,* ed 2, Philadelphia, 1989, WB Saunders.

29. Ortin TTS, Shostak CA, Donaldson SS: Gonadal status and reproductive function following treatment for Hodgkin's disease in childhood: the Stanford experience, *Int J Radiat Oncol Biol Phys* 19:873-880, 1990.

30. Pektasides B, Rustin GJS, Newlands ES: Fertility after chemotherapy for ovarian germ cell tumours, *Br J Obstet Gynaecol* 94:477-479, 1987.

31. Perez CA: *Basic concepts and clinical implications of radiation therapy.* In Sutow WW, Vietti TJ, Fernbach DJ, editors: *Clinical pediatric oncology,* St Louis, 1977, Mosby–Year Book.

32. Ross GT: Congenital anomalies among children of mothers receiving chemotherapy for gestational trophoblastic neoplasms, *Cancer* 37:1043-1047, 1976.

33. Rubin P, Casarett GW: *Clinical radiation pathology,* vol 1, Philadelphia, 1968, WB Saunders.

34. Rubin P, Cooper RA, editors: *Radiation biology and radiation pathology syllabus,* Chicago, 1975, American College of Radiology.

35. Sanders JE: The impact of marrow transplant preoperative regimens on subsequent growth and development, *Semin Hematol* 28:244-249, 1991.

36. Shenkenberg TD, von Hoff DD: Possible mitoxantrone-induced amenorrhea, *Cancer Treat Rep* 70:659-661, 1986.

37. Siris ES, Leventhal BG, Vaitukaitis JL: Effects of childhood leukemia and chemotherapy on puberty and reproductive function in girls, *N Engl J Med* 294:1143-1146, 1976.

38. Varsos G, Yahalom J: Lactation following conservation surgery and radiotherapy for breast cancer, *J Surg Oncol* 46:141-144, 1991.

39. Wallace WHB et al: Ovarian failure following abdominal irradiation in childhood: the radiosensitivity of the human oocyte, *Br J Radiol* 62:995-998, 1989.

40. Warne GL et al: Cyclophosphamide-induced ovarian failure, *N Engl J Med* 289:1159, 1973.

41. Waxman JH et al: Failure to preserve fertility in patients with Hodgkin's disease, *Cancer Chemother Pharmacol* 19:159-162, 1987.

42. Wentz AC: *Amenorrhea: evaluation and treatment.* In Jones HW III, Wentz AC, Burnett LS, editors: *Novak's textbook of gynecology,* ed 11, Baltimore, 1988, Williams & Wilkins.

12

The Testes

Brigid G. Leventhal
Edward C. Halperin
Angel E. Torano

Overall, the effect of cancer treatment on male fertility is more damaging than the effect on female fertility. In one large series of childhood cancer survivors, the adjusted relative fertility of male survivors was 0.76 compared with controls.[18] Baseline studies of male fertility pretreatment have shown underlying abnormalities in patients with Hodgkin's disease[78] and testicular cancer.[36] In addition, spermatogenesis in cancer patients may be reduced in relation to general factors such as poor nutrition[49] and performance status.[1] Surgery alone may interfere with male fertility. Ejaculatory failure caused by damage to the thoracolumbar sympathetic plexus during retroperitoneal lymph node dissection is a major contributor to infertility in males who have had this procedure for germ cell or other testicular tumors.[57] Radiation to the testicle and chemotherapy, particularly with alkylating agents, may have a dramatic effect on spermatogenesis, with sterility a not infrequent consequence of therapy. Testosterone production by Leydig cells is less often affected, and so progression through puberty and maintenance of normal male sexual phenotype is the rule. Little is known about Sertoli cell function in man following cytotoxic damage to the germinal epithelium. On testicular biopsy at the end of treatment for acute leukemia, ultrastructural damage to Sertoli cells was seen[3]; and serum inhibin levels have been elevated in patients treated with radiation to the testis.[74] Therefore, the male patient is at significant risk of infertility after treatment; however, despite an increased number of morphologically abnormal sperm in ejaculates, those who do manage to father children do not appear to have an increased risk of anomalies in the offspring.[63]

PATHOPHYSIOLOGY

Brief Overview of Normal Gonadal Development

The indifferent gonadal anlage develops as a thickening of the coelomic epithelium on the medioventral surface of the urogenital ridge during the fifth week of gestation.[69] By the end of the sixth week, the primordial germ cells have seeded the gonadal anlage. Once in the gonads, the germ cells undergo mitosis and rapidly multiply; most of those that do not reach the gonad disappear, but a minority are postulated to serve as precursors for extra gonadal germ cell tumors postnatally.[29]

Testicular differentiation of the totipotential gonad is effected by a gene on the distal short arm of the Y chromosome, the testis determining–factor gene. The gonads can be recognized as testes 7 to 9 weeks postfertilization. The first stage of testicular differentiation is the formation of testicular cords consisting of Sertoli precursors packed tightly around germ cells (at 6 to 7 fetal weeks). The diploid germ cells, the prespermatogonia, undergo meiosis in the fetal testis and remain in meieotic arrest until puberty. Sertoli cells, which provide a location for support and proliferation of spermatogonia, are derived from the mesonephros and proliferate only during fetal life and in the neonatal period.[71] After the eighth week of fetal life, testosterone is secreted by the Leydig cell of the fetal testis. Luteinizing hormone (LH) release is suppressed, and masculinization of the external genitalia and urogenital sinus of the fetus results. By the third month, the penis and prostate form.[22] Normal testes descend by the seventh month of gestation with little likelihood of continuing spontaneous descent after 9 months.[24] Lack of descent of the testis, or cryptorchidism, is associated with a tenfold increase in the incidence of neoplasia in the testis.[59] LH and follicle-stimulating hormone (FSH) concentration reach pubertal levels in boys until 6 months of age, when testosterone secretion occurs. After this, serum concentrations of gonadotropins and sex steroids reach low values until the peripubertal period (just before secondary sexual development begins).

Male Pubertal Development

The reawakening of gonadal function at puberty is known as gonadarche, and the increased adrenal secretion is adrenarche. Gonadotropin-releasing hormone (GnRH) or luteinizing hormone–releasing hormone (LHRH) is released episodically into the pituitary portal system in a pulsatile fashion, at first just at night, and then finally in the adult pattern where no diurnal variation remains. The pulsatile nature of gonadotropin secretion and the diurnal variation in early puberty makes interpretation of a single value difficult.[7,42] Because of the presence of sex hormone–binding globulin (SHBG), sex steroid concentrations are more constant throughout the day than are gonadotropin concentrations.[71]

Serum concentrations of adrenal androgens begin to increase at 7 to 8 years of age, several years before the peripubertal rise in gonadotropin secretion. The control of adrenarche is separate from the mechanisms of gonadotropin stimulation, and LH and FSH have no effect on secretion of the weak androgen dehydroepiandrosterone (DHEA) or its sulfate DHEAS. Adrenocorticotropin must be present for adrenarche to occur, but other unknown factors must also be operative to precipitate adrenarche.[44]

In a normal male the first sign of puberty is enlargement of the testis to larger than 2.5 cm.[71] This is mainly because of seminiferous tubule growth, but Leydig cell enlargement contributes as well. Androgens from the testes are the driving force behind secondary sexual development, although adrenal androgens play a role in normal puberty. The range of onset of normal male puberty extends from 9 to 14 years. Boys complete pubertal development in 2 to 4.5 years (mean 3.2 years).[71]

The development of the external genitalia and pubic hair has been described in stages by Marshall and Tanner[48] (Tables 12-1 and 12-2). The first appearance of spermatozoa in early morning urinary specimens (spermarche) occurs at a mean age of 13.4 years, at gonadal stages 3 and 4, and at pubic hair stages 2 and 4. The impressive increase in growth rate (known as the pubertal growth spurt) occurs late in puberty in boys at gonadal stages 3 and 4 around the time of the bar mitzvah, making it hard to buy a suit that fits.

The adult testis is an oblongoid, approximately 4.5-cm-long organ weighing 34 to 45 g.[68] The testicular parenchyma consists of seminiferous tubules embedded in a connective tissue matrix containing interspersed Leydig cells, blood vessels, and lymphatics. The seminiferous tubules form loops that terminate in a single duct, which eventually enters the epididymis. The seminiferous tubules are surrounded by a basement membrane (tunica propria). The seminiferous epithelium rests on this membrane. Spermatogenesis, or the process of formation of spermatozoa from immature germ cells, takes place in the seminiferous epithelium within the tubules. The least differentiated germ cells, the spermatogonia, divide to form spermatocytes. These cells, immediately after formation, undergo meiosis or reduction division resulting in the formation of haploid cells, the spermatids, which then metamorphose into flagellate motile spermatozoa. This process may require up to 74 days.[66] Since spermatozoa are continuously produced in adult men, a constant supply of germ cell precursors is essential; however, in the human the stem cell

Table 12-1
Genital Development Stages

		Age at Onset (yr) Mean (Range 95%)
Stage 1	Preadolescent. Testes, scrotum, and penis are about the same size and proportion as in early childhood.	
Stage 2	The scrotum and testes have enlarged; there is a change in the texture and also some reddening of the scrotal skin. Testicular length >2 cm <3.2 cm.	11.6 (9.5-13.8)
Stage 3	Growth of the penis has occurred, at first mainly in length but with some increase in breadth; there is further growth of the testes and scrotum. Testicular length > 3.3 cm <4.0 cm.	12.9 (10.8-14.9)
Stage 4	The penis is further enlarged in length and breadth with development of the glans. The testes and scrotum are further enlarged. The scrotal skin has further darkened. Testicular length >4.1 cm <4.9 cm.	13.8 (11.7-15.8)
Stage 5	Genitalia are adult in size and shape. No further enlargement takes place after stage 5 is reached. Testicular length >5 cm.	14.9 (12.7-17.1)

Data from Marshall WA, Tanner JM: Variation in pattern of pubertal changes in boys, *Arch Dis Child* 45:13-23, 1970; and ODell WD: *Puberty.* In DeGroot LJ, editor: *Endrocrinology,* ed 2, Philadelphia, 1989, WB Saunders.

Table 12-2
Pubic Hair Developmental Stages

		Age at Onset (yrs) Mean (Range 95%)
Stage 1	Preadolescent. The vellus over the pubes is no further developed than that over the abodminal wall (i.e., no pubic hair).	
Stage 2	Sparse growth of long, slightly pigmented downy hair, straight or only slightly curled appearing chiefly at the base of the penis.	13.4 (11.2-15.6)
Stage 3	Hair is considerably darker, coarser, and curlier and spreads sparsely over the junction of the pubes.	13.9 (11.9-16.0)
Stage 4	Hair is now adult in type but the area it covers is still considerably smaller than most adults. There is no spread to the medial surface of the thighs.	14.4 (12.2-16.5)
Stage 5	Hair is adult in quantity and type, distributed as an inverse triangle. The spread is to the medial surface of the thighs but not up the linea alba or elsewhere above the base of the inverse triangle. Most men will have further spread of pubic hair.	15.2 (13.0-17.3)

Data from Marshall WA, Tanner JM: Variation in pattern of pubertal changes in boys, *Arch Dis Child* 45:13-23, 1970; and ODell WD: *Puberty.* In DeGroot LJ, editor: *Endrocrinology,* ed 2, Philadelphia, 1989, WB Saunders.

renewal process is poorly understood. The newly formed spermatozoa are transported through the lumen of the seminiferous tubules into the epididymis where they are stored after completing their physiologic maturation.

Leydig cells are the primary androgen-secreting cells and are found in the interstitial tissue of the seminiferous tubules. Normal secretion of LH by the pituitary gland is essential for Leydig cell function and the production of androgens.[70] If Leydig cell function is inadequate, negative feedback control will not occur and LH levels will rise.

The physiologic role of FSH in spermatogenesis is to trigger an event in the immature testis that is essential for the completion of spermiogenesis (differentiation of spermatids) during the first wave of spermatogenesis. Lack of negative feedback from germinal epithelium results in an elevated FSH level. Once the process of spermatogenesis has been established, it will proceed continuously as long as an adequate and uninterrupted supply of testosterone is available. FSH is delivered to the interstitial area of the testis by way of the arterial system. It passes through the basement membrane of the seminiferous tubule and binds to specific plasma membrane receptors on the Sertoli cells. The production of ABP (an androgen transport protein) by Sertoli cells can be induced and maintained by FSH. Sertoli "nurse" cells also have androgen receptors. The Sertoli cells line the basement membrane of the seminiferous tubules. These nongerminal cells proliferate only during the early stages of testicular development. They have phagocytic activity, and the tight junctions between adjacent cells may form the anatomic basis for the blood-testis barrier. Sertoli cells are also believed to participate in secreting the seminiferous tubule fluid in which the spermatozoa are transported out of the testis and into the epididymis.[70]

Testosterone is the major androgen secreted by the testis and is essential for spermatogenesis. Its actions include stimulation of male secondary sex characteristics and sex-accessory structures as well as control of pituitary LH secretion by a negative feedback mechanism. Measurement of testosterone production by the testis is therefore of major significance in the evaluation of testicular function. However, since intact Leydig cell function is required for normal spermatogenesis, these measurements may not be necessary when sperm production is found to be normal.

CYTOTOXIC EFFECTS OF THERAPY

Effect of Testicular Irradiation

The testes may be irradiated by a combination of direct, scattered, and/or transmitted radiation. Direct irradiation refers to that dose of radiation administered by a primary beam directly impinging upon the testes with no attempt at blocking or organ protection.[34] The scatter dose is the dose provided to a point by all the scattered primary radiation. The amount of dose scattered to a point outside the field of radiation is a function of the distance of that point from the edge of radiation field, the field size and shape, the beam energy, and the depth of tissue. Small children, because of their short trunk length, may be at greater risk from scattered radiation from any source. The transmission dose is the dose reaching a point by transmission through a shielding block, usually made of lead alloy. Such blocks are not, however, completely impervious, and some transmitted dose is unavoidable.[9,10]

Germinal epithelium is most sensitive to radiation effects, and some effect on spermatogenesis will be seen at doses of radiation less than 1 Gy[5] (Table 12-3). Permanent sterilization may be seen with doses as low as 10 Gy.[5] The time-dose-fractionation relationships for azoospermia indicate that complete sterilization may occur with fractionated radiation to a total dose of 1.0 to 2.0 Gy.[58] Regaud demonstrated that protracted brachytherapy was more effective at producing depression of spermatogenesis in the ram testicle than equivalent doses with acute exposure.[54] This finding was later confirmed using fractionated external beam treatment.[23] The observation that multiple small fractions of radiation are more toxic to spermatogenesis than large, single fractions has been termed the reverse fractionation effect.

More attention has been focused on the effects of radiation on spermatogenesis than on its effects on Leydig cell function. The limited data available, however, indicate that chemical changes in Leydig cell function (e.g., hypogonadism) are observable following direct testicular irradiation with the effect more pronounced with 24 Gy than with 12 Gy.[65] The severity of the effect is more marked the younger the patient at the time of radiotherapy.[19] Sertoli cell function may also be

Table 12-3
Effect of Fractionated Testicular Irradiation on Spermatogenesis and Leydig Cell Function

Testicular Dose in Gy (100 rad)	Effect on Spermatogenesis	Effect on Leydig Cell Function
<0.1	No effect	No effect
0.1-0.3	Temporary oligospermia Complete recovery by 12 months	No effect
0.3-0.5	Temporary azoospermia at 4-12 months following irradiation 100% recovery by 48 months	
0.5-1.0	100% temporary azoospermia for 3-17 months from irradiation Recovery beginning at 8-26 months	Transient rise in FSH with eventual normalization
1-2	100% azoospermia from 2 months to at least 9 months Recovery beginning at 11-20 months with return of sperm counts at 30 months	Transient rise in FSH & LH No change in testosterone
2-3	100% azoospermia beginning at 1-2 months Some will suffer permanent azoospermia, others show recovery starting at 12-14 months Reduced testicular volume	Prolonged rise in FSH with some recovery Slight increase in LH No change in testosterone

affected at doses of 30 Gy.[74] In general, however, testosterone production and progression through puberty proceed normally in many males subjected to radiation therapy (RT).

Cytotoxic Effects of Chemotherapy

Germinal epithelium is particularly susceptible to injury by cytotoxic drugs owing to the high mitotic rate. Impairment of spermatogenesis, however, may be reversible in the months to years after chemotherapy. Leydig cells and Sertoli cells, in contrast, appear relatively resistant to the effects of chemotherapy.[74] The testicular effects of alkylating agents were first recognized in 1948 in men treated with nitrogen mustard for lymphoma,[67] and since then it has become apparent that

Table 12-3
Effect of Fractionated Testicular Irradiation on Spermatogenesis and Leydig Cell Function—cont'd

Testicular Dose in Gy (100 rad)	Effect on Spermatogenesis	Effect on Leydig Cell Function
3-4	100% azoospermia No recovery observed up to 40 months All have reduced testicular volume	Permanent elevation in FSH Transient rise in LH Reduced testosterone response to HCG stimulation
12	Permanent azoospermia Reduced testicular volume	Elevated FSH and LH Low testosterone Decreased or absent testosterone response to HCG stimulation Testosterone replacement may be needed to ensure pubertal changes
>24	Permanent azoospermia Reduced testicular volume	Effects more severe and profound than at 12 Gy Prepubertal testes appear more sensitive to the effects of radiation Replacement hormone treatment probably needed in all prepubertal cases

FSH = Follicle-stimulating hormone; LH = luteinizing hormone; HCG = human chorionic gonadotropin. Modified with permission from Ash P: The influence of radiation on fertility in man, *Br J Radiol* 53:271-278, 1980.

alkylating agents in general have similar effects on the gonad.[26] Early reports based on histologic findings from small numbers of patients and normal basal FSH levels suggested that the immature testis was relatively resistant to chemotherapy.[8,55] More recently, however, it has become apparent that both the prepubertal and pubertal testes are vulnerable to cytotoxic drugs.[15] Late recovery of spermatogenesis up to 14 years after chemotherapy has been reported.[17,76] Combination therapy with alkylating agents for Hodgkin's disease (e.g., MOPP) also shows a dose-dependent effect on testicular function,[15] and boys may also show Leydig cell dysfunction after such therapy.[62] Antimetabolite therapy in general, such as that used for acute lymphoblastic leukemia (ALL), does not have an adverse impact on male fertility. Cisplatin-based regimens including velban, bleomycin, and etoposide for treatment of testicular cancer results in temporary impairment of spermatogenesis in all patients but with recovery in a significant percentage.[35]

CLINICAL MANIFESTATIONS

Effects of Radiation

Adult spermatogonia are exquisitely sensitive to radiation (Table 12-3). Studies of single-dose radiation exposure in normal male volunteers show marked but transient suppression of sperm production with doses as low as 0.15 Gy.[63] Depression of sperm counts evolves over 3 to 6 weeks following irradiation, and, depending upon the dose, recovery may take 1 to 3 years. Higher doses will cause more rapid depletion in sperm counts and may slow or abolish recovery.[31] Hahn and colleagues demonstrated that after testicular irradiation to a dose of 0.19 to 1.48 Gy in 12 adult males undergoing treatment for seminoma, the recovery time from azoospermia was dose-dependent.[33] Sklar and colleagues examined 60 long-term survivors of childhood ALL.[65] All patients received identical chemotherapy and either 18 or 24 Gy to one of three fields: cranial alone, craniospinal (estimated gonadal dose 0.36 to 3 Gy), or craniospinal plus 12 Gy abdominal RT to a field including the gonads (estimated gonadal dose 12 Gy). The incidence of primary germ cell dysfunction as judged by raised levels of FSH or reduced testicular volume was significantly associated with field; 0% of those with cranial RT only, 17% of those with CSI, and 55% of those with 12 Gy to gonads were abnormal. Semen analysis was performed by Castillo and colleagues on several late-pubertal/young-adult male patients (aged 15 to 20) who received 12 Gy of testicular irradiation and chemotherapy for ALL.[19] Irradiation was administered when the patients were 5 to 12 years old. All the patients were azoospermic.

Shapiro and colleagues examined testicular function in 27 male patients (aged 14 to 67) with soft-tissue sarcoma who were treated with surgery and high-dose radiation to the tumor bed.[61] The testicular dose from scatter radiation ranged from 0.01 to 25 Gy. There was a dose-dependent increase in the median per patient difference from baseline in serum FSH values following irradiation, with the maximal difference seen at 6 months. Patients who received less than 0.5 Gy had less of an elevation than those who received 0.5 to 2.0 Gy or more than 2.0 Gy. Recovery of serum FSH level occurred gradually after 12 months. Only patients receiving less than 0.5 Gy show early complete recovery 12 months after radiation therapy. Littley and colleagues studied 11 male patients who were treated with whole-body radiation with 10 Gy in five fractions or 12 to 13.2 Gy in six fractions over 3 days.[45] Severe oligospermia or azoospermia was noted in six men tested 5 to 70 months after irradiation, and testicular volume was below the normal adult range in five of seven men assessed. Serum testosterone levels were normal. Two men have fathered two children each, and another has a sperm count of 7×10^6 per ml (60% motile, 20% abnormal forms). Therefore, although depression in spermatogenesis after radiation to the testicle appears to be the rule, late recovery can occur even after relatively high doses. Sy Orton and colleagues assessed gonadal function following treatment for Hodgkin's disease in 20 boys, eight of whom were treated with RT alone.[73] Four of the boys, irradiated at 13 to 15 years of age and receiving pelvic doses of 0, 40, 44, and 44 Gy have fathered children 3 to 19 years after RT. Three had azoospermia 10 to 15 years postirradiation, and one other child had testicular atrophy at biopsy 1 year postirradiation.

In the study by Sklar and colleagues with testicular doses ranging from 0 to 12 Gy, Leydig cell function as assessed by plasma concentrations of LH and testosterone and pubertal development was unaffected in the majority of subjects regardless of RT field.[65] Blatt and colleagues studied four patients with relapsed ALL who received 24 Gy bilateral testicular radiation[12]; three of the four demonstrated delayed sexual maturation, elevated FSH concentrations, low testosterone levels, and elevated LH levels compared with controls. Brauner and colleagues, in 1988, reported on 21 boys who received 24 Gy of testicular irradiation evaluated, on average, 3.8 years following irradiation.[16] In the 12 prepubertal patients the basal serum concentrations of testosterone were normal, but in 10 of the 12 the testosterone response to human chorionic gonadotropin (HCG) was diminished. Basal serum concentrations of LH were normal in nine and increased in three. Among nine pubertal patients, basal serum concentrations of testosterone were diminished in six, testosterone response to HCG was diminished in seven, and basal serum LH concentrations were elevated in seven. There was a correlation between age at the time of testicular irradiation and response to HCG. Several patients had evidence of incomplete pubertal development. In the study by Shapiro and colleagues, only those patients receiving more than 20 Gy showed statistically significant LH changes from baseline levels at each time interval up to 30 months with the maximal median difference from baseline level occurring at 6 months.[61] No significant changes were observed in total testosterone values. Therefore, Leydig cell function appears resistant to direct testicular irradiation with doses as high as 12 Gy, although children who receive testicular irradiation with doses of more than 20 Gy frequently develop both clinical and hormonal evidence of Leydig cell failure. The influence of the radiation itself upon depression of Leydig cell function, as opposed to the late effects of infiltrative disease or testicular biopsy, is not completely defined.

Sertoli cell function has been difficult to assess owing to lack of a measurable biochemical marker; however, the elevated FSH levels in association with spermatogenic failure have been thought to reflect Sertoli cell dysfunction. The recent isolation and characterization of inhibin have provided a possible means of evaluating Sertoli cell function. Tsatsoulis and colleagues studied 18 men 1 to 4 years after treatment for testicular seminoma by unilateral orchiectomy and postoperative RT with 30 Gy to the remaining testis.[74] They found low median inhibin levels and high median FSH levels. Testicular volume was reduced, and 10 of the 18 showed azoospermia. They concluded that Sertoli cell damage had occurred after this therapy.

Effects of Chemotherapy

The effects of alkylating agents on testicular function have been most extensively studied. Cyclophosphamide has been used alone for treatment of nephrotic syndrome, and these patients have been examined for later fertility. Testicular biopsies show damage predominantly to the germinal epithelium with apparently normal Leydig and Sertoli cells, and this is reflected in a reduced sperm count with normal testosterone levels. The extent and reversibility of this damage generally depends on the cumulative dose received, but there is much individual variation. A reduction in sperm count may be seen as early as 3 weeks after commencing chemotherapy, and counts may continue to fall for 2 to 3 months after stopping treatment with an agent such as cyclophosphamide.[8] Doses of cyclophosphamide of 3.5 to 3.7 mg/kg/day for 3 months or longer (i.e., 350 mg/kg total dose) cause sterility in adult males.[8] These same doses in pubertal and prepubertal boys cause oligospermia and azoospermia with elevated gonadotropins in adulthood or late adolescence, but the progression of puberty is unaffected. Aubier and colleagues describe fifteen patients treated in childhood for solid tumors with combinations including cyclophosphamide.[6] Thirteen received a dose of more than 9 g/m^2, and only two were found to have normal testicular function. The effects of chlorambucil on the testis are similar to those of cyclophosphamide. Recovery from oligospermia may be possible if treatment is discontinued before a total dose of 400 mg,[54] but azoospermia appears to be irreversible with total doses of 25 mg/kg or greater.[32]

Nitrosoureas, used in the treatment of brain tumors in childhood, may also cause gonadal damage in boys. In nine children treated for medulloblastoma with craniospinal radiation and a nitrosourea (carmustine or lomustine plus vincristine in four and procarbazine in three) there was clinical and biochemical evidence of gonadal damage with elevated serum FSH and small testes for the stage of pubertal development (compared with eight children similarly treated but without chemotherapy). Ahmed and co-workers concluded that nitrosoureas were responsible for the gonadal damage with procarbazine also contributing in the three children who received this drug.[2] In another series of children with brain tumors that did not arise in the hypothalamic-pituitary axis there was primary gonadal damage in three of nine boys treated with chemotherapy and craniospinal irradiation but in no boy given craniospinal irradiation alone. The only common chemotherapeutic agent here was also a nitrosourea.[46]

Hodgkin's disease patients treated with six or more courses of mechlorethamine, oncovin, procarbazine, and prednisone (MOPP) as well as cyclophosphamide replacing mechlorethamine (COPP) chemotherapy have shown persistent (more than 5 years), if not permanent, azoospermia.[20,21] This effect is apparently dose related, with recovery in the majority of patients who have received up to three courses (in a median of 40 months after therapy).[25] Some of the effect is attributable to the mechlorethamine; however, the alkylating agent procarbazine is also a significant factor in the sterility that is observed after MOPP-based combination therapy. Bramswig and colleagues evaluated 75 boys treated for Hodgkin's disease with involved field or extended field irradiation and stage-dependent chemotherapy with vincristine, prednisone, procarbazine, doxorubicin, and cyclophosphamide (OPPA/COPP).[15] Although pubertal development and testosterone levels were normal in all patients, 18 of the 75 (24%) had elevated basal LH levels, demonstrating chemotherapy-induced Leydig cell damage. In addition, there was a 40.5% incidence of elevated basal FSH values, indicating severe impairment of spermatogenesis as confirmed by azoospermia in four patients. Testicular dysfunction was observed in patients treated before as well as during puberty. The incidence of elevated basal FSH and LH values was significantly higher in patients who had received higher cumulative doses of chemotherapy, that is, 28.9% and 13.2% with two OPPA, 45.5% and 36.4% with two OPPA/two COPP, and 62.5% and 43.8% with two OPPA/4-6 COPP, respectively. When later patients were evaluated after treatment with a similar regimen without the procarbazine (OPA), gonadal function was normal.[37] Nine patients who received two OPA and two to four COMP (with methotrexate substituted for procarbazine) and mean cyclophosphamide doses ranging from 2004 to 3722 mg/m^2 showed no major testicular damage, although some patients had increased stimulated LH levels, possibly indicating compensated Leydig cell insufficiency. Leydig cell damage was also seen by Sherins and colleagues, who studied 19 Ugandan boys with Hodgkin's disease treated with MOPP alone.[62] Nine of 13 pubertal boys (aged 11 to 16) had moderate to severe gynecomastia and germinal aplasia with elevated FSH and LH levels and reduced serum testosterone levels. Six prepubertal boys (3 to 10 years of age) similarly treated showed no change in serum gonadotropins, and gynecomastia did not develop. Therefore, Leydig cell damage of some degree appears to be the rule in boys treated with MOPP-like combination therapy for Hodgkin's disease. In contrast, in adult patients treated with doxorubicin, bleomycin, velban, and dacarbazine (ABVD) for Hodgkin's disease azoospermia was found in only 33%[13] and after temporary oligospermia, full recovery of spermatogenesis was observed in 67% of patients treated with ABVD.[4] Abnormalities of Leydig cell function have not been reported in these patients.

Chemotherapy for germ cell tumors does have deleterious effects on the testis, but it is less severe and there is greater potential for recovery than in patients with Hodgkin's disease. In these patients, ejaculatory failure caused by damage to the thoracolumbar sympathetic plexus during retroperitoneal lymph node dissection (RLND) is a major contributory factor to the infertility of survivors of germ cell tumors.[56] In addition, there may be preexisting germ cell defects in these patients. Hansen and colleagues evaluated gonadal function in 21 patients treated with orchiectomy alone versus 25 patients treated with orchiectomy plus chemotherapy with cisplatin, vinblastine, and bleomycin (PVB). Sperm production was similar in the two groups of patients 1.5 years after treatment and beyond, although approximately half the patients in each group showed sperm counts below the reference level. Fossa and colleagues reported that 50% to 60% of their patients regained active spermatogenesis 1 to 3 years after treatment for testicular cancer with or without RLND, using PVB.[27] Fourteen patients, nine of whom had had RLND, impregnated their wives. Recovery of spermatogenesis was decreased in patients with low pretreatment total sperm counts[36] or with highly increased pretreatment serum FSH.[28] Patients younger than 25 at the time of treatment appear to have fewer abnormalities of LH and FSH than those older than 25.[14,36] Heyn and colleagues described the late effects of therapy in patients with paratesticular rhabdomyosarcoma.[38] These patients were 10 months to 19 years of age at the time of treatment. The majority of these patients also had RLND or sampling. Eight had loss of normal ejaculatory function. The testicular size was small in children whose testes were irradiated and in some who received cyclophosphamide. Tanner staging was normal in 45 patients for whom it was recorded. Elevated FSH values or azoospermia occurred in more than half the patients for whom the data were available.

Male fertility appears to be normal after treatment with actinomycin and vincristine for Wilms' tumor.[6] Perrone and colleagues reported on six male subjects who received chemotherapy only and four male subjects who received abdominal radiation (15 to 30 Gy) in addition.[52] In those patients who had received only chemotherapy endocrine function was normal, but in group 2 (combined modality) LH levels were elevated and FSH and testosterone levels were normal.

Treatment of acute leukemia relies heavily on the use of antimetabolites. The folic acid antagonist methotrexate has been shown to adversely affect tissues with high mitotic activity such as the rapidly dividing spermatogonia and spermatocytes. A rapid decrease in sperm count may occur within 2 to 3 weeks of the onset of chemotherapy owing to inhibition of the early steps of spermatogenesis with progressive increase of early and late spermatids with continued use of the drug.[72] Alkaloids, such as vincristine, are associated with mitotic arrest of spermatogenesis and binding to microtubular proteins, altering the flagella of mature sperm.[30] Corticosteroids cause oligospermia and low sperm motility after 30 mg/day for 15 days, with testicular biopsy specimens showing spermatogenic arrest, sloughing of germinal cells, and a decrease in spermatogonia numbers (reviewed in 26).[47] It is therefore not surprising that 10 of 10 men treated for ALL showed elevated FSH levels and azoospermia after completion of induction and consolidation therapy that contained these drugs as well as cyclophosphamide in modest doses. Recovery of spermatogenesis, as indicated by normalization of serum FSH values and sperm density, occurred in the second year of maintenance therapy with 6-mercaptopurine and methotrexate in all men.[43] In general, testicular function is normal in boys after chemotherapy for ALL.[11] Wallace and colleagues studied 37 adult males at two points after their treatment of ALL. The initial assessment was made by a wedge testicular biopsy after completion of treatment (median age 9.7 years) and the subsequent assessment was performed at a median of 18.6 years. All 37 men completed pubertal development normally and had a testosterone concentration within the normal adult range. Six men showed evidence of severe damage to the seminiferous epithelium with azoospermia or elevated FSH. All six men with germ cell damage had received either cyclophosphamide or both cyclophosphamide and cytosine arabinoside as part of their chemotherapy regimen. All 37 men had undergone a testicular biopsy approximately 10.7 years earlier, and at that time damage to the seminiferous epithelium had been calculated by the estimated tubular fertility index (TFI), that is, the percentage of seminiferous tubules containing identifiable spermatogonia (age matched normal = 100%). Eleven males had a TFI of less than 50%, consistent with severe germ cell damage, and five recovered normal germ cell function more than 10 years later. Twenty-six had a TFI of more than 50% at testicular biopsy and 23 showed completely normal testicular function when reassessed subsequently. Therefore, the testicular biopsy was not a good predictor of fertility in any single individual because of the prognosis for fertility that improves with time.

Other reports of abnormality in testicular function after therapy for acute leukemia generally involve patients who have had either cyclophosphamide or irradiation to the testicle as part of their treatment regimen.

DETECTION AND SCREENING

Delayed puberty may be used to refer to the condition in a boy who has not initiated secondary sexual development by age 14 (i.e., whose testicular length does not exceed 2.5 cm),[44] although the cause may well be constitutional delay in maturation. A careful history should be taken with attention paid to parental height, weight, and age at sexual maturation. It is important to remember that other causes of hypogonadism may not be ruled out merely because one has had a diagnosis of malignancy and treatment. Hypothyroidism may cause developmental delay, and so attention should be paid to history of cold intolerance, constipation, and so on. A detailed growth chart to assess growth rate throughout life should be developed. If a patient is hypogonadotropic, he will probably show normal growth throughout childhood and then miss his adolescent growth spurt. In the older male patient who is being evaluated for fertility, nocturnal ejaculation, erectile function, and libido should be evaluated. A careful history of medication administration, particularly androgens for bodybuilding or other drugs that might affect spermatogenesis, potency, or libido should be elicited. Physical examination should include a search for signs of chronic disease or malnutrition as well as signs of puberty including acne, comedones, mustache, axillary hair, stages of pubic hair, stretched penile length, length and width of testes, stages of genital development, gynecomastia, and tone of voice. Specific measurement of testicular size may be most effectively done by the use of calipers or with Prader orchiometers.[7] The stages of development of secondary sexual characteristics have been described by Marshall and Tanner.[48] Remember that in the majority of patients pubertal development will be normal, but fertility may still be affected.

Laboratory Assessment

Spermatogenesis. If the patient is old enough to produce a semen sample, this is the best test of testicular function.[66] It should be a fresh sample, properly collected. This usually involves abstaining from sex for 3 to 5 days and collecting the specimen by masturbation. It may be necessary to collect several semen samples over 3 to 6 months for precise information. The sperm density should be at least

20×10^6 per ml. Sperm morphology and motility should also be assessed as the latter may be related to functional capacity. If the sperm count is more than 10×10^6 per ml or the total sperm count more than 26×10^6 per ejaculate, it is unlikely that any abnormality of blood levels of testosterone FSH or LH will be found. Patients who have failure of spermatogenesis because of damage to germinal epithelium may progress through puberty normally and have normal erectile ejaculatory function without actually being capable of producing sperm. All adult males, therefore, who have received cancer therapy should have sperm counts performed to evaluate fertility, even if their secondary sexual characteristics are normal. Since recovery from damage to germinal epithelium may occur 5 to 10 years (or even later) after therapy, these counts should be repeated from time to time if such evaluation is indicated.

Bone age. This should be assessed in all patients to assess the contribution of possible constitutional growth delay or hypothalamic abnormality. In addition, GH therapy may be recommended along with other treatment given to initiate pubertal development.

Blood tests. Our patients may suffer from hypogonadism either on a central or a peripheral basis. It is important to determine whether the defect in end organ function is due to damage to the hypothalamus, for example from cranial radiation, or to direct damage to the testicle itself. It is also possible that a patient who has had combined modality therapy may have suffered damage from both causes (Table 12-4). It is important to remember that FSH, LH, and testosterone levels in the blood oscillate during the day, thereby complicating the interpretation of a single value. Initial screening should include the evaluation of basal levels of FSH, LH, and testosterone. In early Leydig cell failure, testosterone levels may remain normal in the face of an elevated LH. Elevated FSH will be present with depression of spermatogenesis. HCG may be given to confirm the diagnosis of end organ failure as a cause of hypogonadism. An abnormal response to HCG is suggestive of disturbed Leydig cell function. Patients with hypogonadotrophic hypogonadism should have a brisk response, although those with decreased Leydig cell function will have little or none. GnRH may be administered to determine whether the primary defect is in the hypothalamus, in which case the pituitary and testicles

Table 12-4
Evaluation of Hypothalamic-Pituitary Axis

	Testosterone	FSH	LH	Response to	
				GnRH	HCG
Primary Leydig cell disease	nl/lo	hi	hi		lo
Primary disease of germinal epithelium	nl	hi	nl		
Hypothalamic disease	nl/lo	nl/lo	nl/lo	nl	
Pituitary disease	nl/lo	nl/lo	nl/lo	lo	

nl = Normal; lo = low; hi = high.

themselves should respond normally to exogenous GnRH, or in the pituitary itself, in which case there will be an inadequate response.[40] An exaggerated response of FSH and LH to GnRH suggests a "failing" testis,[39] so this test may be useful in detecting early testicular failure. Depressed gonadotropins may also be found in patients after the administration of exogenous androgen. Determination of elevated FSH along with small testicular size may offer the most practical approach for predicting subsequent testicular damage in boys with malignancies.[64]

Testicular biopsy. This test can be done under local anesthetic but should involve collecting tissue, not just a needle biopsy. A cross-section of normal seminiferous tubule shows several generations of germ cells. The younger generations are near the basement membrane, and the more differentiated cells are near the lumen. Sertoli cell nuclei can be observed near the basement membrane. Leydig cells are located in capillaries in the interstitial space between tubules. Thickening of the basement membrane and fibrosis or hyalinization of seminiferous tubules can be detected. Spermatogenic arrest at a specific cell generation or complete absence of germ cells can be observed. Many patients with acute leukemia have had elective testicular biopsies at the end of therapy to look for occult disease. In general, because testicular biopsies have been negative in patients who later had testicular relapses, this procedure is no longer performed routinely.[53] Biopsies at the end of therapy have not been particularly good predictors of later fertility because of the late recovery of fertility after chemotherapy (up to 10 years).[75]

MANAGEMENT OF ESTABLISHED PROBLEMS

Pretreatment Fertility

In male patients, banking sperm before treatment seems the logical way to tackle the problem of posttreatment infertility. Unfortunately oligospermia may be present at the time of initial diagnosis, and following "freezing" for artificial insemination, additional defects postthawing have been seen with reduced sperm motility. Overall 66% of patients have shown quantitative or qualitative defects in sperm.[60] In addition, of course, many pediatric patients are too young for this method to be of value.

The realization that retroperitoneal lymph node dissection may lead to ejaculatory failure has led to attempts to avoid this complication by careful preservation of at least part of the sympathetic plexus at the time of operation for staging.[41] The surgeon should also be consulted for insertion of testicular prosthesis at the time of puberty in patients who have required orchiectomy.

Some male patients recover spermatogenesis after testicular irradiation. Since the severity and duration of oligospermia/azoospermia is dose dependent, care must be taken to minimize the dose received at the onset. Even with doses up to 2 Gy, recovery can occur in a proportion of patients up to 4 years later.[31] Careful field collimation and routine use of testicular shielding can decrease the testicular dose of radiation. Pedrick and Hoppe[51] have shown that gonadal shielding speeds recovery of spermatogenesis following irradiation.

There is an attempt to develop chemotherapeutic regimens that are less damaging to male fertility than those commonly in use. Attempts to "down-regulate" the gonad to render it less vulnerable to the effects of cytotoxic chemotherapy by administration of an agonist analog of GnRH, Buserelin, during chemotherapy have been ineffective.[77] Therefore, it is still unfortunately true that a number of men will be rendered sterile by current chemotherapeutic regimens and a smaller number of boys will fail to go through puberty at the appropriate age. For many male patients, hormone replacement therapy may be required. Testosterone enanthate given intramuscularly every 4 weeks at 25 to 50 mg at an age when puberty normally begins and with doses increased by 50 mg every 6 months to a dose of 200 to 300 mg every 4 weeks will cause development of the genitalia.[44] Now that FSH and LH are also available for administration, they are usually given as well to aid in seminiferous tubule development and increase in testicular size. In addition, the regimen is coordinated with GH therapy to assure maximal growth before epiphyseal fusion. Methyl testosterone should not be given, as it may be toxic to the liver. Side effects of testosterone administration may include gyneco-mastia and, with very high doses, decrease in libido. Therefore, the process of inducing puberty in a boy should be coordinated by a pediatric endocrinologist and extends over several years.

Male patients who are azoospermic as a result of direct testicular damage can only wait for recovery of their germinal epithelium. Their Leydig cell function should be evaluated with testosterone and LH levels. Testosterone replacement may increase the sense of well-being in some hypogonadal males.[44] Male patients who are azoospermic as a result of hypothalamic or pituitary injury may be treated with FSH and LH. Several months of therapy will be required before spermatogenesis can be expected to begin.

REFERENCES

1. Aasebo U et al: Gonadal endocrine dysfunction in patients with lung cancer: relation to responsiveness to chemotherapy, respiratory function and performance status, *J Steroid Biochem Mol Biol* 39:375-380, 1991.
2. Ahmed SR et al: Primary gonadal damage following treatment of brain tumors in childhood, *J Pediatr* 103:562-565, 1983.
3. Anelli G et al: Responsiveness of testis morphology to chemotherapy in childhood leukemia, *Anat Rec* 209:491-500, 1984.
4. Anselmo AP et al: Risk of infertility in patients with Hodgkin's disease treated with ABVD vs MOPP vs ABVD/MOPP, *Haematologica* 75:155-158, 1990.
5. Ash P: The influence of radiation on fertility in man, *Br J Radiol* 53:271-278, 1980.
6. Aubier F et al: Male gonadal function after chemotherapy for solid tumors in childhood, *J Clin Oncol* 7:304-309, 1989.
7. August GP, Grumbach MM, Kaplan SL: Hormonal changes in puberty. III. Correlation of plasma testosterone, LH, FSH, testicular size and bone age with male pubertal development, *J Clin Endocrinol Metab* 34:319, 1972.
8. Barton C, Waxman J: Effects of chemotherapy on fertility, *Blood Rev* 4:187-195, 1990.
9. Bentel GC: *Radiation therapy planning,* New York, 1992, MacMillan.

10. Bentel GC, Nelson CE, Noell KT: *Treatment planning and dose calculation in radiation oncology,* Elmsford, 1989, Pergamon.

11. Blatt J, Poplack DJ, Sherins RJ: Testicular function in boys after chemotherapy for acute lymphoblastic leukaemia, *N Engl J Med* 304:1121-1124, 1981.

12. Blatt J et al: Leydig cell function in boys following treatment for testicular relapse of acute lymphoblastic leukemia, *J Clin Oncol* 3:1227-1231, 1985.

13. Bonadonna G et al: Gonadal damage in Hodgkin's disease from cancer chemotherapeutic regimens, *Arch Toxicol Suppl* 7:140-145, 1984.

14. Bosl GJ, Bajorunas D: Pituitary and testicular hormonal function after treatment for germ cell tumours, *Int J Androl* 10:381-384, 1987.

15. Bramswig JH et al: The effects of different cumulative doses of chemotherapy on testicular function, *Cancer* 65:1298-1302, 1990.

16. Brauner R: Leydig cell insufficiency after testicular irradiation for acute lymphoblastic leukemia, *Horm Res* 30:111-114, 1988.

17. Buchanan JD, Fairley KF, Barrier JU: Return of spermatogenesis after stopping cyclophosphamide therapy, *Lancet* 2:156-157, 1975.

18. Byrne J et al: Effects of treatment on fertility in long-term survivors of childhood or adolescent cancer, *N Engl J Med* 317:1315-1321, 1987.

19. Castillo LA et al: Gonadal function after 12 Gy testicular irradiation in childhood acute lymphoblastic leukemia, *Med Ped Oncol* 18:185-189, 1990.

20. Chapman RM et al: Cyclical combination chemotherapy and gonadal function: retrospective study in males, *Lancet* 1:285-289, 1979.

21. Charak BS et al: Testicular dysfunction after cyclophosphamide-vincristine-procarbazine-prednisolone chemotherapy for advanced Hodgkin's disease: a long-term follow up study, *Cancer* 65:1903-1906, 1990.

22. Conte FA, Grumbach MM: *Pathogenesis, classification, diagnosis and treatment of anomalies of sex.* In De Groot LJ, editor: *Endocrinology,* ed 2, Philadelphia, 1990, WB Saunders.

23. Cox JD: The testicle. In Moss WT, Cox JD, editors: *Radiation oncology: rationale, technique, results,* ed 6, St. Louis, 1989, Mosby–Year Book.

24. Czeizel A, Erodi E, Toth J: Genetics of undescended testes, *J Urol* 126:528, 1981.

25. daCunha MF et al: Recovery of spermatogenesis after treatment for Hodgkin's disease: limiting dose of MOPP chemotherapy, *J Clin Oncol* 2:571-577, 1984.

26. Damewood MD, Grochow LB: Prospects for fertility after chemotherapy or radiation for neoplastic disease, *Fertil Steril* 45:443-459, 1986.

27. Fossa SD et al: Post treatment fertility in patients with testicular cancer. II. Influence of cisplatin-based combination chemotherapy and of retroperitoneal surgery on hormone and sperm cell production, *Br J Urol* 57:210-214, 1985.

28. Fossa SD et al: Recovery of impaired pretreatment spermatogenesis in testicular cancer, *Fertil Steril* 54:493-496, 1990.

29. Friedman NB, Van de Velde RL: Germ cell tumors in man, pleiotropic mice and continuity of germplasm and somatoplasm, *Hum Pathol* 12:772, 1981.

30. Greenwald ES: *Cancer chemotherapy,* New York, 1979, Medical Examination.

31. Griffin JE, Wilson JD: *Disorders of the testes and the male reproductive tract.* In Wilson JD, Foster DW, editors: *Williams textbook of endocrinology,* Philadelphia, 1992, WB Saunders.

32. Guesry P, Lenoir G, Broyer M: Gonadal effects of chlorambucil given to prepubertal and pubertal boys for nephrotic syndrome, *J Pediatr* 92:299-303, 1970.

33. Hahn EW: Recovery of aspermia induced by low-dose radiation in seminoma patients, *Cancer* 50:337-340, 1982.

34. Halperin EC: *Pediatric radiation oncology,* New York, 1989, Raven Press.

35. Hansen PV, Hansen SW: Gonadal function in men with testicular germ cell cancer: the influence of cisplatin based chemotherapy, *Eur Urol* 23:153-156, 1993.

36. Hansen PV et al: Testicular function in patients with testicular cancer treated with orchiectomy alone or orchiectomy plus cisplatin-based chemotherapy, *J Natl Cancer Inst* 81:1246-1250, 1989.

37. Hassel JU et al: Testicular function after OPA/COMP chemotherapy without procarbazine in boys with Hodgkin's disease: results in 25 patients of the DAL-HD-85 study, *Klin Padiatr* 203:268-272, 1991.

38. Heyn R et al: Late effects of therapy in patients with paratesticular rhabdomyosarcoma, Intergroup Rhabdomyosarcoma Study Committee, *J Clin Oncol* 10:614-623, 1992.

39. Hudson RW, McKay DE: The gonadotropin response of men with varicoceles to gonadotropin-releasing hormone, *Fertil Steril* 33:427-432, 1980.

40. Illig R et al: Effect of synthetic LH-RH on the release of LH and FSH in children and adolescents, *Schweiz Med Wochenschr* 103:840-842, 1973.

41. Javadpoor N, Morley J: Alternative to retroperitoneal lymphadenectomy with preservation of ejaculation and fertility in stage I non-seminomatous testicular cancer, *Cancer* 55:1604-1606, 1985.

42. Jenner MR et al: Hormonal changes in puberty. IV. Plasma estradiol, LH and FSH in prepubertal children, pubertal females, and in precocious puberty, premature thelarche, hypogonadism and in a child with a feminizing ovarian tumor, *J Clin Endocrinol Metab* 34:521-530, 1972.

43. Kreuser ED et al: Reproductive and endocrine gonadal functions in adults following multidrug chemotherapy for acute lymphoblastic or undifferentiated leukemia, *J Clin Oncol* 6:588-595, 1988.

44. Kulin HE: Disorders of sexual maturation: delayed adolescence and precocious puberty. In De Groot LJ, editor: *Endocrinology,* ed 2, Philadelphia, 1989, WB Saunders.

45. Littley MD et al: Endocrine and reproductive dysfunction following fractionated total body irradiation in adults, *Q J Med, New Series* 78:265-274, 1991.

46. Livesey EA, Brook CGD: Gonadal dysfunction after treatment of intracranial tumours, *Arch Dis Child* 63:495-500, 1988.

47. Mancini RE et al: Effect of prednisolone upon normal and pathologic human spermatogenesis, *Fertil Steril* 17:500-513, 1966.

48. Marshall WA, Tanner JM: Variation in pattern of pubertal changes in boys, *Arch Dis Child* 45:13-23, 1970.

49. Matus-Ridley M, Nicosia SV, Meadows AT: Gonadal effects of cancer therapy in boys, *Cancer* 55:2353-2363, 1985.

50. ODell WD: *Puberty.* In DeGroot LJ, editor: *Endocrinology,* ed 2, Philadelphia, 1989, WB Saunders.

51. Pedrick TJ, Hoppe RT: Recovery of spermatogenesis following pelvic radiation for Hodgkin's disease, *Int J Radiat Oncol Biol Phys* 12:117-121, 1986.

52. Perrone L et al: Prepubertal endocrine follow-up in subjects with Wilms' tumor, *Med Pediatr Oncol* 16:255-258, 1988.

53. Pui CH et al: Elective testicular biopsy during chemotherapy for childhood leukaemia is of no clinical value, *Lancet* 2:410-412, 1985.

54. Regaud C: Influence de la durée d'irradiation sur les effets determinès dans la testicule par le radium, *C R Soc Biol* 86:787-790, 1922.

55. Richter P et al: Effects of chlorambucil on spermatogenesis in the human with malignant lymphomas, *Cancer* 25:1026-1030, 1970.

56. Rivkees SA, Crawford JD: The relationship of gonadal activity and chemotherapy-induced gonadal damage, *JAMA* 259:2123-2125, 1988.

57. Roth BJ, Ironhorn KH, Greist A: Long-term complications of cisplatin-based chemotherapy for testis cancer, *Semin Oncol* 5:345-350, 1988.

58. Rubin P, Cooper RA, editors: *Radiation biology and radiation pathology syllabus,* Chicago, 1975, American College of Radiology.

59. Rutgers JL, Scully RF: Pathology of the testis in intersex syndromes, *Semin Diagn Pathol* 4:275, 1987.

60. Sanger WG, Armitage JO, Schmidt MA: Feasibility of semen cryopreservation in patients with malignant disease, *JAMA* 244:789-790, 1980.

61. Shapiro E et al: Effects of fractionated irradiation on endocrine aspects of testicular function, *J Clin Oncol* 3:1232-1239, 1985.

62. Sherins RJ, Olweny CLM, Ziegler JL: Gynecomastia and gonadal dysfunction in adolescent boys treated with combination chemotherapy for Hodgkin's disease, *N Engl J Med* 299:12-16, 1978.

63. Sherins RJ, Mulvihill JJ: *Gonadal dysfunction.* In deVita VT Jr, Hellman S, Rosenberg SA, editors: *Cancer: principles and practice of oncology,* ed 3, Philadelphia, 1989, JB Lippincott.

64. Simes MA, Rautonen J: Small testicles with impaired production of sperm in adult male survivors of childhood malignancies, *Cancer* 65:1303-1306, 1990.

65. Sklar CA et al: Effects of radiation on testicular function in long-term survivors of childhood acute lymphoblastic leukemia: a report from the Childrens Cancer Study Group, *J Clin Oncol* 8:1981-1987, 1990.

66. Smith KD, Rodriguez-Rigau LJ: *Laboratory evaluation of testicular function.* In DeGroot LJ, editor: *Endocrinology,* ed 2, Philadelphia, 1989, WB Saunders.

67. Spitz S: The histological effects of nitrogen mustards on human tumors and tissues, *Cancer* 1:383-398, 1948.

68. Steinberger E: *Structural consideration of the male reproductive system.* In DeGroot LJ, editor: *Endocrinology,* Philadelphia, 1989, WB Saunders.

69. Steinberger E, ODell WD: Genetics, anatomy, fetal endocrinology. In DeGroot LJ, editor: *Endocrinology,* ed 2, Philadelphia, 1989, WB Saunders.

70. Steinberger E, Steinberger A: *Hormonal control of spermatogenesis.* In De Groot LJ, editor: *Endocrinology,* ed 2, Philadelphia, 1989, WB Saunders.

71. Styne DM: *The testes: disorders of sexual differentiation and puberty.* In Kaplan SA, editor: *Clinical pediatric endocrinology,* Philadelphia, 1982, WB Saunders.

72. Sussman A, Leonard J: Psoriasis, methotrexate and oligospermia, *Arch Dermatol* 116:215-217, 1980.

73. Sy Orton TT, Shastak CA, Donaldson SS: Gonadal status and reproductive function following treatment for Hodgkin's disease in childhood: the Stanford experience, *Int J Radiat Oncol Biol Phys* 19:873-880, 1990.

74. Tsatsoulis A et al: Immunoactive inhibin as a marker of Sertoli cell function following cytotoxic damage to the human testis, *Horm Res* 34:254-259, 1990.

75. Wallace WHB et al: Male fertility in long-term survivors of childhood acute lympho-blastic leukaemia, *Int J Androl* 14:312-319, 1991.

76. Watson AR, Rance CP, Bain J: Long-term effects of cyclophosphamide on testicular function, *Br Med J* 291:1457-1460, 1989.

77. Waxman JH et al: Failure to preserve fertility in patients with Hodgkin's disease, *Cancer Chemother Pharmacol* 19:159-162, 1987.

78. Whitehead E et al: The effects of Hodgkin's disease and combination chemotherapy on gonadal function in the adult male, *Cancer* 49:418-422, 1982.

13

Late Effects of Cancer Therapy on the Genitourinary Tract in Children

Beverly Raney
Ruth Heyn
Robert Cassady
Lawrence B. Marks

This chapter addresses the long-term effects of the treatment of childhood cancer on the genitourinary (GU) tract, primarily focusing on the kidneys, ureters, bladder, prostate, vagina, and uterus. The effects on ovaries and testes are reviewed in Chapters 11 and 12. The most common pediatric cancers that occur in the GU tract include Wilms' tumor, neuroblastoma, and rhabdomyosarcoma. The median age of children affected with these tumors ranges from 3 years (Wilms' tumor, neuroblastoma) to 6 years (rhabdomyosarcoma). Growth and development of the GU tract in the ensuing years may be compromised by the therapeutic modalities employed (surgery, radiation therapy [RT], or chemotherapy; Table 13-1). Furthermore, GU organs may be incidentally damaged by therapies used to treat tumors in non-GU organs (Table 13-2). For example, many of the chemotherapeutic agents used to treat both GU and non-GU tumors are potentially toxic to the bladder or kidney. In addition, radiation fields designed to treat the liver or pelvic bones usually include portions of the kidney or bladder, respectively.

PATHOPHYSIOLOGY

Normal Organ Development

Normal fetal development of the GU structures begins with successive development of pronephric, mesonephric, and, finally, metanephric tubules around the third, sixth, and twelfth weeks of gestation in the embryo, respectively. After 12 weeks the urinary bladder has developed and separated from the rectum. The prostate and testes in boys and the ovaries and uterus in girls are also formed by approximately 12 weeks' gestation. The vagina is developed somewhat later.[12] After birth, prostatic and vaginal-uterine growth proceeds very slowly until adolescence, when the organs enlarge during pubertal growth.

Table 13-1
Summary of Late Organ Damage

Organ	Surgery	Radiation Therapy	Chemotherapy
Kidney	Unilateral loss of renal function due to surgery or RT is generally not a problem if the remaining kidney is normal. Bilateral injury can lead to renal failure.		Glomerular and tubular injury can lead to variable degrees of renal dysfunction (platinum and ifosfamide are major agents).
Ureter	Urinary diversion may be necessary after resection or injury.	Fibrosis is unusual and occurs only after high doses or after intraoperative irradiation.	
Bladder	Dysfunction due to partial or total organ loss may occur. Reconstructive procedures may be needed.	Fibrosis and loss of capacity after irradiation of a large fraction of the organ. Focal ulcerations are possible. Cancer induction possible.	Hemorrhagic cystitis, contracture, and functional loss can occur. Cancer induction is possible (primarily from cyclophosphamide-like agents).
Urethra	Stricture requiring dilation may occur following surgery or RT.		
Vagina	Dysfunction due to partial or total organ loss may occur.	Fibrosis, ulceration, fistula, and maldevelopment are possible.	
Uterus	Dysfunction due to partial or total organ loss may occur.	Maldevelopment is possible.	
Prostate	Dysfunction due to partial or total organ loss may occur.	Loss of glandular function is possible.	

RT = radiation therapy.

Table 13-2
Summary of Methods of Evaluating Organ Function

Organ	History	Physical	Laboratory	Radiologic

Kidney	Hematuria
	Fatigue
		Blood pressure
		Growth
		  parameters
			BUN,
			Creatinine
			Creatinine
			  clearance,
			Urinalysis,
			Serum and urine
			  chemistries,
			Beta-2
			  microglobulin
			  levels,
			HCT.
				Ultrasound, IVP,
				CT, MRI,
				Nuclear medicine
				  scans

Ureter				IVP Retrograde ureterograms

Bladder	Urinary
	  frequency
	Hematuria
			Urinalysis
			Cystoscopy
			Volumetrics
				IVP
				Retrograde
				  studies
				Ultrasound

Urethra	Urinary stream
	Urinary
	  frequency
	Hematuria
				Voiding
				  cystogram

Vagina	Painful intercourse	Pelvic exam		
Uterus	Menstrual issues	Pelvic exam		
Prostate	Ejaculatory function			Ultrasound

BUN = blood urea nitrogen; IVP = intravenous pyelogram; CT = computed tomography; MRI = magnetic resonance imagery; HCT = hematocrit.

Organ Damage and Developmental Problems

The multimodal treatment of cancers with surgery, RT, and multiagent systemic chemotherapy may cause structural or functional impairment of the genitourinary organs and tissues.

Surgery. Removal of a paired structure such as a kidney or a gonad is not usually associated with subsequent functional impairment, unless the remaining organ is damaged from either therapy or the tumor. Conversely, removal of a nonpaired structure such as the bladder, prostate, or uterus can produce severe and life-long impairment such as urinary incontinence or infertility. Urinary diversion after total cystectomy for bladder sarcoma in childhood can be associated with infection and eventual renal impairment from pyelonephritis, ureteral or stomal obstruction, or both.[60,79] In addition, ureterocolic diversion and bladder augmentation have occasionally been associated with early development of colon cancer.[23] However, the recent introduction of so-called continent diversion techniques using repeated catheterization of an indwelling ileal or colonic bladder may provide better results.[29]

Radiation therapy. Organ injury following RT is generally classified as acute (occurring during or soon after therapy) and late (occurring months to years following therapy). Whereas acute effects are usually transient, late effects are usually progressive. Acutely, RT frequently causes irritation of the mucosa of the bladder (causing cystitis) or the vagina and vulva (causing itching and discomfort). These symptoms usually occur after approximately 20 Gy of radiation. Because almost all children receiving genitourinary tract irradiation are receiving concurrent chemotherapy, normal tissue toxicities are seen earlier in the course of RT with chemotherapy than would occur after RT alone. Occasionally, some morbidity is seen after doses as low as 8 to 10 Gy. Acute injury of the kidney, prostate, and uterus is generally not clinically apparent. The late effects of RT are dose dependent and are due to progressive vascular and parenchymal cell damage, generally leading to scarring, fibrosis, and perhaps necrosis. A discussion of late effects for each organ follows.

Kidney. Irradiation appears to cause renal dysfunction secondary to tubular damage. Nephropathy generally occurs when doses in excess of 20 to 25 Gy are delivered to the entire kidney. When chemotherapeutic agents are used as well, lower doses (10 to 15 Gy) can cause significant injury.[33] In general, if only a portion (less than one half to one third) of the kidney is irradiated, then higher doses may be tolerated without demonstrable functional deficits. The sequelae may be more prominent and occur at lower doses in infants. For example, 12 to 14 Gy administered to the kidneys in an infant may cause severe damage. Hyperrenin hypertension can also occur secondary to radiation-induced renal artery narrowing. This phenomenon has been noted most often in children (especially infants) and should be distinguished from other types of renal radiation-induced hypertension. Irradiation to the remaining kidney following nephrectomy may hinder the normal hypertrophic response.

Bladder. Radiation can induce fibrosis and cause dysfunction due to a reduction in bladder capacity and contractility. Although it is not certain, the underlying etiology seems to be radiation-induced vascular ischemia of the muscular wall.[2,3,48,75] The risk of developing bladder dysfunction is related to both the radiation dose and the percentage of the bladder wall irradiated.[16,48] In data compiled for adults, it is clear that a small volume of the bladder can tolerate fairly high doses of radiation.[16,48] However, high doses may cause focal injury to part of the bladder wall resulting in bleeding and stone formation.[51,52,53,56] When the entire bladder is irradiated, doses in excess of 50 Gy may result in severe contraction and secondary whole-organ dysfunction. Consequently, both the radiation dose and volume of organ irradiated must be considered in assessing the risk of injury. Similarly, scarring and fibrosis may occur in the urethra and ureter, causing dysfunction of these structures.[49] Lower doses of radiation may slow or hamper the full development of the bladder.

Pelvic soft tissues and bones. Failure of development of the bones of the pelvis and/or pelvic soft tissues may occur after fairly low doses of radiation. In general, a minimum dose of 15 to 25 Gy is required to reduce major growth retardation or arrest.[21,57,76] The degree of growth arrest is a function of patient age at irradiation, as well as radiation dose, with younger children being more seriously affected. Higher doses of radiation may cause scarring and fibrosis of soft tissues such as the vagina.

Malignant tumors can be seen following irradiation, generally occurring a minimum of 4 to 5 years following completion of radiation.[49]

Chemotherapy

Kidney. Some antineoplastic agents can also cause direct injury to the kidney. Chief among these are cisplatin and ifosfamide. Cisplatin can cause both renal tubular and glomerular damage with prominent loss into the urine of divalent and monovalent cations, particularly magnesium, calcium, and potassium. Elevated serum concentrations of creatinine and decreased glomerular infiltration rate (GFR) with azotemia also occur and are usually dose related. These effects vary in both severity and chronicity.[6,74,78] At present, there are no reports of delayed onset (over 1 year) cisplatin-induced nephropathy. Prior cisplatin administration (more than 360 mg/m^2 cumulative dose) may delay renal clearance of methotrexate.[14]

In addition, there is evidence that prior treatment with cisplatin makes the kidney more susceptible to damage by ifosfamide.[71,78] The acute effects of ifosfamide, seen most commonly in young (less than 3 years old) children with prior renal dysfunction or nephrectomy, include renal tubular damage with hyperphosphaturia, glycosuria, and aminoaciduria, followed by an inability to acidify the urine — the so-called renal Fanconi syndrome.[71,78] Hypophosphatemia and acidosis can lead to inhibition of statural growth as well as bone deformity (renal rickets) in prepubertal or intrapubertal children. Glomerular damage may accompany the tubular damage[11] and lead to a diminished GFR with increased serum creatinine and azotemia, another cause of growth failure. The long-term outcome for affected patients is unknown, because ifosfamide has only recently come into widespread use; however, there appears to be slow improvement after the discontinuation of therapy in some patients.[61] High doses of cyclophosphamide can cause similar renal effects, but this has been uncommon with the dose schedules used in recent years.

Bladder. Bladder damage, including hemorrhagic cystitis, fibrosis, and occasional bladder shrinkage, can occur following chronic administration of alkylating agents such as cyclophosphamide[43] and ifosfamide.[68] The metabolic by-products of these drugs include acrolein, which irritates the bladder mucosa. Fortunately drug-induced hemorrhagic cystitis and the related fibrosis can nearly always be prevented by the use of increased hydration during drug administration and the concomitant administration of intravenous or oral mercaptoethane sulfonate (MESNA).

MESNA serves as a chemical sponge that binds the metabolites, thereby inactivating them and preventing their toxic action on the urothelium. Cyclophosphamide has also been associated with the induction of bladder tumors.[13,22,66]

Combined chemotherapy and radiation therapy. Radiation may interact with a number of chemotherapeutic agents in either an additive or a synergistic fashion. Notable for the organs of the GU tract, particularly the kidneys, is the interaction of radiation with the antibiotics actinomycin D and doxorubicin.[76] In this interaction, significant enhancement of radiation effects is characteristically seen when the agents are given concurrently, but may also occur when the modalities are used sequentially. Radiation may also interact with cyclophosphamide, increasing the severity and chronicity of hemorrhagic cystitis. Therefore, great care is necessary when evaluating patients who have received RT to fields including the kidney or bladder and who have also received these chemotherapeutic agents. This is of particular concern in patients who have had nephrectomy or have a fused or ectopic kidney. In these patients, the functional renal tissue may have been purposefully or inadvertently irradiated. It is therefore critical to have precise information on the definition of the radiation portals.

CLINICAL MANIFESTATIONS

Kidney

Surgery. Following removal of one kidney in childhood, the other normal kidney will ordinarily undergo some degree of hyperplasia. Normal renal function can continue with only as little as one third of one kidney remaining.[31] Radiation in moderate doses (14 to 15 Gy in 9 to 10 fractions) may decrease the amount of renal hyperplasia that otherwise would have taken place in the remaining kidney.[9] As shown in Table 13-3, normal kidney function is usually seen following resection of one of the two kidneys.*

Radiation. Acute radiation nephropathy is an extremely uncommon occurrence, requiring generally more than 30 to 40 Gy to the kidney. Presenting features include hematuria, pyuria, and proteinuria. Dyspnea on exertion, edema, headache, moderate hypertension, and a normochromic and normocytic anemia may also occur. Subacute radiation nephropathy, characterized by hypertension and a decreased glomerular filtration rate, may occur 6 to 8 weeks to several months after lower doses (greater than or equal to 15 Gy) of radiation to both kidneys.

Significant late renal dysfunction occurs following radiation doses over 20 Gy.[17,19,28,33] In children, lower doses (5 to 20 Gy) can cause renal dysfunction.[50,77,81] If a significant volume of renal tissue is left unirradiated, the damage may not be clinically significant. In these cases, regional dysfunction within the irradiated portions of the kidney can be demonstrated. However, if all or the majority of the patient's renal tissue is irradiated, clinical renal dysfunction will result. The data from several studies are listed in Table 13-4. Following therapy for Wilms' tumor (generally with nephrectomy, chemotherapy, and irradiation of the residual renal tissue), renal function remains fairly normal in most patients as long

---

*References 4, 10, 45, 46, 62, 73, 77, 80, 81, 83.

Table 13-3
Renal Function Following Unilateral Nephrectomy

Author	Patient Number	Age at Nephrectomy (Years)	Follow-up (Years)	End-point Studied*	Result
Wilms' tumor patients					
Makipernaa	30	0-7	11-28	Hypertension	17%
Thomas	24	0-11	5-20	Clinical renal function	Normal
Barrera	16	0-7	13-26	Mild proteinuria;	12%
				Tubular function;	Normal
				Diastolic BP >90	25%, one renal artery stenosis
Other					
Wikstad	15	1-15	5-31	Total GFR	92% of normals
Wikstad	36	00-12	7-40	GFR	Slowly declining with long f/u
				Microalbuminuria	47%
Cassidy	12	25-60	3-10	Creatinine clearance after meat load	Normal
Williams	38	29-74	>10	Incidence of HTN	Normal
				Serum creatinine	High by ≈20%
				Creatinine clearance	Low by ≈20%
				Proteinuria	Mildly increased in all
Sobh	45	≈20-62	1-10	Serum creatinine	Mildly elevated by ≈50%
				Creatinine clearance	Mildly increased by ≈25%
				Microscopic hematuria	17% of patients vs 10% of controls
				Hypertension	None
				Proteinuria	Mildly increased
Liu	32	9-61	0-56	GFR	≈80-90% of normal
Robitaille†	27	0-12	17-33	Creatinine clearance	74% of normal, no HTN or proteinuria

*GFR = glomerular filtration rate, HTN = hypertension, BP = blood pressure.
†Includes four patients with Wilms' tumor.

251

Table 13-4
Renal Function Following Renal Irradiation

Author	Patient Number	Radiation Dose (Gy)	Age at RT (Years)	Follow-up (Years)	End-point Studied	Result
*Wilms' patients**						
Kirkbride	3	10-12	2-5	6-8	Growth, renal function	"Normal"
Thomas†	3	≈15-20		>5	Low-grade renal failure	33% transiently after 20 Gy
Wikstad	22	5-15	0-5	5-32	Glomerular filtration rate	82% of normals
Cassady	11	12		≈2	Renal growth after nephrectomy	Normal
Mitus	70	<12	0-10	0-18	Creatinine clearance	Normal in 59%
	27	12-24			Creatinine clearance	Normal in 44%
	11	>24			Creatinine clearance	Normal in 9%
Mitus‡	2	9-14			Creatinine clearance	"Normal"
	3	13-16			Creatinine clearance	"Borderline" (55-63 ml/min/m^2)
	3	13-45			Creatinine clearance	Below 54 ml/min/m^2
Other§						
Dewit	5	40		3-5	Ipsilateral glomerular filtration	30-40% of pretreatment value
	7	40		3-5	Ipsilateral tubular function	30% of pretreatment value
	12	40		3-5	Concentrating capacity	Normal
	12	40		3-5	Hypertension	42%
Birkhead‖	17	40	10-70	>3	BUN, Serum creatinine	Normal
Willett	31	>25	30-86	>1	Creatinine clearance	≈24% reduction

*Patients generally had unilateral nephrectomy and RT to the remaining kidney, plus chemotherapy.
†These 3 patients had bilateral disease. Transient renal failure followed bilateral irradiation.
‡Bilateral irradiation for bilateral Wilms' tumor.
§Generally, RT was delivered to the majority of one kidney +/- some of the other kidney.
‖Partial renal irradiation during splenic RT for Hodgkin's disease.

as the radiation dose is low (less than 15 Gy). Higher doses frequently cause dysfunction. The lower portion of Table 13-4 includes data from non-Wilms' patients whose irradiation fields did not include the total renal volume. In these instances, overall renal function is generally satisfactory.[5]

Chemotherapy. Children who have been treated with nephrotoxic agents such as cisplatin and ifosfamide are only recently becoming classified as long-term survivors. Thus, the late effects of these agents are not well characterized. Long-term glomerular injury secondary to cisplatin may improve slowly; 1½ to 7 years after completing cisplatin therapy, a median improvement in GFR of 22 ml/min/1.73 m^2 was noted in 22 of 24 children with an end-of-treatment GFR less than 80 ml/min/1.73 m^2.[8] However, tubular injury, manifested by hypomagnesemia, appeared to persist. It is not yet known whether ifosfamide-induced tubular dysfunction will also be irreversible.

The influence of aging on the expression of damage is primarily related to growth of the patient. Renal functional impairment may not become prominent until the growing child reaches a size that exceeds the ability of the remaining renal tissue to accommodate the need for metabolic adjustments and excretion. The child may therefore outgrow the kidney and require management for renal failure.

Bladder

Manifestations of radiation injury and of cyclophosphamide and ifosfamide damage are similar and may be quite severe. Both modalities may cause mucosal irritation, bleeding, severe fibrosis, and ultimately an incontinent bladder.

Radiotherapy. RT alone or in combination with chemotherapy can cause severe late bladder injury in both adults and children. Although the data in children are limited, multiple studies have been reported in adults. Following RT for adenocarcinoma of the prostate in adults, approximately 1% to 5% develop severe bladder symptoms.* In these patients only a small volume of the bladder is exposed to a very high dose of radiation (greater than 60 Gy), and the majority of the bladder receives a lesser dose (approximately 45 to 50 Gy). Following RT for carcinoma of the bladder in adults, during which the entire bladder is usually treated with a fairly high dose (55 to 65 Gy), a larger fraction of patients experience severe late toxicity.† Bladder injury has also been observed following pelvic irradiation in children.

Jayalakshmamma and Pinkel retrospectively reviewed the records of 50 children who received both cyclophosphamide and pelvic irradiation (26 to 50 Gy).[35] Nine (18%) developed severe chronic toxicities, including hematuria, fibrosis, and dysuria. However, similar toxicities were not observed in 60 children who received cyclophosphamide and extrapelvic irradiation.[35] Some of the clinical data are summarized in Table 13-5. As shown, the bladder complication rates are higher when the entire bladder is irradiated, especially with a high dose. The limited data available regarding childhood irradiation are also included.

---

*References 1, 7, 32, 41, 42, 54, 64, 65, 67, 69, 72.
†References 11, 19, 20, 30, 47, 48, 58, 59, 70, 84.

Table 13-5
Risk of Serious Late Bladder Injury Following Pelvic Irradiation*

Disease Treated	Minimum Dose to the Entire Bladder (Gy)	Maximum Dose to a Part of the Bladder (Gy)	Number of Patients	Reported Complication Rate or Range (%)	References†
Prostate cancer, Adults	30-50	62-77	3057	0-10 (Average 5)	a
Bladder cancer, Adults	50-70	50-70	726	2-30 (Average 16)	b
Cervical cancer, Adults‡	≈40-50	>60-75	1558	2-13 (Average 5)	c
	≈40-50	75->80	403	9-28 (Average 17)	c
Pelvic tumors, Children (with cyclophosphamide)		26-50	50	18	d

*The doses listed in the tables are approximate. Risks are generally calculated in a crude manner, rather than actuarially.
†The data from some series with unusual fractionation schemes were included in the review.
   a: Sandler, Lawton, Greskovich, Sack, Pilepich, Shipley, Rounsaville, Leibel, Amdur
   b: Shipley, Quilty, Duncan, Yu, Goodman, Corcoran, Marcial
   c: Montana, Pourquier, Perez
   d: Jayalakshmamma
‡Some of the dose is delivered with interstitial implants.

Chemotherapy. The timing and onset of hemorrhagic cystitis secondary to chemotherapeutic agents are variable, with some patients experiencing this complication during therapy, and others developing it several months following cessation of therapy.[34,43,68,78] The hematuria may be microscopic or macroscopic, including clot passage, and can even result in significant anemia. Urgency, frequency, and difficulty voiding can also occur with or without hematuria and proteinuria. Cyclophosphamide appears to be associated with the development of transitional cell carcinoma of the bladder as well.[13,22,66]

The impact of aging on the bladder is similar to the effects of aging on the kidney: a small bladder may be adequate for a 3-year-old patient, but a bladder that does not grow with a child, or actually shrinks owing to fibrosis, may be inadequate for the same patient 5 years later.

Prostate

Because the prostate is a quiescent structure until puberty, clinical manifestations of radiation or surgical injury are not noted until puberty. Atrophy of the normal glandular tissue in the prostate can be seen following moderate or high doses of radiation.[26,36] Impaired growth of the seminal vesicles with consequent decreased production of, and storage capacity for, seminal fluid may result in a diminished ejaculum.[54] Because the normal ejaculate is a combination of fluids derived from the gonads, seminal vesicles, and prostate, dysfunction of any of these structures theoretically can lead to abnormalities in ejaculate volume and function.

Vagina

Fibrosis and diminished growth secondary to surgical procedures or RT have been described.[21,24,25,35] Vaginal mucositis can occur acutely during RT or following chemotherapy, notably with methotrexate, actinomycin D, and doxorubicin. In patients who have received prior RT, the administration of actinomycin D or doxorubicin can result in a "radiation recall" reaction with vaginal mucositis. Significant fibrosis of the vagina can occur after high-dose RT or after more modest doses of radiation when combined with chemotherapy. These therapies interfere with the normal development of the vagina and therefore have a negative impact on sexual function. Both the size and the flexibility of the vagina may be adversely affected. At extremely high doses of RT, soft tissue necrosis of the vaginal wall can occur. In adults, this appears to be more common in the posterior and inferior portions of the vagina.[63]

Uterus

Decreased uterine growth can be seen following exposure to 20 Gy of radiation.[25,44,55] Scarring may be produced at higher doses of radiation. The resultant decreased uterine size may prevent the successful completion of pregnancy or result in low-birth-weight babies.[44] Decreased uterine blood flow has been seen in women who received pelvic irradiation as children.

Ureter

The sparse data available regarding ureteral injury in adults suggest that the ureter is fairly resistant to the effects of radiation.[48] However, ureteral injury is occasionally seen when very high doses of radiation are delivered to the ureter.[48] The length of the ureter included within the radiation field appears to be important.[39] A higher incidence of ureteral injury is seen when the ureter is included in the radiation field during intraoperative RT. In these circumstances, a portion of the ureter receives a fairly high dose of radiation (approximately 15 to 20 Gy in a single fraction).[27,37]

Urethra

The limited information available in adults suggests that ureteral stricture occurs very infrequently (approximately 0 to 4%) following RT alone. However, stricture is seen more commonly (approximately 5 to 16%) in patients who have surgical manipulation of the urethra in addition to RT.[1,32,48,65,69]

DETECTION AND SCREENING

Evaluation of Overt Sequelae

Structure and function of the GU tract can be assessed by a variety of techniques. Simple screening methodologies include the history, with particular attention to urinary incontinence, urine volumes and urine character (bloody or foamy), and the urinalysis. A creatinine clearance (12 or 24 hours) is a simple, cost-effective screen of kidney function. Structural abnormalities can be investigated by several tests, including ultrasound (least invasive), IVP, CT scan, and MRI. Retrograde studies may be useful for structural and functional evaluation of the ureters and bladder. Cystoscopy may be necessary to evaluate hematuria in the long-term survivor. Consultation with an experienced radiologist is recommended in planning individualized investigations for each patient. (See Table 13-2.)

For those young girls who have had pelvic tumors, gynecologic examinations may be necessary at a young age. The vagina, cervix, and uterus are best examined under direct visualization using a speculum. In young girls, general anesthesia may be required to produce adequate relaxation and to decrease motion. The uterus' corpus can be examined by ultrasonography, CT, and MR; injection of contrast-enhancing dye is not generally necessary.

Young boys with pelvic tumors may also need imaging studies to evaluate the growth of their pelvic organs. The bladder and prostate are especially easy to visualize ultrasonographically because of the difference in echogenicity afforded by the contrasting substances of the urine in the bladder and the solid tissue in the prostate.

Screening for Preclinical Injury

Because the kidneys have a large functional reserve, clinical renal function usually remains normal until there is serious derangement of glomerular or tubular function. Urinalysis is not very quantitative, but it is the cheapest, simplest, and most useful test, along with assessment of blood pressure, for periodically reevaluating patients for the development of nephropathy. Elevation of serum concentrations of blood urea nitrogen (BUN) and creatinine suggest a need for more accurate measurement of glomerular function. Although glomerular function may be accurately evaluated by radionuclide scanning, the creatinine clearance, which requires a timed collection of urine and one serum sample, is easier and less expensive. Tubular dysfunction may be identified by quantitative tests of urine glucose, phosphate, amino acids, bicarbonate, magnesium, and potassium. Urinary beta-2 microglobulin levels are good indicators of tubular dysfunction. Injury to the bladder wall can be screened by urinalysis.

Guidelines for Follow-Up of Asymptomatic Patients

All patients who have received therapies with known renal toxicities should undergo simple screening tests such as hemoglobin or hematocrit, urinalysis, BUN, creatinine, and blood pressure monitoring annually. Determination of serum electrolyte concentrations and more definitive tests of renal function (creatinine clearance) may be indicated in selected patients, especially when statural growth is not proceeding at the expected velocity judged by premorbid progress.

After nephrectomy, preservation of the residual kidney is essential. Participation in contact sports, especially football, is not advised owing to risk of renal trauma. Kidney guards are often recommended, although there are no data regarding efficacy in injury prevention. More likely, the appliance serves to remind the individual of vulnerability. Urinary tract infection should be treated aggressively in all patients, particularly those with a single kidney or renal dysfunction. Patients with anatomic alterations of the GU tract will need periodic imaging studies to rule out obstruction and also urine cultures to assess urine sterility. The role of chronic urinary antimicrobial prophylaxis in patients with urinary diversion is still controversial. Urinalysis is a good screening tool to assess for bladder wall damage following therapy.

MANAGEMENT OF ESTABLISHED PROBLEMS
Therapy

Kidney. If any preclinical abnormalities are found, serial follow-ups at 6- to 12-month intervals should be initiated. Such patients should be followed closely by a pediatric nephrologist. Although little evidence is available that improvement in renal plasma flow or GFR occur with time, tubular function does appear to undergo some recovery, and, therefore, efforts to support and treat the patient until such recovery can occur is appropriate. In the event of severe renal failure, the choice between dialysis and renal transplantation should rest with the patient, the family, and the nephrologist after discussions with the oncologist. For children who have undergone irradiation to one kidney and who develop renal-vascular hypertension, unilateral nephrectomy is potentially curative if no contralateral renal changes have occurred. The pediatric renal specialist should also prescribe medications for control of the hypertension and electrolyte imbalance.

Bladder. Hemorrhagic cystitis can occur during or after therapy. In patients acutely affected, a number of interventions have been used, including intravesicular installation of formalin or alum solutions,[18,43] and cauterization of bleeding sites. Partial or total cystectomy may be necessary. The former can be followed by bladder augmentation, allowing for the possibility of urinary continence.[26] In patients with late-onset hemorrhagic cystitis, cystoscopy is useful to assess the degree of mucosal damage and to confirm the etiology of the hematuria. Patients with late-onset hemorrhagic cystitis are at risk for transitional cell carcinomas of the bladder that may be accompanied by hematuria. An IVP or retrograde study of the upper tracts may be necessary to identify other abnormalities that can cause bleeding.

Ureter and urethra. Strictures of the urethra are usually dealt with by dilatation. Obstruction of the ureter can usually be treated with a stent. Urinary diversion is, at times, necessary.[79]

Prostate, vagina, and uterus. Management of established problems in these structures almost always includes some form of surgical revision such as plastic reconstruction of the fibrosed vagina or relief of the constriction in some portion of the lower urinary tract. When gonadal hypofunction is present, replacement hormone therapy may favorably affect the status of these tissues.

REHABILITATION

Rehabilitation efforts may well be needed both for physical and psychologic problems as the patient matures. For example, children undergoing urinary diversion will need education and psychosocial support in dealing with their stoma and its proper hygiene. As the children grow older and learn that they are physically different from their peers, careful discussion of this problem with the pediatric oncologist, the surgeon, and a psychologist will be of paramount importance in defining rehabilitative treatments and allaying the patient's anxiety about the future. We have learned through following such patients over several decades that there is no substitute for a warm, caring primary physician as captain of the team. Internists should be involved in the care of patients who reach adulthood (age 18 to 21). Ideally, these physicians will be knowledgeable about pediatric cancer patients,[15] but more commonly the pediatric oncologist will need to provide information about the late effects of treatment to the patient's other physicians. Good communication between the initial treatment team and follow-up clinic and consultant should lead to optimum care for the long-term survivor of childhood cancer.

ACKNOWLEDGMENTS

Thanks to Julia McDonald for her skillful assistance in the preparation of this manuscript. Dr. Lawrence B. Marks is the recipient of an American Cancer Society Career Development Award, #92-53.

REFERENCES

1. Amdur RJ et al: Adenocarcinoma of the prostate treated with external-beam radiation therapy: 5-year minimum follow-up, *Radiother Oncol* 18:235-246, 1990.
2. Antonakapoulos GN et al: Early and late morphological changes (including carcinoma of the urothelium) induced by irradiation of the rat urinary bladder, *Br J Cancer* 46:403-416, 1982.
3. Antonakapoulos GN, Hicks RM, Berry RJ: The subcellular basis of damage to the human urinary bladder induced by irradiation, *J Pathol* 143:103-116, 1984.
4. Barrera M, Roy LP, Stevens M: Long-term follow-up after unilateral nephrectomy and radiotherapy for Wilms' tumor, *Pediatr Nephrol* 3:430-432, 1989.
5. Birkhead BM, Dobbs CE, Beard MF et al: Assessment of renal function following irradiation of the intact spleen for Hodgkin's disease, *Radiology* 130:473-475, 1979.
6. Blachley JD, Hill JB: Renal and electrolyte disturbances associated with cisplatin, *Ann Intern Med* 95:628-632, 1981.
7. Bostwick DG, Egbert BM, Fajardo LF: Radiation injury of the normal and neoplastic prostate, *Am J Surg Pathol* 6:541-551, 1982.
8. Brock PR et al: Partial reversibility of cisplatin nephrotoxicity in children, *J Pediatr* 118:531-534, 1991.

9. Cassady JR et al: Effect of low dose irradiation on renal enlargement in children following nephrectomy for Wilms' tumor, *Acta Radiol Oncol* 20:5-8, 1981.

10. Cassidy MJD, Beck RM: Renal functional reserve in live related kidney donors, *Am J Kidney Dis* 11:468-472, 1988.

11. Corcoran MO et al: Invasive bladder cancer treated by radical external radiotherapy, *Br J Urol* 57:40-42, 1985.

12. Corliss CE: *Patten's human embryology: elements of clinical development,* New York, 1976, McGraw-Hill.

13. Cox PJ: Cyclophosphamide cystitis and bladder cancer. A hypothesis, *Eur J Cancer* 15:1071-1072, 1979.

14. Crom WR et al: The effect of prior cisplatin therapy on the pharmacokinetics of high-dose methotrexate, *J Clin Oncol* 2:655-661, 1984.

15. D'Angio GJ: The child cured of cancer: a problem for the internist, *Semin Oncol* 9:143-149, 1982.

16. Dewit L, Ang KK, Vanderschueren E: Acute side effects and late complications after radiotherapy of localized carcinoma of the prostate, *Cancer Treat Rep* 10:79-89, 1983.

17. Dewit L et al: Radiation injury in the human kidney: a prospective analysis using specific scintigraphic and biochemical endpoints, *Int J Radiat Oncol Biol Phys* 19:977-983, 1990.

18. Donahue LA, Frank IN: Intravesical formalin for hemorrhagic cystitis: analysis of therapy, *J Urol* 141:809-812, 1989.

19. Duncan W, Quilty PM: The results of a series of 963 patients with transitional cell carcinoma of the urinary bladder primarily treated by radical megavoltage x-ray therapy, *Radiother Oncol* 7:299-310, 1986.

20. Duncan W et al: An analysis of the radiation related morbidity observed in a randomized trial of neutron therapy for bladder cancer, *Int J Radiat Oncol Biol Phys* 12:2085-2092, 1986.

21. El-Mahdi AM et al: Sequelae of pelvic irradiation in infancy, *Radiology* 110:665-666, 1974.

22. Fairchild WV et al: The incidence of bladder cancer after cyclophosphamide therapy, *J Urol* 122:163-164, 1979.

23. Filmer RB, Spencer JR: Malignancies in bladder augmentations and intestinal conduits, *J Urol* 143:671-678, 1990.

24. Flamant F et al: Embryonal rhabdomyosarcoma of the vagina in children. Conservative treatment with curietherapy and chemotherapy, *Eur J Cancer* 15:527-532, 1979.

25. Flamant F et al: Long-term sequelae of conservative treatment by surgery, brachytherapy, and chemotherapy for vulvar and vaginal rhabdomyosarcoma in children, *J Clin Oncol* 8:1847-1853, 1990.

26. Gill WB et al: Sandwich radiotherapy (3,000 and 4,500 rads) around radical retropubic prostatectomy for stage C prostatic carcinoma, *Urology* 16:470-475, 1980.

27. Gillette SL et al: Ureteral injury following experimental intraoperative radiation, *Int J Radiat Oncol Biol Phys* 17:791-798, 1989.

28. Goldberg ID, Garnick MB, Bloomer WD: Urinary tract toxic effects of cancer therapy, *J Urol* 132:1-6, 1984.

29. Golomb J, Klutke CG, Raz S: Complications of bladder substitution and continent urinary diversion, *Urology* 34:329-338, 1989.

30. Goodman GB et al: Conservation of bladder function in patients with invasive bladder cancer treated by definitive irradiation and selective cystectomy, *Int J Radiat Oncol Biol Phys* 7:569-573, 1981.

31. Graham SD Jr: *Partial nephrectomy.* In Glenn JF: *Urologic surgery, 3e,* Philadelphia, 1983, JB Lippincott.

32. Greskovich FJ et al: Complications following external beam radiation therapy for prostate cancer: an analysis of patients treated with and without staging pelvic lymphadenopathy, *J Urol* 146:798-802, 1991.

33. Halperin EC et al: *Pediatric radiation oncology,* New York, 1989, Raven Press.

34. Heyn R et al: Late effects of therapy in patients with paratesticular rhabdomyosarcoma, *J Clin Oncol* 10:614-623, 1992.

35. Jayalakshmamma B, Pinkel D: Urinary-bladder toxicity following pelvic irradiation and simultaneous cyclophosphamide therapy, *Cancer* 38:701-707, 1976.

36. Kagan AR: *Bladder, testicle, and prostate irradiation injury.* In Vaeth JM, Meyer JL, editors: *Frontiers of radiation therapy and oncology: radiation tolerance of normal tissues, vol 23,* Basel, 1989, Karger.

37. Kinsella TJ et al: Tolerance of the canine bladder to intraoperative radiation therapy: an experimental study, *Int J Radiat Oncol Biol Phys* 14:939-946, 1988.

38. Kirkbride P, Plowman PN: Radiotherapy to the surviving kidney after unilateral nephrectomy in bilateral Wilms' tumour, *Br J Radiol* 65:510-516, 1992.

39. Knowles JF, Trott KR: Experimental irradiation of the rat ureter: the effects of field size and the presence of contrast medium on incidence and latency of hydronephrosis, *Radiother Oncol* 10:59-66, 1987.

40. Krivit W et al: Prevention of cyclophosphamide-induced hemorrhagic cystitis by use of ascorbic acid to reduce urinary pH, *Proc Am Soc Clin Oncol* 2:27a, 1983.

41. Lawton CA et al: Long-term treatment sequelae following external beam irradiation for adenocarcinoma of the prostate: analysis of RTOG studies 7506 and 7706, *Int J Radiat Oncol Biol Phys* 21:935-939, 1991.

42. Leibel SA, Hanks GE, Kramer S: Patterns of care outcome studies: results of the national practice in adenocarcinoma of the prostate, *Int J Radiat Oncol Biol Phys* 10:401-409, 1984.

43. Levine LA, Richie JP: Urological complications of cyclophosphamide, *J Urol* 141:1063-1069, 1989.

44. Li FP et al: Outcome of pregnancy in survivors of Wilms' tumor, *JAMA* 257:216-219, 1987.

45. Liu P-L et al: Renal function in unilateral nephrectomy subjects, *J Urol* 147:337-339, 1992.

46. Makipernaa A et al: Renal growth and function 11-28 years after treatment of Wilms' tumor, *Eur J Pediatr* 150:444-447, 1991.

47. Marcial VA et al: Split-course radiotherapy of carcinoma of the urinary bladder, stages C and D_1. A Radiation Therapy Oncology Group study, *Am J Clin Oncol* 8:185-199, 1985.

48. Marks LB et al: The response of the urinary bladder to radiation (submitted for publication).

49. Meadows AT et al: Second malignant neoplasms in children: an update from the Late Effects Study Group, *J Clin Oncol* 3:532-538, 1985.

50. Mitus A, Tefft M, Fellers FX: Long-term follow-up of renal functions of 108 children who underwent nephrectomy for malignant disease, *Pediatrics* 44:912-921, 1969.

51. Montana GS, Fowler WC: Carcinoma of the cervix: analysis of bladder and rectal radiation dose and complications, *Int J Radiat Oncol Biol Phys* 16:95-100, 1989.

52. Perez CA et al: Radiation therapy alone in the treatment of carcinoma of the uterine cervix. II. Analysis of complications, *Cancer* 54:235-246, 1984.

53. Perez CA et al: Radiation therapy alone in the treatment of carcinoma of the uterine cervix: a 20-year experience, *Gynecol Oncol* 23:127-140, 1986.

54. Pilepich MV et al: Complications of definitive radiotherapy for carcinoma of the prostate, *Int J Radiat Oncol Biol Phys* 7:1341-1348, 1981.

55. Piver MS, Rose PG: Long-term follow-up and complications of infants with vulvovaginal embryonal rhabdomyosarcoma treated with surgery, radiation therapy, and chemotherapy, *Obstet Gynecol* 71:435-437, 1988.

56. Pourquier H et al: A quantified approach to the analysis and prevention of urinary complications in radiotherapeutic treatment of cancer of the cervix, *Int J Radiat Oncol Biol Phys* 13:1025-1033, 1987.

57. Probert JC, Parker BR: The effects of radiotherapy on bone growth, *Radiology* 114:155-162, 1975.

58. Quilty PM, Duncan W, Kerr GR: Results of a randomized study to evaluate the influence of dose on morbidity in radiotherapy for bladder cancer, *Clin Radiol* 36:615-618, 1985.

59. Quilty PM, Duncan W: Primary radical radiotherapy for T3 transitional cell cancer of the bladder: an analysis of survival and control, *Int J Radiat Oncol Biol Phys* 12:853-860, 1986.

60. Raney B Jr et al: Sequelae of treatment in 109 patients followed for five to fifteen years after diagnosis of sarcoma of the bladder and prostate: a report from the Intergroup Rhabdomyosarcoma Study (IRS) Committee, *Cancer* (in press).

61. Raney B et al: Renal toxicity in patients treated with ifosfamide on Intergroup Rhabdomyosarcoma Study (IRS)-IV pilot regimens, *Med Pediatr Oncol* 20:429, 1992.

62. Robitaille P et al: Long-term follow-up of patients who underwent unilateral nephrectomy in childhood, *Lancet* i:1297-1299, 1985.

63. Rotman M, Aziz H, Choi KN: *Radiation damage of normal tissues in the treatment of gynecological cancers.* In Vaeth JM, Meyer JL, editors: *Frontiers of radiation therapy and oncology: radiation tolerance of normal tissues, vol 23,* Basel, 1989, Karger.

64. Rounsaville MC et al: Prostatic carcinoma: limited field irradiation, *Int J Radiat Oncol Biol Phys* 13:1013-1020, 1987.

65. Sack H, Nosbuesch H, Stuetzer: Radiotherapy of prostate carcinoma: results of treatment and complications, *Radiother Oncol* 10:7-15, 1987.

66. Samra Y, Hertz M, Lindner A: Urinary bladder tumors following cyclophosphamide therapy: a report of two cases with a review of the literature, *Med Pediatr Oncol* 13:86-91, 1985.

67. Sandler HM et al: Dose escalation for stage C (T3) prostate cancer: minimal rectal toxicity observed using conformal therapy, *Radiother Oncol* 23:53-54, 1992.

68. Sarosy G: Ifosfamide — pharmacologic overview, *Semin Oncol* 16:2-8, 1989.

69. Shipley WU et al: Radiation therapy for localized prostate carcinoma: experience at the Massachusetts General Hospital (1973-1981), *NCI Monogr* 7:67-73, 1988.

70. Shipley WU et al: Full-dose irradiation for patients with invasive bladder carcinoma: clinical and histological factors prognostic of improved survival, *J Urol* 134:679-683, 1985.

71. Skinner R et al: Nephrotoxicity after ifosfamide, *Arch Dis Child* 65:732-738, 1990.

72. Smit WGJM et al: Late radiation damage in prostate cancer patients treated by high dose external radiotherapy in relation to rectal dose, *Int J Radiat Oncol Biol Phys* 18:23-29, 1990.

73. Sobh M et al: Long-term follow-up of the remaining kidney in living related kidney donors, *Int Urol Nephrol* 21:547-553, 1989.

74. Stewart DJ et al: Renal and hepatic concentrations of platinum: relationship to cisplatin time, dose, and nephrotoxicity, *J Clin Oncol* 3:1251-1256, 1985.

75. Stewart FA: Mechanism of bladder damage and repair after treatment with radiation and cytostatic drugs, *Br J Cancer* 53:280-291, 1986.

76. Tefft M et al: Acute and late effects on normal tissues following combined chemo- and radiotherapy for childhood rhabdomyosarcoma and Ewing's sarcoma, *Cancer* 37:1201-1213, 1976.

77. Thomas PRM et al: Late effects of treatment for Wilms' tumor, *Int J Radiat Oncol Biol Phys* 9:651-657, 1983.

78. Vogelzang NJ: Nephrotoxicity from chemotherapy: prevention and management, *Oncology* 5:97-112, 1991.

79. Wespes E, Stone AR, King LR: Ileocaecocystoplasty in urinary tract reconstruction in children, *Br J Urol* 58:266-272, 1986.

80. Wikstad I et al: Kidney function in adults born with unilateral renal agenesis or nephrectomized in childhood, *Pediatr Nephrol* 2:177-182, 1988.

81. Wikstad I et al: A comparative study of size and function of the remnant kidney in patients nephrectomized in childhood for Wilms' tumor and hydronephrosis, *Acta Paediatr Scand* 75:408-414, 1986.

82. Willett CG et al: Renal complications secondary to radiation treatment of upper abdominal malignancies, *Int J Radiat Oncol Biol Phys* 12:1601-1604, 1986.

83. Williams SL, Oler J, Jorkasky DK: Long-term renal function in kidney donors: a comparison of donors and their siblings, *Ann Intern Med* 105:1-8, 1986.

84. Yu WS et al: Bladder carcinoma: experience with radical and preoperative radiotherapy in 421 patients, *Cancer* 56:1293-1299, 1985.

14

Long-Term Effects on the Musculoskeletal and Integumentary Systems and the Breast

Robert B. Marcus, Jr.
Bryan McGrath
Kathy O'Conner
Mark Scarborough

Musculoskeletal System
PATHOPHYSIOLOGY
Normal Organ Development

The musculoskeletal system develops from the mesoderm and the neural crest. The mesoderm forms a series of tissue blocks on each side of the neural tube that differentiate into the sclerotome (ventromedially) and the dermomyotome (dorsolaterally). By the end of the fourth week of gestation, the sclerotome cells form a loose tissue called the mesenchyme, which then migrates and differentiates into fibroblasts, chondroblasts, or osteoblasts.[40] Cells from the myotome region of the dermomyotomes become elongated, spindle-shaped cells called myoblasts. These embryonic muscle cells fuse to form multinucleated muscle cells called muscle fibers. The dermatome regions of the dermomyotomes give rise to the dermis of the skin.[23]

In the flat bones of the skull and face the mesenchyme develops directly into bone (membranous ossification); however, most of the remainder of the skeleton first forms hyaline cartilage, which in turn ossifies (endochondral ossification). Most of the ossification in the long bones occurs during fetal life.

The axial skeleton consists of the skull, the vertebrae, the sternum, and the ribs. The bones of the limbs make up the appendicular skeleton. The bones of the axial skeleton are flat or irregularly shaped. Most of the bones of the appendicular skeleton are long bones (Fig. 14-1),[41] which have a shaft (diaphysis), a medullary cavity, and two enlarged ends (epiphyses). The epiphysis at each end extends from articular cartilage to the epiphyseal growth plate. The metaphysis is the region between the epiphyseal plate and the diaphysis. After initial ossification in utero, longitudinal growth of the bone occurs only at the epiphyseal plate (physis). The mechanism of growth at the physis is from the proliferation of a layer of

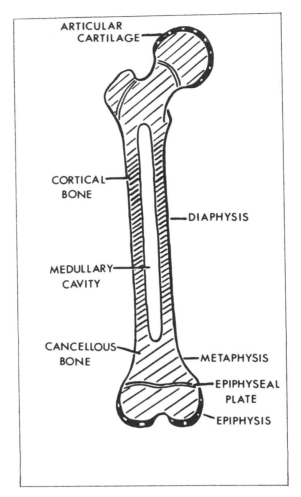

Fig. 14-1. Schematic of a growing long bone. The shaft of the bone is called the diaphysis and contains the medullary cavity filled with bone marrow. The two expanded ends are the epiphyses. The epiphysis at each end extends from the articular cartilage to the epiphyseal growth plate. The metaphysis is the region between the epiphyseal plate and the diaphysis. (From Salter RB: *Textbook of disorders and injuries of the musculoskeletal system,* ed 2, Baltimore, 1983, Williams & Wilkins.)

chondroblasts, which forms a layer of cartilage (Fig. 14-2). Small blood vessels invade the cartilage, causing demineralization and stimulating the formation of osteoblasts. The osteoblasts create osteoid, which calcifies into bone.[37,38]

Most skeletal muscle also develops before birth, although some muscle formation continues until the end of the first year of life. No new muscles cells are created after that time; muscle tissue enlarges because of increases in the number of

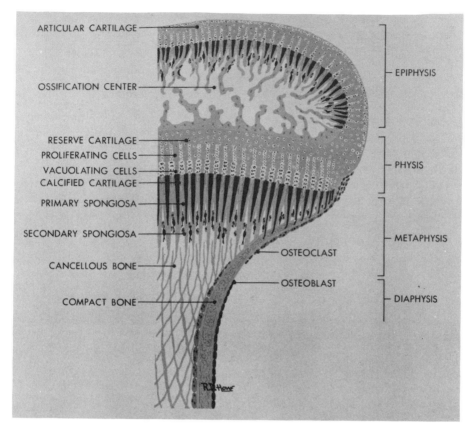

Fig. 14-2.   A closeup of the region of the metaphysis and epiphysis. The proliferating cells (chondroblasts) are shown in the region of the physis. (From Rubin P et al: Radiation induced dysplasias of bone, *Am J Roentgenol* 82:206-216, 1959.)

myofilaments within each fiber, thereby increasing the diameter of the individual muscle cells.

Organ Damage Induced by Cytotoxic Therapy

Direct damage to the developing musculoskeletal system from cytotoxic therapy is most often caused by irradiation. The cells most sensitive to irradiation appear to be the chondroblasts, particularly the very active ones in the epiphyseal plate.[11,37,53] Low total doses reduce cell mitosis and completely disrupt cytoarchitecture. Surviving clones of chondroblasts repopulate the physis (though not always completely) if the total dose is below 20 Gy. Above that level, little repopulation occurs.

Osteoblasts are damaged only by high doses of radiation, but radiation quickly increases vascularity of the bone, particularly in the metaphysis. The increased vascularity increases the resorption of bone, thereby increasing the porosity and demineralization of the immature metaphysis.[27]

The major risk factors for producing late musculoskeletal effects secondary to irradiation are age at the time of treatment; quantity of radiation, dose per fraction, and total dose; volume irradiated; growth potential of the treated site; individual genetic and familiar factors; and coexisting therapy—surgery and chemotherapy.[9]

There are too many variables to determine the effect of each individually. In general, though, if the radiation dose is fractionated normally (1 to 2 Gy per day), the total dose is one of the most important factors. The epiphyseal plate is the most sensitive structure, although for total doses less than 10 Gy, there are few detectable long-term changes. Doses of 10 to 20 Gy produce partial growth arrest of the epiphysis. Doses of greater than 20 Gy will usually result in complete arrest. However, the response to radiation is not an all-or-nothing phenomenon; the higher the total dose and the lower the age at treatment, the greater the ultimate deficit. This is probably because the epiphyseal plate appears to close more quickly with increasing levels of radiation.

Many models have been created to predict growth deficits secondary to irradiation. One of the most recent is shown in Fig. 14-3 from Silber and

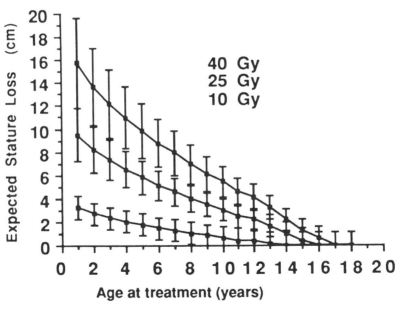

Fig. 14-3.   An example of the model for expected stature loss after RT to the spine during childhood as proposed by Silber and co-workers. The hypothetical male patient was treated from T10-11 to L4-5, and his ideal adult stature was 176.8 cm. Each point corresponds to an age when irradiated, a dose in Gy, and stature loss ±1 standard deviation. (From Silber JH, Littman PS, Meadows AT: Stature loss following skeletal irradiation for childhood cancer, *J Clin Oncol* 8: 304-312, 1990.)

co-workers, based on conclusions derived from their own experience. The reader is referred to the article for details of the multivariate linear regression model presented.[44]

One of the goals of hyperfractionated irradiation (the use of small doses 2 or more times a day) is to decrease the extent of late effects. Studies are only now beginning to accumulate data, but early data from Marcus and associates in the treatment of Ewing's sarcoma indicate that fractions of 1.2 Gy twice a day (total 50.4 Gy to 63.2 Gy) produce fewer musculoskeletal late effects than would be expected from similar doses using fractions of 1.8 to 2.0 Gy once a day (Fig. 14-4).[20] However, most of the patients in this study were teenagers. More data are needed before any strong conclusions can be drawn about younger patients.

Other factors influence late sequelae. Orthovoltage radiation, dose for dose, causes more growth deficits in the bone than megavoltage irradiation, because of the increased bone absorption. The larger the field of irradiation, the more significant the late effects.

Similar dose levels apply to muscle development as well. Doses of less than 10 Gy cause virtually no detectable defect, and doses of 10 to 20 Gy produce some hypoplasia. Higher doses produce more significant problems.

Although high single doses of radiation can cause necrosis of muscle cells, in clinical practice such an event is extremely rare.[53] More commonly, radiation damages the small vessels in muscles, preventing the full development of the muscle because of relative ischemia. Higher doses can give rise to atypical fibroblasts that lay down excessive fibrin in the tissues, causing fibrosis.

There are few data on the pathophysiology of damage to growing muscle and bone by cytotoxic drugs. However, high or prolonged courses of steroids can cause the development of avascular necrosis of the femoral head. In addition, high doses of cyclophosphamide can produce poor chest wall growth.

Chemotherapy often retards growth during the course of treatment, but after the end of active therapy, most reports indicate that patients return to their normal growth rate or even exhibit catch-up growth.[30] Is there a final deficit, however? This is more controversial. Evidence now seems to indicate that growth deficits do occur, but that they are most likely due to endocrine dysfunction rather than to a direct effect on the developing musculoskeletal system.[3,5] Further studies are needed.

CLINICAL MANIFESTATIONS

Surgery, radiation therapy (RT), and chemotherapy can all produce long-term sequelae in the developing musculoskeletal system. The effects of surgery and radiation have been more thoroughly studied than those of chemotherapy.

Most of the following text will focus on the late effects of irradiation; however, it is important to remember that the surgical removal of a portion of the musculoskeletal system can result in the same physical and psychologic late effects as damage to the same portion from RT or chemotherapy. The loss of a muscle group in the proximal lower extremity will cause weaknesses and gait disturbances; the amputation of an entire extremity will require the abrupt need for extensive

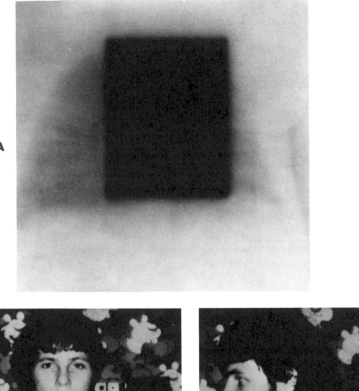

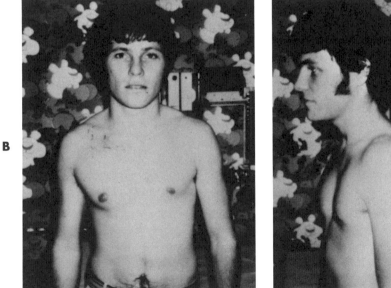

Fig. 14-4.   A 3-month-old boy was treated in 1962 for a thoracic neuroblastoma with approximately 20 Gy in 10 fractions to the mediastinum and much of the left chest. **A,** An anteroposterior-posteroanterior technique with 2 MV photons was used. **B** and **C** show the patient 20 years later. Mild hypoplasia of the left chest is present.

rehabilitation. The fact that the deficit is planned does not imply that the late effects should be discounted.

Bone

The adverse effects of irradiation on growing bone are physeal injuries, pathologic fractures, and osteonecrosis, most commonly of the femoral head.

Physeal injury. Physeal effects are secondary to damage to the chondroblasts. This results in slowing or arrest of physeal growth, producing abnormal development of the involved bone. This can give rise to spinal abnormalities, leg or arm length discrepancies, angular deformities at joints, slipped capitofemoral epiphyses, and osteocartilaginous exostoses.

Spinal abnormalities. Spinal abnormalities most commonly consist of decreased stature or scoliosis, although lordosis or kyphosis also occur.[27] Except for decreased growth, severe spinal complications are less common after megavoltage irradiation compared with orthovoltage irradiation, if the entire vertebral body is within the treatment field.[33] However, marked curvature can occur at times. On standard radiographs, vertebral bodies show subcortical lucent zones within 9 to 12 months after the end of RT. These progress over the next year or two and form growth arrest lines that parallel the epiphysis of the vertebral body.[39] Following the development of these arrest lines, little or no further growth occurs. The higher the dose, the quicker growth arrest occurs. Other changes are seen on radiographs at times. During the first few months after irradiation, vertebral bodies may have a more bulbous contour.[16] Scalloping of the physeal cartilage plates may also be observed, and not infrequently the final appearance is that of rounded vertebral bodies with central beaking.[39]

Clinically, the deleterious effect of radiation on growing bone has been recognized for a long time. Neuhauser and colleagues[27] reported on 24 children who received orthovoltage irradiation to the spine during their treatment for Wilms' tumor or neuroblastoma. Doses below 10 Gy (using orthovoltage irradiation) caused no detectable vertebral abnormality regardless of the age at treatment. Higher doses did cause more severe late effects in the spine. Mayfield and co-workers[21] reported on 28 children with neuroblastoma who received irradiation to their spines. Scoliosis was the most common sequela and occurred most severely at doses above 30 Gy with orthovoltage irradiation. Probert and Parker were the first investigators to attempt to evaluate bone growth alterations secondary to megavoltage irradiation. They noted a deficit in sitting height for patients who received radiation to the spine for medulloblastoma, leukemia, and Hodgkin's disease.[31,32] Doses of greater than 35 Gy were found to produce a significantly greater deficit in sitting height (as compared with 15,000 normal controls) than doses of less than 25 Gy. Silber and co-workers,[44] using data from a study of 36 children whose spines or pelvises were irradiated, have developed a mathematic model to predict stature loss. The model is based on the radiation dose in Gy, the location of the therapy (including whether or not the capitofemoral epiphysis is treated); the patient's gender, and the ideal adult height. Figure 14-3 shows an example of the model, based on different radiation doses.

Limb length discrepancy and angular deformity. Irradiation of the extremities or hip usually produces more long-term symptomatic sequelae than irradiation of the spine, particularly when an epiphysis is treated. Radiographic changes first reveal metaphyseal irregularities and epiphyseal widening. Later changes include sclerosis around the physis and eventually sclerosis and closure of the epiphyseal plate. Such premature closure can cause a discrepancy in ultimate length between the irradiated and nonirradiated extremity. In addition, if the entire physis is not included in the radiation port, then juxtaarticular angular deformities can result.

Slipped capitofemoral epiphysis. The presenting symptom of patients with slipped capitofemoral epiphyses is pain in the hip or knee (referred from the hip). The pain can be either of acute onset or chronic in nature, because slippage of the capitofemoral epiphysis often proceeds slowly. There are a number of causes for this condition. Wolf and associates[52] first reported cases of slipped capitofemoral epiphysis as a result of childhood irradiation. These occurred 1 to 6 years posttherapy after doses of 28.5 to 54 Gy. Children developing a slipped epiphysis after irradiation were generally 2 to 3 years younger than the average patient with idiopathic slipped capitofemoral epiphysis, had a twice greater risk of bilateral involvement (20% to 50%) if both proximal femurs were exposed to radiation, and did not usually fit the generally obese body habitus of the average patient presenting with the idiopathic variety.[4,48,52] Slippage of the physis is thought to occur as a result of excess stress, either from obesity or from a weakening of the bone and physis secondary to RT.

Exostosis. Osteocartilaginous exostoses are benign outgrowths of the physis. They have been reported to occur in up to 18% of children treated with RT,[1] although the incidence in the megavoltage era is much less. The etiology is unknown, but it is thought that exostoses are due to an injury to the periphery of the growth plate. The lesion is a combination of a radiolucent cartilaginous cap with areas of ossification and calcification. It has a typical cauliflower appearance, and the base may be narrow or broad. On physical examination a hard mass is palpable adjacent to a joint.[46] Lesions may continue to grow slowly throughout childhood, although growth should cease by the third decade.

There is a small incidence of malignant degeneration that causes pain and occurs after skeletal maturation.

Pathologic fracture. Irradiation of the metaphyseal portion of the bone may temporarily cause increased porosity and demineralization. Radiographs show cortical thinning and irregularities during this time. The irradiated segment of bone therefore acts as a stress concentrator and predisposes the bone to fracture. This is particularly true in patients in whom the irradiated bone has been weakened by tumor involvement such as in Ewing's sarcoma of the humerus and femur. Pathologic fractures usually occur within 3 years after treatment.

Osteonecrosis. Osteonecrosis of the femoral head is an unusual late effect occurring primarily in adults, but occasionally in children. It occurs primarily at doses above 60 Gy and is caused by radiation damage to the tenuous blood supply to the femoral head. The presenting symptom is pain, either acute in onset or more chronic. The typical radiographic picture is shown in Fig. 14-5.

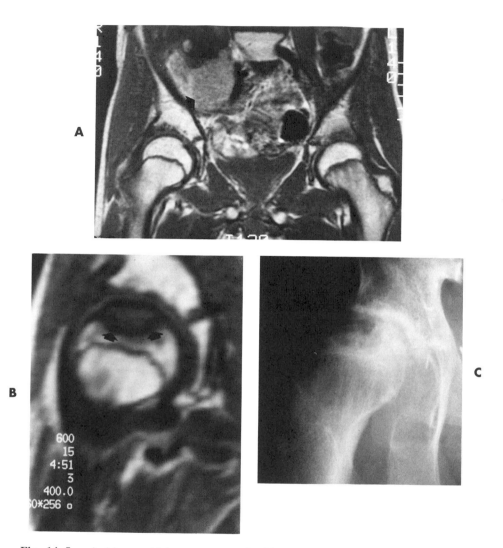

Fig. 14-5.   A 14-year-old boy was treated with preoperative irradiation (61 Gy) and chemotherapy for a synovial cell sarcoma of the right iliopsoas muscle. **A,** Tumor *(arrows)* and normal femoral heads. **B,** A magnetic resonance scan 6 months later showing a close-up of the right femoral head. The scalloped, nonenhancing lesion in the femoral head is typical for an osteonecrosis. **C,** A plain radiograph 1 year later showing healing of the femoral head.

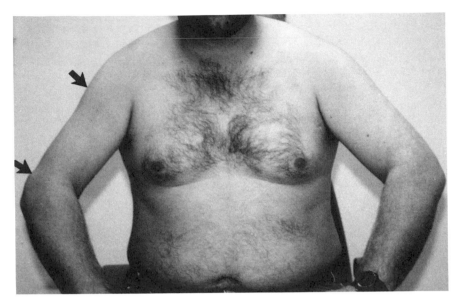

Fig. 14-6.   A 14-year-old boy was treated for a Ewing's sarcoma of the right humerus with 50.4 Gy using a fractionation scheme of 1.2 Gy twice a day. There was little noticeable difference between the muscle development of both upper arms until he started weightlifting. The left (untreated) arm responded, but the muscles in the radiation field did not increase as much in size or strength. In a picture taken 11 years after treatment, the area of hypoplasia from the field of irradiation can be clearly seen (the proximal and distal end of the field are marked with arrows).

Muscle

The most common late effect secondary to irradiation of developing muscle tissues is diminished development (hypoplasia). The muscles treated are smaller and functionally not as strong as the patient's nonirradiated muscle tissues. Nevertheless, the differences in strength are not pronounced, and for the majority of patients it is more of a cosmetic problem than a functional one. However, at times these tissues can develop marked fibrosis, which can produce stiffness, a decrease in range of motion of a joint, and even pain. In mild cases, the stiffness or pain occurs primarily in the early morning and is improved by use of the involved muscles. Occasionally, the patient may have pain that is more persistent, lasts all day, and does not improve with use.

Impact of Aging

In general, growth deficits of the musculoskeletal system from irradiation are amplified with increasing years after treatment. Obviously, when all epiphyses are closed, further bone growth deficits do not occur. However, other late effects on bone continue to occur, and muscular hypoplasia may become more significant, as will fibrosis.

DETECTION AND SCREENING

A good history and physical examination are critical in the evaluation of musculoskeletal treatment sequelae. It is necessary to know the time a deformity became symptomatic, the symptom complex, and the details of the previous cytotoxic treatment related to the deformity. Attention should be given to the types of surgical procedures, the location of radiation fields and doses used, and the details (including doses) of the chemotherapy regimen.

The physical examiner should look for skin changes from the cytotoxic treatment, as well as any obvious deformity. The musculoskeletal assessment should include serial measures of weight, height, and sitting height (crown to rump). These measurements should be plotted on growth velocity charts to assess whether growth rate is within normal limits. Most normal children will grow a minimum of 5 cm per year between age 3 and puberty. A patient in that age group who grows less than 5 cm per year, or whose serial heights on growth charts begin to fall into lower percentiles, may be experiencing growth failure.[25]

Any joints involved in the radiation fields or affected by surgery can be put through passive and active ranges of motion, and comparisons can be made with the contralateral side. Joint measurements can be taken if indicated by abnormalities in performances of range of motion. For example, if the active motion of a particular joint is noted to be less than the passive range of motion, further assessment is indicated. Other pertinent joint problems include pain, crepitation, swelling, loss of mobility, or weakness.[19]

Observation of gait and posture are included in the musculoskeletal assessment. As indicated by treatment received, the muscles to be examined can be assessed by functional groups, and comparisons can be made bilaterally for symmetry, tone, size, and strength. Any areas of deformity, swelling, atrophy, or weakness should be noted.[19]

The patient should be assessed for level of functioning and participation in normal daily activities, such as school and home life. Normal growth and development parameters should be incorporated into this assessment, as developmental stages may influence the patient's participation in some activities. Another influence on level of functioning or decreased participation in activities could be the lack of adjustment to body image changes.

There is no current method of completely preventing the development of late musculoskeletal effects from surgery or RT. The patient who has experienced an amputation or a significant growth deficit due to RT may or may not have incorporated this long-term effect into a new, positive body image. Many other factors contribute to general growth and development, such as nutritional deficits, other tissue damage, and hormonal influences. The examiner should not rush to attribute the entire problem to the cytotoxic treatment.[25] If the right assessment is made, intervention can sometimes prevent an asymptomatic or mildly symptomatic problem from becoming more clinically significant, or it may at least be possible to assist the patient in adapting to body image changes (see the discussion of rehabilitation later in this chapter).

Spinal Sequelae

The evaluation of spinal sequelae should include the region of curvature, the magnitude of the curve, the deviation from vertical, the degree of shoulder asymmetry, the position of any rib humps or rib flare, and the type and degree of any gait abnormality. Usually the best way to examine the back is with the patient bending over with the arms touching the toes and the knees straight. At each visit, measurements should be taken of the standing and sitting heights. Although spinal shortening does occur as a result of irradiation, it is not correctable, and except for an ultimate decrease in height, does not usually cause major problems unless spinal curvature develops. Anteroposterior and lateral films of the entire spine should be performed to screen for this. It is also important to be able to inform patients of the height deficit to be expected. Figure 14-3 shows a model of expected stature loss by age at treatment for three radiation dose levels for a hypothetical male patient receiving radiation from T10-T11 to L4-5.[44]

If the spine has been irradiated, standard scoliosis radiographs should be done every 1 to 2 years until skeletal maturity to detect early scoliosis or kyphoscoliosis (Fig. 14-7). After that, films should still be taken every 1 to 2 years if some curvature is already present. It is rare that curvature develops after skeletal maturity if none was present before.

The most common method for measuring spinal curvature is the Cobb technique. The two end vertebrae of the curvature, the ones most tilted from the horizontal on the upright film, are selected. A line is drawn along the upper end plate of the upper end vertebra and along the lower end plate of the lower end vertebra. The angle of intersection of the perpendiculars from these lines is the angle of the curvature (Fig. 14-8). It is extremely important to perform these measurements carefully and accurately. In the event of a double curvature, both should be measured. Because progression of any defect may be more important than the occurrence of the defect, the amount of curvature should always be measured from the same two vertebrae to ensure accurate comparison.[51,53]

Leg Length Discrepancy

Limb length discrepancies are usually more significant. Differences in length between upper extremities are not often a problem, but leg length discrepancies can cause significant functional deficits. It is therefore important to be able to predict the ultimate outcome when RT is chosen. To do so, a knowledge of the future growth of all epiphyses is necessary. In the lower extremity, 65% of future growth comes from the knee, 37% from the distal femoral physis, and 28% from the proximal tibial physis. Only 15% occurs at the proximal femoral plate and 20% from the distal tibial plate.[24,53] Table 14-1 provides rough estimates, by age of the patient, of the growth remaining for the four major lower extremity epiphyses.[2] Information such as this can be used to calculate the probable discrepancy that will develop, assuming no growth of the irradiated physis after treatment. This is not completely accurate, because some growth may occur for a short time, and other untreated growth plates in the same extremity may partially compensate for the closed physis.

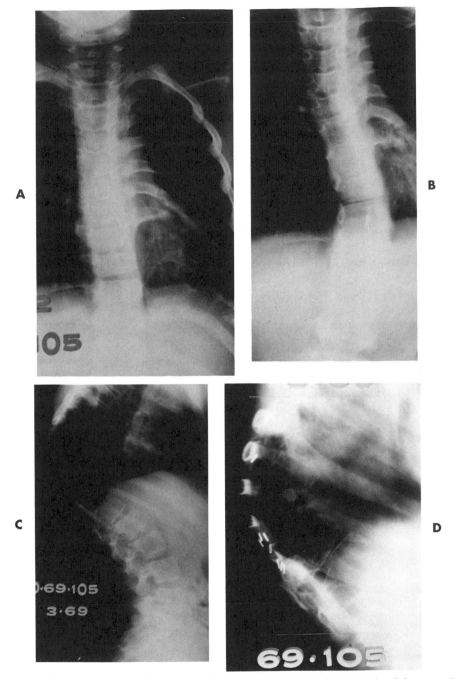

Fig. 14-7. A 2-year-old girl was treated with orthovoltage irradiation to the abdomen and spine (dose unknown) for a neuroblastoma in 1960. **A,** Mild scoliosis developed 2 years after treatment. **B** and **C,** Progression of kyphoscoliosis occurred over the next 7 years. **D,** A close-up of the spine 9 years posttherapy shows osteoporosis of vertebral bodies and wedge-shaped compression fracture.

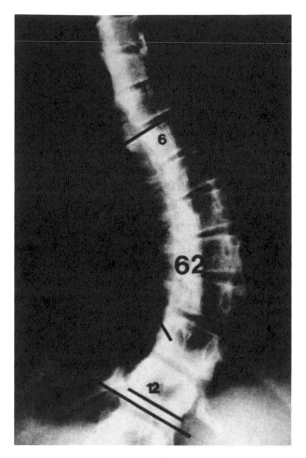

Fig. 14-8.   Cobb technique for measuring the angle of spinal curvature. See text for a description. (From Winter RB: *Spinal problems in pediatric orthopaedics.* In Lovell WW, Winter RB, editors: *Pediatric orthopedics,* ed 3, Philadelphia, 1990, J. B. Lippincott.)

Table 14-1

Average Growth (in cm) Remaining for Each Lower Extremity Epiphysis by Age and Sex

Epiphysis	Boys—Age in Years					Girls—Age in Years				
	8	10	12	14	16	8	10	12	14	16
Proximal femur	3.5	3.0	2.0	0.8	<0.5	2.8	1.9	0.8	<0.5	0
Distal femur	8.5	7.5	5.0	2.0	0.5	7.0	4.7	2.0	0.8	0
Proximal tibia	6.0	5.0	3.5	1.0	<0.5	4.5	3.0	1.0	<0.5	0
Distal tibia	4.2	3.7	2.5	1.0	<0.5	3.4	2.3	1.0	<0.5	0

(Adapted from Anderson M, Green WT, Messner MB: Growth and predictions of growth in the lower extremities, *J Bone Joint Surg* 45A:1-14, 1963, p 11.)

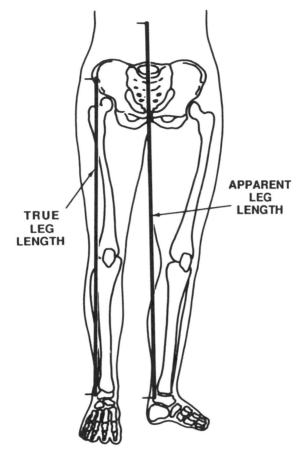

Fig. 14-9.   Measurement of leg length discrepancy. See text for details. (From Mosely CF: *Leg-length discrepancy.* In Lovell WW, Winter RB, editors: *Pediatric orthopedics,* ed 3, Philadelphia, 1990, JB Lippincott.)

The evaluation of a limb length discrepancy on physical examination is also primarily based on accurate measurements. The patient should be undressed completely for the measurements to avoid tenting of the tape around folds in the patient's clothes. The *real* length of each leg is measured from the anterior superior iliac spine to the tip of the medial malleolus (Fig. 14-9). The *apparent* length is measured from the umbilicus to the tip of the medial malleolus. The real length is the more important measurement because pelvic obliquity does not influence this measurement. Measurement of the apparent length allows the evaluating physician to determine whether the patient is compensating for the limb length discrepancy. To detect developing leg length discrepancies, measurements should also be taken at least once a year to follow the extent of the evolving discrepancy. If there is a high chance of a significant discrepancy developing, then film measurements should be taken as well.

There are several accepted radiographic methods of evaluating limb length differences, and mistakes are easy to make in such measurements. It is therefore ideal if the same physician is able to evaluate the patient repetitively; as this is not always possible, it is important for any evaluating physician to carefully review the previous films (not just the reports) before using surgery to correct the defect. To evaluate the radiographic difference, a single exposure is taken of both legs on a long film, usually with the patient standing and a radiographic ruler placed on the cassette. The real length can then be measured from the anterior iliac spine to the medial malleolus.[24,53]

Other Bony Sequelae

Other bony sequelae are usually acutely symptomatic. A slipped capitofemoral epiphysis causes pain and can be diagnosed using a radiograph of the involved hip (Fig. 14-10). A pathologic fracture also will be symptomatic and readily apparent on radiograph.

Muscle

To evaluate a deficit in muscle development, measurements of the circumferences of the involved extremity should be performed and the range of motion of all joints in the involved limb should be determined. Measurements of the opposite normal extremity should be taken as well for comparison.

MANAGEMENT OF ESTABLISHED PROBLEMS

Management

It is not possible to prevent many of the late effects of irradiation. Of the common deficits that develop, scoliosis and leg length discrepancies necessitate intervention most often.

Scoliotic curve progression beyond 30 degrees (or curves over 20 degrees with rapid progression) generally require bracing. Curves greater than 40 degrees, particularly in skeletally immature patients, should be instrumented and fused.

Table 14-2 shows the recommended treatment for categories of leg length discrepancies.[24,53] Small differences (zero to 2 cm) usually require no intervention. Greater differences require an orthopedic evaluation. Differences of 2 to 6 cm can be corrected with a shoe lift or a contralateral epiphysiodesis, an operation creating a premature fusion of an epiphysis in the contralateral limb to arrest growth. This prevents further exaggeration of the deficit. Greater inequality (6 to 15 cm) requires more aggressive management. Contralateral limb shortening or ipsilateral lengthening procedures are usually necessary to restore a functional gait. Differences of greater than 15 to 20 cm are difficult to manage.

Other less common late effects may also need intervention. Partial epiphyseal plate injury results in juxtaarticular angular deformities of long bones. These uncommon growth aberrations are difficult to treat and often require complete physeal arrest and osteotomies for correction. That they occur infrequently now is ascribed to more careful attention to irradiation technique such that the entire physis is incorporated within the portal.

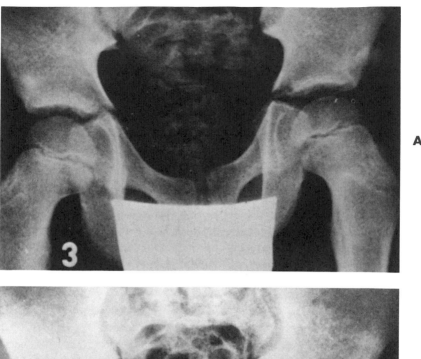

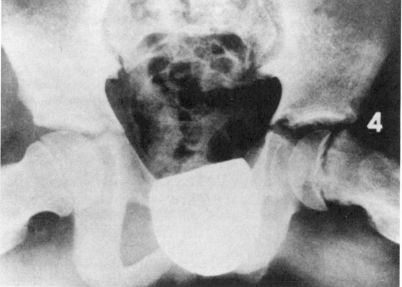

Fig. 14-10.   A 4-year-old patient was treated for a lymphoma of the testicle. **A,** Routine follow-up radiograph of patient at age 9 shows hypoplasia of the left ischium and pubis, with a normal left femoral head and neck. **B,** At age 11, 2 years later, patient developed slippage of the left femoral capital epiphysis. (From Wolf EL et al: Slipped femoral capital epiphysis as a sequela to childhood irradiation for malignant tumors, *Pediatr Radiol* 125:781-784, 1977.)

Table 14-2
Recommended Treatment for Categories of Leg Length Discrepancies

Leg Length Discrepancy	Treatment
0-2 cm	None required
2-6 cm	Shoe lift, epiphysiodesis
6-15 cm	Leg lengthening
>15 cm	Prosthetic fitting

(From Mosely CF: *Leg-length discrepancy.* In Lovell WW, Winter RB, editors: *Pediatric orthopedics,* Philadelphia, 1990, JB Lippincott.)

The occurrence of a slipped capitofemoral epiphysis is a medical emergency requiring immediate referral to an orthopedic surgeon. Slipped capitofemoral epiphyses require an in situ pin fixation. Because there is an increased incidence of a slipped capitofemoral epiphysis in the other leg if it also has been irradiated, consideration should be given for prophylactic pinning of it as well. Severe slips (greater than 60 degrees) may require a proximal femoral osteotomy and osteoplasty.[4]

A few exostoses may require excision because of symptoms or malignant degeneration.

Pathologic fractures in the irradiated field, more common if the irradiated bone was biopsied or involved with tumor, will rarely heal without internal fixation. The concomitant radiation changes in the surrounding soft tissue envelope of the bone further complicate the management of these fractures. These compromised tissues greatly increase the risk of postoperative infection. Some authors advocate bone grafting, as well as internal fixation, to decrease the risk of nonunion (Fig. 14-11).[45] In the event of severe wound complication and nonunion, an amputation should be considered.

Fig. 14-11.   A 10-year-old girl was treated with 55 Gy in 31 fractions (1.77 Gy per fraction) for a large Ewing's sarcoma of the left femur. **A,** Bone destruction at the time of diagnosis. A fracture occurred 9 months after treatment in the femoral neck. Four pins were placed across the femoral neck. Six months after this a subtrochanteric fracture occurred just beyond the site of the pins. **B,** An AP radiograph of the proximal femur with four pins placed across the femoral neck fracture *(small arrow).* The subtrochanteric fracture is marked by the large arrow. **C,** Internal fixation of the subtrochanteric fracture using a sliding hip screw device. One year after this procedure, the femur fractured in the midshaft, again beyond the device. **D,** Lateral radiograph of the proximal femur showing healed femoral neck and subtrochanteric fractures. An intramedullary nail was placed through the midshaft fracture *(arrow).* Since this device was placed in position in 1983, no further events have occurred, and the femur is stable, although shorter than normal.

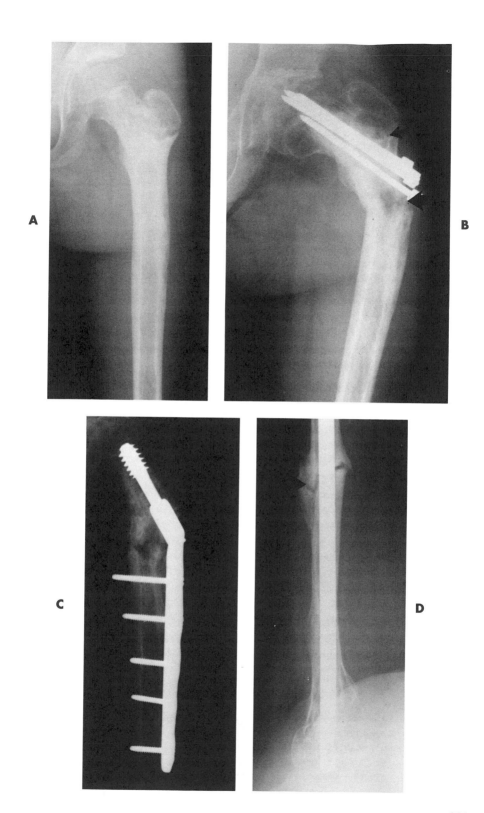

Muscular atrophy is usually a cosmetic problem for which there is no treatment. Even patients who strenuously pursue weightlifting or similar activities to build muscle strength find that the irradiated area rarely responds. However, appropriate exercise will prevent contractures and further decreases in muscle strength, as well as loss of the range of motion of joints.

Rehabilitation

In most cases, late effects from cytotoxic therapy involve both the muscles and the bones of an anatomic region. Although it is possible to prevent major problems, this cannot always be done, and moderate to severe sequelae do develop (Fig. 14-12). Whether or not surgery is required, one necessary portion of the management is a good exercise program. Range-of-motion exercises should progress slowly to weight-bearing, then muscle-strengthening exercises. The battle with sequelae may be lifelong, and a proper exercise program is one of the few means of combating the progression of damage, or regaining function previously lost. However, caution should be used in recommending vigorous exercise regimens for patients who have received high cumulative doses of doxorubicin, because cardiac decompensation may result.

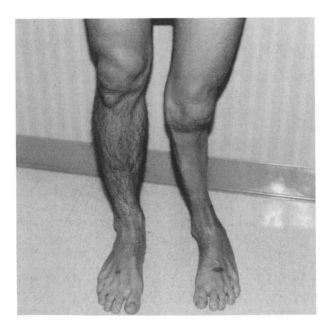

Fig. 14-12.   An 18-month-old boy was treated postoperatively with 50 Gy in 25 fractions for a primary rhabdomyosarcoma of the left calf. His leg is shown 16 years after treatment. The muscles are extremely hypoplastic, the distal leg is shortened and alopecic. An epiphysiodesis was performed on the other leg to prevent the occurrence of too large a limb length discrepancy.

The psychologic adaptation to the long-term sequelae of treatment also needs attention. Novotny stated that one's body image is composed of fluctuating physical, psychologic, and social aspects.[29] A positive adjustment to changes in body image requires discarding the previously held perception of one's body and incorporating the changes into a new perception. If the previous body image cannot be put aside so that the changes can be integrated and accepted, a negative body image may result.

Medical personnel can assist patients and their families in making a positive adaptation to changes in body image. Strategies for promoting acceptance of treatment-related body-image changes must be individualized according to the situation.[29] The initial approach should begin with facilitating open, honest communication within the family about previous experiences, current and antici- pated concerns, and educational needs. This information is the foundation on which to build a plan of care.

Novotny provided general guidelines on which to build an individualized plan to assist the patient and family in positively coping with body image changes.[29] The guidelines include:

1. Assessing the level of knowledge and adaptation
   a. encouraging patient and family to verbalize fears, concerns, and questions
   b. providing anticipatory guidance for the expected physical changes
2. Promoting family unity and coping skills
   a. including parents, siblings, significant friends, and school personnel in creating a supportive environment
   b. providing education and emotional support to significant others in the patient's life
3. Reaffirming adaptive behaviors
   a. promoting participation in the "normal" activities of the peer group to meet developmental and psychosocial needs
   b. advocating school attendance and participation
4. Changing maladaptive behaviors
   a. supporting the initiative and independence of the patient
   b. encouraging the maintenance of usual family roles and discipline
   c. emphasizing abilities instead of disabilities

These strategies can be implemented on an ongoing basis, but as the patient grows older, adjustments will need to be continually made. Alteration in body image is a fluid process, and assisting the patient with coping during the various stages of life may be necessary.

Another ongoing process is meeting the educational needs of the patient and family. Patients who were diagnosed at a young age should be educated and reeducated at age-appropriate levels about their diseases, treatments, and actual and potential late effects.[7] The musculoskeletal physical examination provides a good opportunity to explain to the patient what the examiner is looking for and why. Patients who have not evidenced musculoskeletal late effects within a short time after treatment may still be at risk for the remainder of their lives. Awareness of potential problem areas may assist the patient in future detection of late effects.

In general, patient and family education about musculoskeletal late effects should include information about the following[22]:

1. Nutritional influences on musculoskeletal growth and nutritional counseling
2. Avoidance of excessive weight gain
3. Participation in noncontact sports and refraining from contact sports
4. Realistic expectations about functional abilities and growth patterns
5. General health education, especially cancer prevention
6. The importance of lifelong surveillance care by knowledgeable health care professionals.

The patient who is biologically cured of cancer must still live with the after-effects of the disease and its treatment. A thorough assessment of the many factors affecting each patient's growth and development, promoting positive coping with changes, and providing ongoing education can result in an overall improved quality of life for the patient and family.

Integument and Breast

PATHOPHYSIOLOGY

Brief Overview of Normal Organ Development

Skin. The skin develops from two sources—the superficial layer (epidermis) from the surface ectoderm and the deep layer (dermis) from mesoderm. Early in development, the fetus is covered with a single layer of ectodermal cells. In the beginning of the second month through the fourth month, the four layers of the epidermis form: the basal layer, responsible for the production of new cells, is known as the germinative layer; a thick spinous layer consisting of large polyhedral cells; the granular layer, the cells of which contain small keratohyalin granules; and the horny layer, forming the tough scalelike surface of the epidermis and made up of closely packed dead cells loaded with keratin. Also, during the first 3 months, cells of neural crest origin invade the epidermis. These cells (melanocytes) synthesize melanin pigment, which can be transferred to other cells of the epidermis through the dendritic processes.

The dermis develops during the third and fourth months. The dermis consists of a layer of connective tissue and fatty tissue and contains a number of structures, including hair. Hair starts as solid epidermal proliferations penetrating the underlying dermis. Nerve endings and blood vessels develop with the hair papillae, and cells from outbuddings of the follicle walls form the *sebaceous glands,* which degenerate, thereby forming a fatlike substance that is secreted into the hair follicle and then to the skin.

Breast. The mammary glands are a specialized skin structure. The first indication is found in the form of a bandlike thickening of epidermis, the *mammary line* or *ridge.* This extends on each side of the body from the base of the forelimb to the region of the hindlimb by week 7. Most of the mammary line disappears quickly, but a small portion in the thoracic region persists and penetrates the underlying mesenchyme, forming the breast bud. The bud sprouts 16 to 24 cords, which ultimately form the *lactiferous ducts* surrounded by the alveoli of the gland. The ducts at first open into a small epithelial pit in the bud, but shortly after birth, this pit matures into the nipple by proliferation of the underlying mesenchyme.[40] At birth, the male and female breast are identical. At puberty the breast bud enlarges first, then the mammary glands enlarge and extensive deposition of fat occurs. The nipple and areola enlarge as well.[23]

Organ Damage Induced by Cytotoxic Therapy

Skin. Both RT and chemotherapy can cause acute and late effects on the skin and subcutaneous tissues. Radiation damage to the skin is primarily due to effects on the germinative layer of the epidermis. Even low doses quickly diminish mitotic activity, so that cell replacement is nearly zero. The cells of the basal layer become swollen and vacuolated, with nuclear pleomorphism and binucleation. The epidermis becomes thin with flattening of the papillae. Epidermal cell maturation no longer occurs, causing incomplete keratinization of the superficial cells, thus producing desquamation. This is caused by intracellular edema with enhancement of the intercellular bridges. With high-enough doses the epidermis may slough, exposing the dermal surface, which becomes coated with a layer of fibrin. After treatment, reepithelialization occurs, although the effectiveness of this process will depend on the extent of the damage. If all the basal cells are not killed, there is a radiation-induced increase in enzyme activity in the melanocytes, which is transmitted to the newly formed squamous cells, causing them to become very dark as they shed.

In the dermis, radiation first causes acute inflammation: edema and a lymphocytic infiltrate. High doses produce nuclear swelling and unequal nuclear divisions of the fibroblasts. The papilla of the hair follicle is easily damaged; radiation will quickly stop mitotic activity in the hair follicle, and the hair root eventually separates from the papilla and is shed. Sweat glands are about 2 to 3 mm below the surface of the skin, have long lives, and only occasionally undergo mitosis. However, the cells can be destroyed by high doses of radiation. Sebaceous glands are more easily destroyed, partially because the normal life cycle includes cell death to produce sebum and therefore there is a need for a continual replacement through cellular proliferation.

Late dermal reactions are caused by the development of subendothelial fibrous hyperplasia in the blood vessels. This causes telangiectasia (a spidery pattern of small blood vessels easily visible beneath the surface) and decreased blood supply to the dermis, which results in increased fibroblastic activity. The skin then takes on a woody texture called fibrosis.[26]

The skin changes resulting from RT are related to the total dose and fractionation of the radiation employed. However, there are differences between acute and late effects. Acute effects are dependent primarily on the total dose and the overall time in which the radiation is delivered, from the beginning to the end of the course of treatment. The higher the total dose and the shorter the overall time, the more significant the acute effects. Late effects are heavily dependent on the dose per fraction as well as the total dose. Doses of greater than 2 Gy per fraction cause increased late effects to the skin and subcutaneous tissues. Most "curative" fractionation schemes include doses per fraction of less than 2 Gy. This is particularly true in treating children, in whom late effects are of even more concern.

Modern megavoltage irradiation is "skin-sparing," which means that the full buildup of irradiation does not occur at the surface of the skin, but rather at some depth below. The higher the energy of the beam used, the deeper the maximum dose occurs in the tissue. Therefore, the severe skin changes seen in orthovoltage irradiation used before 1960 to 1970 (depending on the institution), in which the maximum dose was at the surface of the skin, do not occur as often now, unless for some clinical reason it is necessary to produce a high dose at the surface of the skin. With the skin-sparing capabilities of high-energy beams and the use of multiple fields to converge on the tumor, thereby further limiting the dose to the skin in each treatment field, the true skin dose usually is not enough to cause severe skin injury. At times, when treating skin lesions or in the event of another unusual situation, the skin receives a dose high enough to cause desquamation. Technical conditions in the delivery of the radiation can also cause a higher dose to be delivered to the skin, for example, if the radiation beams are arranged tangentially if bolus (tissue-equivalent material) is used on the skin, or if the lead blocks and blocking tray used to shape the radiation fields are too close to the patient.

A number of chemotherapy-induced skin changes occur, because antineoplastic drugs interfere with nucleic acid formation, ribosomal function, and other protein synthesis. Rapidly dividing tissues are the most sensitive; the skin damage is therefore primarily to the germinative layer, the hair follicles, and the melanocytes. Certain drugs, bleomycin in particular, occasionally cause increased melanogenesis. Biopsies of the epidermis after bleomycin administration have shown larger melanocytes with larger and more complex dendritic processes.[6]

CLINICAL MANIFESTATIONS

Effects on the skin can be categorized as acute or late. During a course of high-dose irradiation of the skin, the first sign of a skin reaction is faint erythema around the hair follicles. If the radiation is fractionated conventionally (less than 2 Gy per fraction), a dose of 20 Gy will usually produce erythema. Higher doses cause a progression to a generalized erythema, epilation, decrease in sweating, and diminished sebaceous gland secretion. The skin next becomes brightly erythematous, warm, and edematous, as well as painful to touch; all of these signs and symptoms are sharply limited to the irradiation field. Dry desquamation occurs at 30 Gy, and moist desquamation follows (occurring at about 40 Gy), leaving the dermis bare, with a layer of fibrin covering it. After treatment, these effects heal, usually within 1 to 2 weeks.[50] Most children never develop such a severe reaction, because usually the dose to any region of skin is considerably less than the dose to the tumor, and a total dose of 40 Gy to the skin is rarely reached. However, any cream or other foreign substance present on the skin during treatment will enhance the skin reaction to radiation.

Doses of even a few Gy will cause temporary alopecia. Recovery takes 8 to 12 weeks after the end of treatment; the hair starts regrowing at that point and usually grows at a normal rate thereafter. The hair can return with a different texture or color; the same phenomenon occurs after chemotherapy. Doses of 40 Gy and above to the hair follicles will cause permanent alopecia.

High doses of radiation may cause a skin necrosis (destruction of tissue in the area treated). This has become extremely rare with the advent of megavoltage therapy.

The first noticeable late effect consists of very slowly progressing atrophy, starting in the first few months after RT. The skin also loses its elasticity. If the injury is severe, telangiectasia will occur. In the dermis, fibrosis develops, with contraction and scarring in the treated field. Epilation can persist and nails will become brittle. Glands will no longer function normally; the involved skin will not sweat, nor produce sebaceous secretions. The formation of comedones has been reported, although this is rare.[49] Related skin structures such as the breast bud will not develop normally or secrete normally. This means that breast development may be hypoplastic (underdeveloped) or may not occur at all.

Radiation effectively accelerates skin aging. Therefore, as the irradiated person grows older, the skin prematurely develops changes consistent with aging. It becomes drier, less flexible and may develop "aging" spots or other discolorations. The extent of these changes is dose related. Doses below 10 Gy (to the skin) rarely cause noticeable problems, although the risk of such late effects increases at doses above 30 Gy.[12]

Another potential late sequela of treatment is the risk of the development of a secondary skin cancer, usually a basal cell carcinoma.[12,34,43] Basal cell carcinomas are observed in patients with no evidence of chronic skin changes secondary to RT.[12] The exact risk of a secondary basal cell carcinoma is small: in one series the excess risk is calculated to be $0.31/10^4$ patient-years per Gy.[34] The latency period is usually at least 20 years. There may be no excessive risk for a skin surface dose of less than 10 Gy for patients receiving standard fractionations, but this conclusion is controversial.

There are at least three skin reactions to chemotherapy: changes related to cytotoxicity, pigment alterations, and rashes and eruptions. Cytotoxic changes related to nucleic acid synthesis, ribosomal function, and so on, rarely appear after chemotherapy alone. However, "radiation recall" may be due to cytotoxic changes in the skin. This phenomenon consists of erythema, blistering, and sometimes moist desquamation in a previously irradiated area. It usually occurs a few weeks to a few months after RT subsequent to a course of chemotherapy containing doxorubicin HCl or dactinomycin (or occasionally a number of other drugs, particularly if given in high doses).[28] These same drugs cause increased radiation reactions if given concomitantly with RT. The etiology is probably renewed damage by chemotherapy to stem cells that have residual injury from irradiation.

Alopecia occurs through damage to the hair follicles. It is the most predictable skin reaction to chemotherapy. Drugs that cause alopecia include cyclophosphamide, doxorubicin, and dactinomycin, but the list of agents is very long. Alopecia does not appear to require a large threshold dose but occurs after each cycle of the drug. In almost all cases, the alopecia induced by chemotherapy is reversible, although permanent alopecia has been noted after a busulfan with cyclophosphamide conditioning regimen for bone marrow transplant.

Drugs reported to cause pigment changes are shown in Table 14-3. Although some, including doxorubicin, have been postulated to have a direct effect on melanocytes,[17] the mechanism essentially remains undefined. Generalized hyperpigmentation from bleomycin therapy is probably the most common of these abnormalities, but other drugs such as busulfan, cyclophosphamide, dactinomycin, 5-fluorouracil, hydroxyurea, and methotrexate can also cause this on occasion.[8] This condition usually resolves slowly with time, but can be permanent.

Antimitotic agents can also cause banding of the nails, either vertical or horizontal, as well as black pigmentation. The latter occurs first at the base of the nails, then moves distally.[28,42] Although these changes usually reverse when the drug is withdrawn, at times the nail hyperpigmentation can be permanent.[42]

Drugs such as 5-fluorouracil, high-dose methotrexate, dactinomycin, and doxorubicin can cause skin eruptions (including urticaria), a generalized erythematous rash, hyperpigmented brawny indurated plaques (particularly of the hands and feet), as well as nodularity of the hands and feet.[6,10] These effects are temporary.

Children receiving chemotherapy have been reported to develop increased numbers of benign melanocytic nevi after treatment.[14]

Table 14-3
Pigment Changes from Chemotherapy

Abnormality	Associated Drugs
Generalized hyperpigmentation	5-Fluorouracil, busulfan
Localized hyperpigmentation	Adriamycin, cyclophosphamide, and other alkylating agents; bleomycin, mithramycin, dactinomycin, various hormones
Hyperpigmentation of nails	Adriamycin, cyclophosphamide, nitrogen mustard, 5-fluorouracil, methotrexate, nitrosoureas, DTIC, others
Linear hyperpigmentation	Most cytotoxics (along veins); bleomycin (on trunk and extremities separate from venous channels)

DTIC = dimethyltriazenyl imidazole carboxamide.
(From Nixon DW et al: Dermatologic changes after systemic cancer therapy, *Cutis* 27:181-194, 1981.)

In the growing breast, the most sensitive structure is the breast bud. Doses of as little as 10 Gy to the breast bud will cause the breast to be hypoplastic; doses above 20 Gy may ablate development altogether.[13,35] Doses of 20 Gy or more to regions of the anterior chest other than the breast bud may prevent breast development in that area. Low doses of radiation may cause failure to lactate.[36]

DETECTION AND SCREENING

It is usually not difficult to predict the extent of the acute changes during treatment based on the dose and fractionation schedule of the course of RT and the chemotherapy regimen used. The patient and parents can therefore anticipate the severity of the reaction. This will usually diminish some of the anxiety that inevitably accompanies the reaction.

Late effects progress with time and may be subtle at first. Careful physical exams checking for cutaneous late effects should be performed by someone who is knowledgeable about the treatment received. Areas of pigmentation changes, dryness, atrophy, telangiectasia, contraction, and scarring should be noted and carefully recorded. If chemotherapy has been given, skin coloration should also be checked, along with the status of the nail beds.

After the completion of treatment, these physical examinations should be performed two to three times a year for at least 2 years, then at least yearly thereafter. If the radiation field included the breast, careful monitoring of that area should occur as well, particularly as puberty approaches. Tanner staging should be done with each follow-up examination to document the expected physical maturation.

Though a reversal of skin changes secondary to irradiation and chemotherapy is not possible (although subcutaneous tissues will occasionally soften with time), education of the patient and family can be effective in decreasing the long-term effects. Because radiation damage and sun damage to the skin are similar, it is important for the patient to avoid severe sun exposure after treatment. Sun exposure will increase the aging process started by irradiation. If heavy sun exposure is anticipated, a strong sunscreen (skin protection factor 15 or above) must be used on the treated region.

Most chemotherapy-related skin changes require no specific care, but it is important to carefully check the status of all benign nevi after treatment with chemotherapy. An increased number of benign melanocytic nevi appears to be one of the strongest risk factors in the development of malignant melanoma. Because it has been reported that children treated with chemotherapy have more nevi than normal, careful assessments are required.[14,47]

MANAGEMENT OF ESTABLISHED PROBLEMS

Management and rehabilitation. Although the acute effects of irradiation are less common now, they can be alarming when they occur. It is important to remember that healing will generally occur spontaneously within 2 to 4 weeks.

There is no effective way to reverse late radiation-induced skin changes. Because of the lack of sebaceous secretions, it may be helpful to use vaseline or a moisturizing cream for patient comfort.

Temporary alopecia from RT or chemotherapy needs no particular treatment and will resolve in time. Permanent alopecia from RT cannot be reversed, but hair transplants have been reported to be effective. A hair transplant can be done only if there remains a large unaffected portion of the scalp from which plugs of normal hair can be harvested and if the area of alopecia involves well-healed scalp.[15]

Breast hypoplasia can be corrected by breast augmentation. This should be done by someone who is familiar with the treatment received, as healing may be retarded or difficult in regions previously irradiated. However, breast augmentation may make follow-up of the region more difficult.

Guidance needs to be provided for the female patient who can expect to develop, or who has developed, breast hypoplasia from irradiation. Development of a positive body image is an especially difficult task for adolescent girls who expect normal development. A female teenager who has the potential for unequal breast development is particularly at risk for developing a negative body image, with accompanying lowered self-esteem. The impact on present and future sexuality cannot be overlooked. Likewise, adolescent boys who develop unilateral gyneco-mastia may become quite concerned and self-conscious. Family and peer support and understanding can be critical for these patients at this time. Anticipatory guidance and suggestions for coping with these late effects may assist the adolescent in positive adaptation. The strategies suggested by Novotny and discussed earlier in this chapter will be helpful here as well.[29]

The female patient who has already experienced breast development when RT is given may be at risk for decreased skin elasticity and fibrosis. In addition, all patients who receive radiation to the breast should be counseled on performing monthly breast self-examinations, as there may be an increased risk of breast cancer if the breast is irradiated. A baseline mammogram should be performed initially between ages 20 and 25 years, with follow-up examinations every 5 years.

If fertility is maintained (depending on sites of previous cancer and the treatments used), the female patient should be informed that the affected breast may not lactate after childbearing. If the other breast was not within the radiation field, the patient can expect to breastfeed normally from the untreated side.

REFERENCES

1. Ackman JD, Rouse L, Johnston CE II: Radiation induced physeal injury, *Orthopaedics* 11:343-349, 1988.
2. Anderson M, Green WT, Messner MB: Growth and predictions of growth in the lower extremities, *J Bone Joint Surg* 45A:1-14, 1963.
3. Bajorunas DR et al: Endocrine sequelae of antineoplastic therapy in childhood head and neck malignancies, *J Clin Endocrinol Metab* 50:329-335, 1980.

4. Barrett IR: Slipped capital femoral epiphysis following radiotherapy, *J Pediatr Orthop* 5:268-273, 1985.

5. Clayton PE et al: Growth in children treated for acute lymphoblastic leukaemia, *Lancet* 1:460-462, 1988.

6. Cohen IS et al: Cutaneous toxicity of bleomycin therapy, *Arch Dermatol* 107: 553-555, 1973.

7. D'Angio G: Cure is not enough: late consequences associated with radiation treatment, *J Assoc Pediatr Oncol Nurses* 5:20-23, 1988.

8. DeSpain JD: Dermatologic toxicity of chemotherapy, *Semin Oncol* 19:501-507, 1992.

9. Donaldson SS: *Effects of irradiation on skeletal growth and development.* In Green DM, D'Angio GJ, editors: *Late effects of treatment for childhood cancer,* New York, 1992, Wiley-Liss.

10. Etcubanas EW Jr: Uncommon side effects of adriamycin, *Cancer Chemother Rep* 58:757-758, 1974 (letter).

11. Fajardo LF: *Pathology of radiation injury,* New York, 1982, Masson.

12. Fragu P et al: Long-term effects in skin and thyroid after radiotherapy for skin angiomas: a French retrospective cohort study, *Eur J Cancer* 27:1215-1222, 1991.

13. Furst CJ et al: Breast hypoplasia following irradiation of the female breast in infancy and early childhood, *Acta Oncol* 28(4):519-523, 1989.

14. Hughes BR, Cunliffe WJ, Bailey CC: Excess benign melanocytic naevi after chemotherapy for malignancy in childhood, *Br Med J* 299:88-91, 1989.

15. Jacobs JB, Monell C: Treatment of radiation-induced alopecia, *Head Neck Surg* 2:154-159, 1979.

16. Katzman H, Waugh T, Berdon W: Skeletal changes following irradiation of childhood tumors, *J Bone Joint Surg* 51A:825-842, 1969.

17. Kew MC et al: Melanocyte stimulating hormone levels in doxorubicin induced hyperpigmentation, *Lancet* I:811, 1977.

18. Maeda M et al: Effects of irradiation on cortical bone and their time-related changes: a biomechanical and histomorphological study, *J Bone Joint Surg* 70A:392-399, 1988.

19. Malasonos L et al: *Musculoskeletal assessment.* In *Health assessment,* ed 2, St Louis, 1981, Mosby–Year Book.

20. Marcus RB Jr et al: Local control and function after twice-a-day radiotherapy for Ewing's sarcoma of bone, *Int J Radiat Oncol Biol Phys* 21:1509-1515, 1991.

21. Mayfield JK et al: Spinal deformity in children treated for neuroblastoma: the effect of radiation and other forms of treatment, *J Bone Joint Surg* 63A:183-193, 1981.

22. Meadows AT: The concept of care for life, *J Assoc Pediatr Oncol Nurses* 5:7-9, 1988.

23. Moore KL: *Essentials of human embryology,* Toronto, 1988, BC Decker.

24. Mosely CF: *Leg-length discrepancy.* In Lovell WW, Winter RB, editors: *Pediatric orthopedics,* ed 3, Philadelphia, 1990, JB Lippincott.

25. Moshang T Jr, Lee MM: Late effects: disorders of growth and sexual maturation associated with the treatment of childhood cancer, *J Assoc Pediatr Oncol Nurses* 5:14-19, 1988.

26. Moss WT, Brand W: *The bone.* In *Therapeutic radiology: rationale, technique, results,* ed 3, St Louis, 1969, Mosby–Year Book.

27. Neuhauser EBD et al: Irradiation effects of roentgen therapy on the growing spine, *Radiology* 59:637-650, 1952.

28. Nixon DW et al: Dermatologic changes after systemic cancer therapy, *Cutis* 27:181-194, 1981.

29. Novotny MP: Body image changes in amputee children: how nursing theory can make the difference, *J Assoc Pediatr Oncol Nurses* 3:8-13, 1986.

30. Pinkel D: Five-year follow-up of "total therapy" of childhood lymphocytic leukemia, *JAMA* 216:648-652, 1971.

31. Probert JC, Parker BR: The effects of radiation therapy on bone growth, *Radiology* 114:155-162, 1975.

32. Probert JC, Parker BR, Kaplan HS: Growth retardation in children after megavoltage irradiation of the spine, *Cancer* 32:634-639, 1973.

33. Riseborough E et al: Skeletal alterations following irradiation for Wilms' tumor, *J Bone Joint Surg* 58A:526-536, 1976.

34. Ron E et al: Radiation-induced skin carcinomas of the head and neck, *Radiat Res* 125:318-325, 1991.

35. Rosenfield NS, Haller JO, Berdon WE: Failure of development of the growing breast after radiation therapy, *Pediatr Radiol* 19(2):124-127, 1989.

36. Rostom AY, O'Cathail S: Failure of lactation following radiotherapy for breast cancer, *Lancet* 1(8473):163-164, 1986 (letter).

37. Rubin P: *Dynamic classification of bone dysplasia,* Chicago, 1964, Mosby–Year Book.

38. Rubin P et al: Radiation induced dysplasias of bone, *Am J Roentgenol* 82:206-216, 1959.

39. Rutherford H, Dodd GD: Complications of radiation therapy: growing bone, *Semin Roentgenol* 9:15-27, 1974.

40. Sadler TW: *Langman's medical embryology,* ed 6, Baltimore, 1990, Williams & Wilkins.

41. Salter RB: *Textbook of disorders and injuries of the musculoskeletal system,* ed 2, Baltimore, 1983, Williams & Wilkins.

42. Shah PC, Rao KRP, Patel AR: Cyclophosphamide induced nail pigmentation, *Br J Dermatol* 98:675-680, 1978.

43. Shore RE et al: Skin cancer incidence among children irradiated for ringworm of the scalp, *Radiat Res* 100:192-204, 1984.

44. Silber JH, Littman PS, Meadows AT: Stature loss following skeletal irradiation for childhood cancer, *J Clin Oncol* 8:304-312, 1990.

45. Springfield DS, Pagliarulo PAC: Fractures of long bones previously treated for Ewing's sarcoma, *J Bone Joint Surg* 67A:477-481, 1985.

46. Springfield DS: *Bone and soft tissue tumors.* In Lovell WW, Winter RB, editors: *Pediatric orthopedics,* Philadelphia, 1990, JB Lippincott.

47. Swerdlow AJ et al: Benign melanocytic naevi as a risk factor for malignant melanoma, *Br Med J* 292:1555-1559, 1986.

48. Walker SJ et al: Slipped capital femoral epiphysis following radiation and chemotherapy, *Clin Orthop* 159:186-193, 1981.

49. Walter JF: Cobalt radiation-induced comedones, *Arch Dermatol* 116:1073-1074, 1980.

50. White DC: *An atlas of radiation histopathology,* Oak Ridge, Tenn, 1924, USERDA Technical Information Center.

51. Winter RB: *Spinal problems in pediatric orthopaedics.* In Lovell WW, Winter RB, editors: *Pediatric orthopedics,* ed 3, Philadelphia, 1990, JB Lippincott.

52. Wolf EL et al: Slipped femoral capital epiphysis as a sequela to childhood irradiation for malignant tumors, *Radiology* 125:781-784, 1977.

53. Zeman W, Solomon M: *Effects of radiation on striated muscle.* In Berdjis CC, editor: *Pathology of irradiation,* Baltimore, 1971, Williams & Wilkins.

15

Late Effects after Bone Marrow Transplant

Jean Sanders

Marrow ablating doses of chemotherapy or chemotherapy combined with radiotherapy (RT) followed by an infusion of hematopoietic stem cells is being used for an increasing number of children and young adults as treatment for malignant or nonmalignant disorders. This practice has resulted in an increasing number of long-term survivors. Understanding the delayed effects that may occur after the bone marrow transplant (BMT) is important in determining appropriate evaluations and therapy for these unique patients. This chapter describes some of the major effects that have been observed to date and suggests an approach for evaluation and management.

EFFECTS RELATED TO THE TRANSPLANT PREPARATIVE REGIMEN

Endocrine System

The agents used in BMT-preparatory regimens are designed to suppress the patient's immune system and to eradicate the abnormal cells. The most common regimens use high-dose cyclophosphamide (CY) given alone or in combination with other agents, such as busulfan (BU) or total body irradiation (TBI). Other chemotherapy agents that have been used include high-dose carmustine (BCNU), melphalan, and etoposide (VP-16), and other RT regimens include thoracoabdominal or total lymphoid irradiation (TLI). Both chemotherapy and RT affect endocrine function.[37]

Thyroid function. Irradiation of the thyroid gland has been associated with development of compensated hypothyroidism, overt hypothyroidism, thyroiditis, and thyroid malignancies.[23] Asymptomatic compensated hypothyroidism occurs within the first year after RT for up to half of children and may progress to overt hypothyroidism over the next several decades. The actuarial risk of developing thyroid disease at 20 and 26 years after 44 Gy mantle RT for Hodgkin's disease has been reported to be 52% and 67%, respectively.[26] The risk of thyroid malignancies was 1.7% after 19 years, which is significantly greater than the expected risk of 0.07% for normal age-matched controls.

Table 15-1
Post–Marrow Transplant Evaluations for Endocrine Effects

	Tests	Frequency
Thyroid	TSH, T_4	Annual
Growth	Height	Annual until age 20
	Bone age*	Annual until maturity
	GH*[†]	Annual until maturity or deficiency present
Sexual development	Tanner score	Annual age 8-18
	LH, FSH	Annual after age 10
	Estradiol (girls)[‡§]	Annual after age 10
	Testosterone (boys)[‡§]	Annual after age 10
	Semen analysis	As indicated
Gonadal function		
Women	Menstrual history	Annual — postpubertal
	PAP smear	Annual — adult
	LH, FSH	Annual
	Estradiol	Annual
Men	LH, FSH	Annual
	Testosterone	Year 1
	Semen analysis[§]	As indicated

TSH = thyroid-stimulating hormone; GH = growth hormone; LH = luteinizing hormone; FSH = follicle-stimulating hormone.
*Not indicated for cyclophosphamide-only preparative regimen.
[†]Not indicated if the patient is receiving GH.
[‡]Not indicated if patient is receiving sex hormone therapy.
[§]Not indicated after recovery to normal levels documented.

Table 15-2
Suggested Treatments for Endocrine Function Disorders

Abnormality	Treatment*
Hypothyroid	Thyroxine
Growth failure with GH deficiency	GH (until maturity)
Delayed puberty	
Girls	Ethinyl/estradiol and medroxyprogesterone
Boys	Testosterone enanthate
Gonadal failure	
Women	Premarin and Provera

GH = growth hormone.
*For details of drug administration see Chapters 4, 11, 12.

Chemotherapy-only preparative regimens including CY or BU plus CY (BU/CY) do not appear to cause thyroid function abnormalities at a frequency greater than could be expected in the normal population.[40,54,57] However, after radiation containing preparative regimens, compensated hypothyroidism and overt hypothyroidism often occur. After 7.5 to 10 Gy single-exposure TBI, 28% to 56% of patients have developed abnormal thyroid-stimulating hormone (TSH) and up to 13% have overt hypothyroidism, whereas after 12 to 15.75 Gy fractionated TBI, 10% to 14% have compensated hypothyroidism and fewer than 5% have overt hypothyroidism.[30,54,66] Although there appears to be a higher incidence following single-exposure TBI, these patients were followed for more than 5 years after TBI, whereas patients given fractionated TBI were followed for a median of 4 years at time of evaluation. The only risk factor associated with the development of abnormal thyroid function after transplant appears to be TBI. At least 6 children are known to have developed thyroid masses, which occurred 4 or more years after TBI. These were determined to be papillary carcinoma (4), toxic goiter (1), and adenoma (1) (Sanders, unpublished data). The adenoma was discovered at autopsy 8 years after TBI, but the other 5 children were treated with either thyroidectomy (4) or radioactive iodine (1). All are receiving thyroxine.

Suggested studies (see Table 15-1)

	Test	Frequency
Screening	TSH, T4	Annual
Abnormal screening:	Free T4, T3, RT$_3$U, TRH	When indicated
Thyroid physical exam:		Annual

Suggested treatment (see Table 15-2). All patients who develop overt hypothyroidism should receive thyroxine. Patients with compensated hypothyroidism are not treated by some investigators, who argue that the benefit is unclear, and some patients have transiently elevated TSH levels.[30] Other investigators do administer thyroid replacement in this setting (see Chapter 7). Patients who develop a thyroid mass require further investigations to determine the etiology and appropriate treatment.

Growth. Height growth is largely regulated in infancy by nutrition, in childhood by growth hormone (GH), and in puberty by the synergistic action of GH and sex steroids.[37] It is unclear whether chemotherapy regimens that are not accompanied by central nervous system (CNS) irradiation are associated with growth impairment.[7,32,51,67] Reported growth rates after conventional therapy have included patients who received chemotherapy with and without CNS irradiation.

Irradiation to the CNS can clearly result in GH deficiency (see Chapter 4). Retardation of growth is related to the child's age at time of RT, the dose received, and the length of follow-up after RT.[62] Many children have received 18 to 24 Gy CNS irradiation prior to BMT. When TBI is included in the preparative regimen, the total CNS irradiation dose will often exceed 30 Gy, which exceeds the estimated threshold for development of GH deficiency.[64] Thus, it may be expected that nearly all children who have received CNS RT plus TBI are at risk to develop GH deficiency.

Normal growth rates and GH levels have been reported after a transplant preparative regimen of CY only.[57,68] Decreased growth rates have been reported after BU/CY preparative regimen for patients with leukemia or thalassemia major.[40,57,82] Some of these patients were documented to have GH deficiency. Height standard deviation (SD) or "Z" scores after BMT for patients receiving BU/CY have demonstrated progressive decrease in standardized height growth, but follow-up does not extend beyond 3 years after transplant.

Height SD "Z" scores among TBI recipients demonstrate progressive negative scores with each additional year after TBI. By 5 years, all patients are more than 2 SD below the mean and at 8 years more than 3 SD below the mean. After preparative regimens that include TBI, more than 50% of patients have been reported to have subnormal GH levels.[54] Direct RT effects on bone growth may account for a component of the growth inhibition.

Suggested studies (see Table 15-1)

Test	Frequency
Height measurement	Annual[1]
Growth hormone	Annual[2]
Bone age	Annual[2]

1. The height should be measured with a Harpenden stadiometer.
2. Growth hormone measurements are valid only for patients receiving less than 0.5 mg/kg prednisone every other day. Patients receiving higher doses or daily prednisone treatment may have low GH levels on the basis of steroid-induced suppression. GH measurements are also valid for consideration of therapy only among patients with open epiphysis on bone age films. Various tests are used for measurement of GH (see Chapter 4). A pediatric endocrinologist should be involved with performance and interpretation of these tests.

Suggested treatment (see Table 15-2). Studies of children with idiopathic hypopituitarism have shown that the final height achieved is related to the patient's height at the start of treatment with GH.[29] The total height gained from treatment appears to be inversely related to patient age at the start of therapy and positively related to the duration of therapy. Growth before puberty appears to be the major determinant of final height. Therefore, treatment with GH during the prepubertal period should be optimized. Data on the use and efficiency of GH therapy after TBI, despite documentation of GH deficiency and decreased growth rates, are sparse. Patients who have been treated have generally not demonstrated the catch-up growth response that has been observed among nonirradiated GH-deficient children, although therapy did improve the height velocity "Z" score for some patients.[8,58] However, no data are available for patients who were treated during the prepubertal period.

GH therapy should be managed by a pediatric endocrinologist. In general, treatment should be initiated as soon as the patient demonstrates growth failure and GH deficiency, although not before 1 year post BMT. The duration of therapy is dependent upon the patient's bone age and should be discontinued when there is evidence of epiphyseal closure. Reports of leukemia occurring in patients treated with GH have been considered by some investigators to suggest a causal relationship between GH therapy and development of leukemia.[18,59] The Lawson Wilkins Pediatric Endocrine Society and the United States Human Growth Foundation's review of 11 suspect cases determined that the incidence of leukemia was about 1 per 21,000 patient-years of risk and the annual leukemia incidence among hypopituitary patients was 1 per 42,000 patient-years.[22] Although there may be a small increase in leukemia incidence associated with GH treatment of GH-deficient patients, it is not clear that this is directly related to GH therapy. Assuming a 10-year GH treatment course, a current estimate of individual risk would be 1 per 2400 (0.042%), which is not different from the Surveillance Epidemiology and End Results (SEER) program estimate of the annual incidence of new cases of leukemia reported in the United States. Therefore, treatment of GH-deficient children after BMT should not contribute significantly to an increased leukemia risk.

Sexual development. Gonadal hormone production and germ cell viability are affected by the high doses of alkylating agents and TBI.[50] Associated variables include patient age, sex, and the type and dose of therapy. Prepubertal boys and girls who received cumulative doses of up to 200 mg/kg CY usually will not experience gonadal failure and will experience development of puberty at a normal age. No data are available with respect to the impact of high-dose BU on the prepubertal gonad, and no data are available regarding the delayed effects of irradiation of the prepubertal ovary. Irradiation of the prepubertal testes results in damage to the germinal epithelium, which does not become apparent until after the time of puberty.[63]

Pubertal development has been evaluated among patients who were prepubertal when given high-dose CY and BMT for aplastic anemia and are now 12 years of age or older.[55,57] All girls demonstrated normal pubertal development. Menarche occurred at a median age of 13 years (range: 11 to 16) and all have normal gonadotropin levels and ovarian function. Currently, 10 of these now mature women have given birth to 14 normal children. Development of secondary sexual characteristics was also normal for 90% of boys. All have normal Leydig cell function with normal levels of luteinizing hormone (LH) and testosterone. Follicle-stimulating hormone (FSH) levels were normal for 90%, but were elevated in 10%, demonstrating Sertoli cell damage. Normal sperm counts were present in 70% of patients, and the remainder had azoospermia. Seven men have fathered 10 normal children.

No data are available for patients who received BU/CY and BMT for leukemia. However, data are available for 15 girls and 15 boys who received BU/CY and BMT for thalassemia.[14] All 15 girls had evidence of gonadal failure, and most boys had evidence of impaired spermatogenesis.

Following TBI, delayed development of puberty has been observed in more than 70% of girls and more than 78% of boys who are now over 12 years of age.[55,58] Those with delayed puberty all had primary gonadal failure with elevated LH and FSH and subnormal estradiol or testosterone levels. All boys who received additional testicular RT have testicular failure. The boys who had normal, age-appropriate progression through puberty had received fractionated TBI. The type of TBI administered, single or fractionated exposure, did not influence whether girls developed normally. Five girls who recovered ovarian function have become pregnant, but all had either spontaneous or elective abortions.

Suggested studies (see Table 15-1)

Test	Frequency[1]
Tanner Developmental Score	Annual
LH, FSH	Annual
Estradiol or testosterone	Annual
Menstrual history	Girls, annual
Semen analysis	Boys, annual

1. Performance of these studies is of little or no value before the patient is 8 to 10 years of age. Testosterone values obtained need to be correlated with the expected values for the patient's age. Studies should be performed annually until evidence of recovery of gonadal function or until sexual hormone therapy is initiated.

Suggested treatment (see Table 15-2). Patients who manifest delayed onset of puberty as determined by standardized Tanner Developmental Scores and hypergonadotropic hypogonadism will probably benefit from appropriate sexual hormone supplementation. Administration of the sexual hormones should be with a pediatric endocrinologist's guidance. Because normal production of sex hormones is necessary for promotion of the pubertal growth spurt in addition to promoting sexual maturation, sex hormones must be carefully administered with gradually increasing doses of the hormone to prevent premature advancement of bone age and premature closure of the epiphysis. Patients should also have growth rates carefully followed during administration of sex hormones.

Gonadal function. Women who receive alkylating agents may have impaired ovarian function. Ovarian atrophy has been observed after BU administration,[6] and ovarian biopsies after CY demonstrate loss of ova.[80] The severity of this ova loss, and, therefore, the potential for fertility, is related to patient age and total dose of CY. Because the number of oocytes normally decreases with increasing age, equivalent CY doses in older patients whose ova are more depleted than younger patients may explain why the likelihood of infertility is greater in older women given CY.

Testicular biopsies from men treated with CY have demonstrated Sertoli cell damage with absent spermatogonia and spermatozoa.[20,21] These men usually have an elevated FSH level and azoospermia. Leydig cell function is spared and patients have normal LH and testosterone levels. Patient age is not a factor, but the total dose of CY appears to be related to the degree of testicular dysfunction. Patients who receive less than 250 mg/kg CY often develop reversible oligospermia; however, recovery may not occur for after a year or more.

Women. Following administration of 200 mg/kg CY and BMT for aplastic anemia, all women younger than 26 years of age at the time of CY administration recovered ovarian function with gonadotropin levels returning to normal and menstruation returning between 0.25 and 3.0 (median 0.75) years after transplant.[55,56] However, among women 26 to 38 years of age, approximately 40% develop permanent primary ovarian failure with elevated LH and FSH and low estradiol levels. Among the women who did recover ovarian function, 18 have had 25 pregnancies that have resulted in 20 live births and 5 abortions. Fifty women have had ovarian function evaluated 1 to 2 years after a preparative regimen with BU/CY. None of these women have recovered ovarian function. All have evidence of primary ovarian failure.

After TBI preparative regimens and BMT, all women developed ovarian failure lasting at least 3 to 6 years.[55,56] Ten of 380 women evaluated have demonstrated ovarian recovery with return of menstruation as well as normal LH, FSH, and estradiol levels. All of these women with ovarian recovery were younger than 26 years of age at time of TBI administration. A total of 10 pregnancies have occurred among 7 women resulting in 4 normal infants and 6 abortions. Most women with primary ovarian failure experience symptoms of menopause with vasomotor instability, insomnia, osteoporosis, vaginitis, and vaginal atrophy.[60]

Men. Among the 82 men evaluated after 200 mg/kg CY and BMT for aplastic anemia, Leydig cell function was normal in 95% with normal LH and testosterone production. Sertoli cell function was normal in 87% with normal FSH levels.[55] Twenty-seven children have been fathered by 18 men. After BU/CY, the majority of 34 men evaluated had normal LH but elevated FSH levels. Semen analysis demonstrated that one of five men who submitted specimens for analysis had return of spermatogenesis. This man fathered a child 2 years after transplant. Therefore, the BU/CY combination seems to have a greater potential than CY alone to impair Sertoli cell functions and fertility.

Evaluation of testicular functions after TBI preparative regimens has demonstrated that, in general, Leydig cell function is preserved with normal LH and testosterone levels.[55] These men had impaired Sertoli cell function with elevated FSH levels, and only 5 of 323 men who submitted semen for analysis had evidence of spermatogenesis. Recovery of Sertoli cell function did not occur earlier than 6 to 7 years after TBI, and then only among men who received 10 Gy single-exposure TBI. These five men have fathered nine normal children. None of the men given fractionated exposure TBI have recovered spermatogenesis. This observation is in keeping with other data on the effects of RT on spermatogenesis.

Suggested studies (see Table 15-1)

Test	Frequency
LH, FSH	Annual
Estradiol or testosterone	Annual
Menstrual history	Annual
Gynecologic examination	Annual
Semen analysis	Annually until recovery

Suggested treatment (see Table 15-2)

WOMEN. Except for the young women transplanted after high-dose CY only, all women should be evaluated initially at least by 3 to 6 months after transplant. Those women with evidence of primary ovarian failure should receive estrogen/progesterone hormone supplementation to prevent symptoms and complications referable to estrogen insufficiency. All women should be evaluated and have hormone supplementation monitored by a gynecologist.

MEN. No specific treatment is indicated. It may be wise to suggest that adult male patients with adequate sperm production store sperm prior to marrow transplant because the probability of recovery for the majority of men is poor.

Central Nervous System

Neurologic complications. Late neurologic complications occurring after marrow transplant may result from prior cranial RT, intrathecal or systemic chemotherapy, or recurrent leukemia. Multifocal leukoencephalopathy after BMT is usually due to the same factors that influence its development in nontransplant treatment settings. Patients with leukemia have often received one or more of these therapeutic modalities. After TBI and BMT for leukemia, a 7% incidence of leukoencephalopathy has been observed among patients who received pretransplant CNS treatment and posttransplant intrathecal therapy.[77] Symptoms often become evident approximately 4 to 6 months after TBI. Reversible neurotoxicity has been occasionally observed in patients treated with high-dose acyclovir or cyclosporine.[79,87]

Neuropsychologic abnormalities. Details of neurocognitive problems after CNS treatment are described in Chapter 2. Intrathecal methotrexate (MTX) and CNS RT have been implicated in the development of neurologic and learning disorders after non-BMT treatment.[47] A preliminary analysis of 145 children studied immediately before and one or more years after TBI and BMT suggests no significant impairment of fine-motor hand-eye coordination occurs. Evaluation of full-scale, performance, and verbal-intelligence quotient (IQ) demonstrates a significant decrease in full-scale and performance IQ with increasing number of years after transplant.[42] Patient age at time of initial CNS RT, number of years after RT, and total dose of CNS RT were all significant factors. These data translate into some very practical problems for patients. For example, a child who was 3 years of age at time of cranial RT and 4.5 years of age at time of TBI and BMT and who is now a 10-year disease-free survivor after BMT is likely to have difficulty with short-term and long-term memory, learning new facts, and performance under

Table 15-3
Posttransplant Evaluations

System	Disorder	Test	Frequency
Neurologic	Leukoencephalopathy	LP	As clinically indicated
		MRI	As clinically indicated
	Neuropsychologic	Psychologic*	Pretransplant
		IQ*	1, 3, 5, 7, 10 years after BMT†
Ophthalmologic	Sicca syndrome	Schirmer's test	As clinically indicated‡
	Cataracts	Complete ophthalmologic examination	Annual‡
Autoimmune	Chronic GVHD		Day 80 and subsequent evaluations as clinically indicated§
	Skin	Exam and biopsy	
	Mouth	Exam and biopsy	
	Eyes	Schirmer's test	
	Liver	Bilirubin, AST, alkaline phosphatase	
Immune	Function	Skin tests to recall antigens	Annual until first positive
		Skin tests to neoantigens	Year 1
		Serum immunoglobulins	Annual until normal
Pulmonary	Routine follow-up	Chest radiograph	Annual
		PFT	Annual
	Suspected OAD (see text)	Sinus radiograph	As indicated
		BAL	As indicated
Hematopoietic	Rejection	Cytogenetics	
		Donor/host DNA analysis (see text)	
		Bone marrow exam	
Original disease	Relapse	Bone marrow	
		Imaging studies	As indicated

LP = lumbar puncture; MRI = magnetic resonance imaging; IQ = intelligence quotient; BMT = bone marrow transplant; GVHD = graft-versus-host disease; AST = aspartate serum transaminase; PFT = pulmonary function test; OAD = obstructed airways disease; BAL = bronchoalveolar lavage; DNA = deoxyribonucleic acid.
*See Chapter 2 for details regarding specific cognitive and IQ tests.
†For all TBI recipients or cranial RT patients.
‡For all TBI, steroid, and chronic GVHD patients as annual screening.
§Patients with chronic GVHD should be reevaluated at least every 9 to 12 months (see text).

Table 15-4
Suggested Treatments

Abnormality	Treatment
Leukoencephalopathy	Supportive/symptomatic
Cognitive dysfunction	Special education
Sicca syndrome (dry eyes)	Artificial tears; if severe, lacrimal duct ligation
Cataracts	Severe — may require corrective surgery
Chronic GVHD	Immunosuppression with corticosteroids with or without cyclosporine (see text)
Immune deficiency	Prophylactic trimethoprim sulfamethoxazole
	IV IgG for IgG-deficient patients monthly until pre-IV IgG serum level normal for 2 months
Obstructed airway disease	Infection prevention, prophylactic oral antibiotic, IV IgG (as indicated)
	Immunosuppressive therapy similar to that administered for chronic GVHD
Graft rejection	Consider second transplant after immunosuppression and marrow infusion
Relapse	Variable depending on clinical condition, donor availability time after initial transplant (see text)

GVHD = graft-versus-host disease; IV = intravenous; IgG = immunoglobulin G.

pressure. A child who performed very well in grade school may begin to have difficulty in junior high and may have more difficulty in high school.

Suggested studies (see Table 15-3)

NEUROLOGIC

Test	Frequency
Computed tomography (CT) or magnetic resonance imaging (MRI) of CNS	As clinically indicated
MRI	If leukoencephalopathy is suspected
Lumbar puncture	As clinically indicated

NEUROPSYCHOLOGIC

Psychologic tests	Certainly when learning disabilities expected, but baseline and periodic testing in all patients is encouraged. (Prospective studies on this point are ongoing.)

Suggested treatment (see Table 15-4)

NEUROLOGIC. Patients who develop leukoencephalopathy should be managed with the assistance of a pediatric neurologist who is familiar with this problem. Supportive care has resulted in clinical improvement for some children. Specific medications are given as clinically indicated.

NEUROPSYCHOLOGIC. Recognition that a child may develop learning disabilities after BMT is important to facilitate appropriate and timely psychologic testing and placement of the child in special education classes if necessary. Parents should be told of this risk before the BMT, and inquiry regarding school performance should occur with each annual posttransplant clinic visit. A pediatric psychologist will be an important individual in the diagnosis and management of this disorder. Annual psychologic tests may be indicated, because it appears that the problem is not static and may worsen with increasing time. Precise frequency of testing is not known because prospective research studies are currently being conducted.

Ophthalmologic Abnormalities

Cataracts are a well-known complication of long-term steroid therapy as well as RT. Approximately 80% of patients given single-exposure TBI develop posterior, subcapsular cataracts by 6 years after TBI. Most have required cataract repair. Patients who received 12 to 15.75 Gy fractionated TBI have a significantly lower incidence of cataracts (20%), and of these only 20% have required cataract repair.[15] Dry eyes due to diminished lacrimal gland function and decreased tear formation may also occur.[27]

Suggested studies (see Table 15-3)

Tests	Frequency
Ophthalmologic examination	Annual

A pediatric ophthalmologist should be involved in the posttransplant care of children. An annual examination including slit-lamp examination and Schirmer's test will be important for this population of patients.

Suggested treatment (Table 15-4). Patients with sicca syndrome (dry eyes) should use artificial tears. Often this is all that is required. However, if the frequency of artificial tear administration becomes a major problem, then punctal ligation of the lacrimal duct may be a helpful adjunct to use of artificial tears. Treatment of cataracts should be as clinically indicated.

Secondary Maligancies

Multiagent CT and RT have both been implicated as causes for development of secondary malignancies (SMN). Results and methods of evaluation of children at risk are described in Chapter 16 and will not be repeated here.

SMNs have been observed after BMT. The etiologies of these secondary tumors is most likely multifactorial. Studies of irradiated and nonirradiated mice given hematopoietic transplants have suggested that graft-versus-host disease (GVHD) was a major contributing factor in the development of secondary lymphoid malignancies.[25] Among dogs given TBI and BMT, the relative risk of developing a malignancy was 5 times higher than among nonirradiated control animals.[16] Among more than 2000 patients transplanted in Seattle, 35 SMNs occurring between 1.5 months and 14 years after BMT have been reported.[83] The age-adjusted overall incidence of these SMNs was 6.69 times higher than the SEER-reported incidence of primary cancers observed in the general population. When

TBI was incorporated in the preparative regimen, the risk of SMN increased by 3.9 times compared with the expected incidences. The types of malignancies observed were non-Hodgkin's lymphomas, usually associated with Epstein-Barr virus in 16 patients; leukemias of different types in six patients; and solid tumors that included gliomas, carcinomas, and melanomas in 13 patients. Multivariate analysis indicated that risk of developing any type of SMN was significantly associated with use of posttransplant immunosuppression with antithymocyte globulin (ATG), anti-CD3 monoclonal antibody, or TBI. Among patients who developed a non-Hodgkin lymphoma, additional significant factors were T-cell depletion of donor marrow and BMT from a nonidentical marrow donor. Among the patients who developed a solid tumor, only use of ATG was significant.[83] A recent update of the SMN from Seattle (January 1, 1992) demonstrates that among 4223 BMT patients at risk, a total of 82 SMNs have occurred. Detailed analysis of this total group is pending.

It is therefore clear that patients undergoing BMT, similar to patients receiving CT or RT in a nontransplant setting, have an increased risk of developing SMN. Although there is currently no convincing evidence that GVHD is a risk factor, as has been suggested by murine studies, treatment of GVHD appears to have a major impact. Conceivably, continuous allogeneic stimulation of donor-derived cells by host antigens in the context of severe immunosuppression associated with GVHD and its treatment probably contributes to uncontrolled lymphoid proliferation. RT increases the risk for certain tumors. Investigations in large animal models suggest a rather long latency period between transplant and the diagnosis of SMN. Among patients transplanted for aplastic anemia, those who received a preparative regimen that included RT had a significantly higher incidence of SMN at 8 years after transplant, compared with those who received CY only.[86] Therefore, it appears possible that with prolonged observation of transplant recipients, a higher incidence of SMN may be seen.

Suggested studies. Although no specific studies can be suggested, the physician must be aware that unusual symptoms or signs should be investigated with appropriate studies. Contact should be made with the center where the transplant was performed to determine if special research studies on the tumor tissue are desired and to register the patient as one developing a SMN.

Suggested treatment. As indicated by the specific tumor discovered.

EFFECTS RELATED TO THE TRANSPLANT PROCESS
Chronic Graft-Versus-Host Disease

Incidence and risk factors. Initial reports demonstrated a 30% incidence of chronic GVHD developing among BMT patients who survived more than 150 days after transplant.[71] More recent analysis of patients with hematologic malignancies has demonstrated that the probability of developing chronic GVHD increases with increased human leukocyte antigen (HLA) disparity between donor and recipient.[4] Current studies in Seattle demonstrate an actuarial risk of developing chronic GVHD of 33% among 1148 recipients of non–T-depleted HLA-identical marrow compared with 49% among 220 recipients of non–T-depleted HLA-nonidentical family member marrow (P = 0.0001) and 64% among 69 recipients of non–T-depleted unrelated donor marrow (P = 0.04 compared with recipients of HLA-nonidentical family marrow).[69] The median day of onset was day 159 for recipients of HLA-nonidentical family marrow, day 133 for unrelated donor recipients, and day 201 for recipients of HLA-identical marrow. Few patients have developed chronic GVHD after 500 days post BMT. The consideration of patient age at transplant along with the type of donor is important in determining chronic GVHD risk. Among recipients of HLA-identical marrow, the actuarial risk of developing chronic GVHD is 13% for patients aged 10 years or younger, 28% for patients 10 to 19 years of age, and 45% for patients aged 20 years or older (P = 0.0001). Among recipients of HLA-nonidentical or unrelated donor marrow, however, the risks are approximately 42% for patients aged 10 years or younger and 50% to 56% for patients older than 11 years of age.

Clinical manifestations. The clinical and pathologic findings of chronic GVHD resemble features of several of the naturally occurring autoimmune diseases, with the exception that chronic GVHD patients do not develop CNS or renal abnormalities.[69] In more than 75% of patients, the skin is involved with erythema, dyspigmentation, poikiloderma, or lichenoid lesions. Without treatment, skin will become progressively indurated and sclerotic, which will result in joint contractures and disability. Hepatocellular dysfunction occurs in 73% of patients. The predominant pattern is cholestatic, but the abnormal liver functions may be difficult to distinguish from those caused by viral hepatitis. Isolated hepatic abnormalities without other target organ involvement has not been observed. Therefore, abnormal liver function is probably due to chronic GVHD if other systems are also involved. Oral lesions occur in 72% of patients.[61] The lesions include atrophy and lichen planus–like findings. Buccal lesions range in appearance from white reticular striae to large plaques. Mucosal atrophy, reduced keratinization, and xerostomia may be present. Increased salivary sodium and decreased or absent secretory immunoglobulin A (IgA) may contribute to increased dental caries. Ophthalmic abnormalities with keratoconjunctivitis sicca, conjunctivitis, and uveitis occur in 47% of patients. Less frequent (less than 15%) manifestations are desquamative esophagitis, polyserositis, vaginal stenosis, and myasthenia gravis.

Diagnosis. An evaluation between 80 and 100 days after BMT is most useful in diagnosing early chronic GVHD.[36] Examination of the skin with biopsies is important. Dermatopathology of early skin involvement reveals eosinophilic bodies, liquefactive degeneration, and basal layer lichenoid reaction.[65] Later, dermal fibrosis and epidermal atrophy may be observed. Oral examination with an oral mucosal biopsy is needed. The oral biopsy findings include squamous cell necrosis and abnormalities similar to Sjögren's syndrome.[53] Liver function tests should be performed. A Schirmer's test to evaluate tear formation is often indicated. Patients with limited chronic GVHD have isolated skin involvement with or without liver abnormalities.[36] Subclinical chronic GVHD patients have characteristic pathologic findings on skin biopsy or oral biopsy in the absence of clinical signs or symptoms.

The diagnosis of clinical extensive chronic GVHD is made if the patient has multiorgan clinical expression with positive skin and oral biopsies.

Treatment. Among patients with subclinical chronic GVHD, none of the treatment efforts to prevent progression to overt chronic GVHD has been successful to date. These trials have included administration of thymic factors and prevention of infection with use of intravenous (IV) Ig.

Without treatment, only 20% of patients with clinical chronic GVHD survive with Karnofsky scores greater than or equal to 70%.[71] Immunosuppressive therapy with antithymocyte globulin (ATG) or corticosteroids administered late in the disease course has not altered the progression of disease. Treatment with thymosin, transfer factor, penicillamine, hydroxychloroquine, and electron beam RT also have been unsuccessful.

Early treatment with administration of prednisone improved 5-year actuarial disability-free survival to 61%, and nonrelapse mortality was decreased to 21%.[73] This trial compared treatment using prednisone alone with combination therapy using prednisone and azathioprine. The combination treatment group had a significantly decreased survival of 47% compared with the prednisone-alone group ($P = 0.0001$) and also a higher nonrelapse mortality of 40% ($P = 0.003$). The differences were largely related to increased infections in the combination treatment group. Patients whose expression of chronic GVHD also included thrombocytopenia had the highest risk of failure, with a long-term survival of 26% when treated with prednisone alone. Treatment of this patient population with prednisone plus cyclosporine has improved survival to 51% at 5 years, although nonrelapse mortality remains high at 40%.[72] Therefore, cyclosporine appears to be an effective agent for treatment of chronic GVHD. Other approaches that have been effective in treating chronic GVHD include thalidomide and psoralen with ultraviolet A radiation (PUVA).[19,78] Neither of these modalities has yet been tested in prospective randomized trials for patients with early chronic GVHD. Other agents that may be useful include the macrolide compound FK-506 and rapamycin.[17,44]

Factors that have been found to be predictive of outcome or response to treatment include the type of onset of chronic GVHD and the skin biopsy obtained 2 months after initiation of chronic GVHD therapy.[36] Patients who developed de novo GVHD (no history of prior acute GVHD) or quiescent GVHD (resolved acute GVHD before onset of chronic GVHD) had an actuarial survival exceeding 55% at 5 years, compared with patients with progressive onset (nonresolved acute GVHD evolving into chronic GVHD) who had an actuarial survival of less than 20% at 5 years. When skin biopsies repeated 2 months after initiation of treatment indicated resolution of dermal activity, patients usually had favorable outcomes. These studies were performed in a setting where all patients received a minimum of 9 months of therapy. It is not known whether a shorter course of treatment would be sufficient.

Suggested studies (see Table 15-3)

Organ system	Test
Skin	Physical exam, biopsy (involved area, if possible)
Mouth	Physical exam, mucosal biopsy

Organ system	Test
Eyes	Schirmer's test
Liver	AST, alkaline phosphatase, bilirubin direct/indirect
Immune	Ig

History
Type of marrow donor
Current immunosuppressive therapy
Acute GVHD

Note: Patients who are receiving immunosuppressive treatment with corticosteroids at the time of evaluation for chronic GVHD at 80 to 100 days after transplant and who have no or subclinical chronic GVHD should be reevaluated for activity of chronic GVHD after immunosuppressive therapy has been discontinued. This is particularly critical for patients with subclinical chronic GVHD who may have full expression of active chronic GVHD after completion of their immunosuppressive therapy.

Suggested treatment (see Table 15-4)

CLINICAL EXTENSIVE CHRONIC GVHD. Immunosuppressive treatment for a minimum of 9 months with reevaluations as clinically indicated. Prednisone, 1 mg/kg every other day with cyclosporine, 6.25 mg/kg twice a day every other day.

REEVALUATION. Every 9 months until all clinical and pathologic manifestations of chronic GVHD have resolved. Additional therapy may be needed or treatment regimen altered for patients who demonstrate progression of chronic GVHD.

SUBCLINICAL CHRONIC GVHD. It is anticipated that at least 60% of these patients will progress to clinical extensive chronic GVHD. Because 40% of these patients do not progress, the risk of developing extensive chronic GVHD should be considered when one is deciding whether to taper immunosuppressive therapy (i.e., cyclosporine or prednisone) or to continue patients on single- or dual-agent therapy. If the risk is high (e.g., HLA-nonidentical or unrelated donor BMT) then treatment should probably be continued for the duration of the first year after BMT. However, if the risk is low (patient under 10 years of age with HLA-identical BMT), then consideration for tapering therapy may be reasonable.

Immunologic Recovery

Repopulation of the immune system after BMT depends upon appropriate proliferation, maturation, and differentiation of cells of donor origin. Time after BMT is the most important factor.[85] All marrow graft recipients have profound impairment of most immune functions during the first 6 to 9 months after transplant, regardless of the type of graft, underlying disease, conditioning regimen, postgrafting immunosuppression, or presence of acute GVHD. Among patients without chronic GVHD the immunologic parameters return to normal about 1 year after grafting, and the majority of these patients remain healthy.

Humoral immunity returns to normal 3 to 4 months after BMT with normal levels of IgG and IgM.[84] Total hemolytic complement levels also become normal about 3 months after BMT. Cellular and humoral responses to recall antigens and neoantigens recover to normal levels by 1 year in healthy recipients, but these responses remain impaired or absent among chronic GVHD patients. These GVHD patients have diminished levels of antibody in response to injections of penumococcal antigen, as well as to the neoantigens bacteriophage 0X174 and keyhole limpit hemocyanin. They also fail to switch from IgM to IgG production in secondary responses.

The absolute numbers of T and B cells return to normal levels early; however, subsets of T lymphocytes repopulate at different rates.[3] Healthy long-term survivors have suppressor cells that appropriately suppress donor responses to host histocompatibility antigens but do not interfere with immune responses to pathogens. Chronic GVHD patients have nonspecific suppressor cells that alter immunologic responses, thereby increasing the patient's susceptibility to infections.[39] These patients have elevated numbers of CD8 suppressor lymphocytes and decreased levels of CD4 helper lymphocytes. In vitro studies demonstrate that T lymphocytes in these patients exert suppressor function and B lymphocytes fail to proliferate or differentiate into immunoglobulin-secreting cells. These abnormalities are present in chronic GVHD patients regardless of treatment.

It is not surprising that infections are a common problem after BMT.[81] The actuarial probability of developing bacteremia or septicemia after 100 days is 20% for recipients of HLA identical marrow and nearly 40% for recipients of unrelated donor marrow.[69] The probability of mortality due to nonrelapse causes after day 100 is 6% for patients without chronic GVHD, but 22% for those with chronic GVHD ($P = 0.001$). Therefore, preventing infections is critical for the long-term survival of BMT patients, especially those with chronic GVHD. The use of oral antibiotic prophylaxis with trimethoprim sulfamethoxazole not only prevents bacterial infections but also provides prophylaxis against *Pneumocystis carinii* interstitial pneumonia.[73] Prolonged administration of monthly IV IgG appears to benefit patients who have developed serum IgG or IgG subclass deficiencies.[70]

It has been demonstrated that immunity is transferred from donor to recipient following marrow grafting and that this immunity may be protective for some time after BMT.[38] The antibody levels to diphtheria and tetanus antigens, however, decline with increasing time (years) after transplant. Periodic booster immunizations will be needed for patients with low levels of serum antibody to these antigens. The use of pneumococcal or other vaccines is of limited value early after transplant. Among patients without chronic GVHD, immunizations with pneumococcal, Salk polio, influenza, and diphtheria-pertussis-tetanus or diphtheria-tetanus (as indicated) vaccine may be given after the first year, and the measles-mumps-rubella vaccine has been safely administered after the second year.

Suggested studies (see Table 15-3)

Test	Frequency
Skin test to recall antigens and neoantigens	Annual until first positive
Serum immunoglobulin levels	At 3 and 12 months for all patients (see treatment)

Suggested treatment (see Table 15-4)

IgG deficient patients   Until pre-IV IgG infusion levels are normal for 2 consecutive months

Supplemental IV IgG should be administered to patients with low levels of IgG or IgG subclass 2 or 4. Prophylactic antibiotics with trimetheoprim sulfamethoxazole should be administered for 6 months for nonchronic GVHD patients or until all therapy for chronic GVHD has been discontinued.

Pulmonary Effects

Abnormal pulmonary function with noninfectious pneumonia has been attributed to lung injury related to preparative regimen toxicity (CT and/or TBI) with resultant diffuse interstitial pneumonia.[43] Symptomatic severe obstructive airways disease (OAD) was first recognized after allogeneic BMT in 1982, and over the next 5 years more than 70 patients with OAD were reported.* One review of 35 recipients of allogeneic BMT with new onset of OAD determined that chronic GVHD was present in 74% of these patients.[11] The time of onset was 50 to 500 days (median: 150). Most patients had pulmonary symptoms: cough, dyspnea, and wheezing. Physical examination and chest radiographs were usually normal, but more than half of the patients had pulmonary or sinus infection or both. Two cases of fatal bronchiolitis were recently described after autologous BMT.[48] Both patients had received extensive chemotherapy and local thoracic RT prior to BMT.

The major risk factor for development of OAD is chronic GVHD, but MTX for GVHD prophylaxis has also been implicated.[11] Patients with low serum IgG levels may also be at increased risk for development of OAD, although this is not clearly established.

The association between new onset OAD and chronic GVHD has led to the hypothesis that host bronchiolar epithelial cells may serve as targets for donor cytotoxic T-lymphocytes (CTL). This theory is supported indirectly by the finding that the bronchiolar surface epithelial cells express class II major histocompatibility complex antigens and therefore could be targets for HLA-unrestricted CTL responses.[13,75] Experimentally, bleomycin-induced lung injury promotes expression of these antigens. Preliminary unpublished data (Crawford, 1992), however, demonstrate no correlation between class II antigen expression in lung tissue samples after BMT and the presence of GVHD. Therefore, there are no direct data to support the hypothesis that OAD is a form of pulmonary GVHD.

Other explanations for OAD include recurrent infection or recurrent aspiration. The varied histopathologies, differentials of bronchioalveolar-lavage (BAL) cells, the varied frequency of associated pulmonary infection, the variable occurrence of OAD after autologous BMT, and the varied clinical courses all suggest a multifactoral etiology of OAD.

---

*References 2, 9-11, 28, 34, 35, 52.

Clinically the rate of progression of OAD is also variable. Patients with severe OAD, defined as a decline in forced expiratory volume in 1 second (FEV_1) of more than 30% between measurements taken 50 days apart, usually have a rapidly progressive course resulting in death due to respiratory failure in 71% of patients.[11] This is in contrast to no deaths due to respiratory failure for the patients with less than 30% decline in FEV_1 in these 50-day intervals. The initial rate of progression of OAD is the major factor predictive of outcome. Time of appearance of OAD after BMT does not seem to influence the disease course.

Appreciation of the relationships between pathology (bronchiolitis), physiology (airway obstruction), and associated conditions (chronic GVHD) are helpful in recognizing patients likely to have OAD. It is important to also have a high index of suspicion in a BMT patient with cough, wheezing, dyspnea, and/or hypoxemia in the presence of a normal chest radiograph. Occasionally patients may present without symptoms but have an obstructive pattern on pulmonary function tests (PFTs). These patients may have a mild case, or it may be very early in the course of the illness. Careful follow-up studies for these as well as all patients are indicated.

Suggested studies (see Table 15-3)

All patients	Physical examination
	History of or presence of chronic GVHD
	Chest radiograph
	PFT[1]
Suspected bronchiolitis[2]	Sinus radiograph
	Lung tissue sample (BAL), open biopsy for bacterial, fungal, viral cultures for histopathology and for other opportunistic infections
	White blood cell count (WBC) with differential

1. Include spirometry, lung volumes, diffusion capacity, and arterial blood gases or oxygen saturation.
2. Additional studies.

Suggested treatment (see Table 15-4). There are no standard treatment approaches or prospective studies for treatment of OAD. Immunosuppressive therapy similar or identical to that administered for chronic GVHD is usually indicated, especially if the patient has active chronic GVHD. Infection prophylaxis with an oral antibiotic (e.g. trimethoprim sulfamethoxazole) may be useful.

EFFECTS RELATED TO THE ORIGINAL DISEASE

Rejection or Graft Failure

Graft rejection almost never occurs when non-T-cell–depleted marrow grafts from HLA-identical sibling donors have been used for patients with hematologic malignancy receiving BMT after a preparative regimen with chemotherapy and TBI.[76] When donors are non-HLA-identical family members, 12% of grafts are rejected.[1] Factors associated with graft rejection were an increasing degree of donor

HLA disparity and prior alloimmunization. Among recipients of T-cell–depleted donor marrow, rejection has occurred with an increased frequency compared with recipients of non-T-cell–depleted marrow. Several investigators have suggested that more intensive preparative regimens appear to decrease the incidence of graft rejection after T-cell–depleted marrow, but no prospective randomized studies have been performed.[41] As an increasing number of unrelated marrow donor transplants are being performed, graft rejection among affected patients has also been observed. The incidence of rejection among recipients of non-T-cell–depleted unrelated donor marrow is similar to that observed among matched sibling transplants.[4,5,31] Those given T-cell–depleted grafts had a significantly higher incidence of graft rejection. The major mechanism of graft rejection appears to be related to residual host immunity, as demonstrated by the presence of host lymphocytes in the majority of patients who reject.

Suggested studies (see Table 15-3). The peripheral blood is examined for the cellular origin of lymphocytes. In the case of opposite sex donor-recipient pairs, this may be easily accomplished by determination of the origin (donor or host) of phytohemagglutinin-stimulated peripheral blood lymphocytes. For patients of same sex, molecular techniques using polymerase chain reaction techniques to evaluate variable nucleotide tandem repeats (VNTR) regions for differences between donor and host DNA have been useful. When the patient and donor are not HLA identical, HLA typing may be helpful if enough lymphocytes can be obtained.

Suggested treatment (see Table 15-4). A uniform or successful method of therapy has not been determined. The majority of patients have failed to achieve successful sustained engraftment using additional immunosuppression and a second marrow infusion.[1] A regimen of ultra–high-dose methylprednisolone and ATG has been reported to be modestly successful. The length of time after initial BMT may be an important factor, although this has not been clearly demonstrated for hematologic malignancy patients in whom the graft is rejected. However, among patients transplanted for aplastic anemia who received CY only as the transplant preparative regimen, none of the seven children given second transplants within 6 months of the original transplant survived, but all of the seven children who received the second transplant after more than 6 months survived with sustained engraftment.[68] Part of any decision to perform a second BMT includes not only the general medical condition of the patient but also the risk-benefit ratio to the donor.

Recurrent Leukemia

Despite marrow ablative doses of CT and TBI, recurrent leukemia after BMT remains a major problem. The incidence varies with the phase of disease at time of BMT. Between 15% and 40% of patients who receive transplants while in remission will relapse, and up to 80% of patients who receive transplants while in relapse will relapse. The optimal treatment strategy for patients who relapse after BMT has not been resolved. Management of the relapsed patient varies depending on the type of relapse and the patient's underlying diagnosis.

Isolated testicular relapse among males transplanted for acute lymphoblastic leukemia has been observed among approximately 16% of males who are disease free more than 1 year after transplant. Treatment with orchectomy, testicular RT, and systemic CT for 1 to 2 years has resulted in subsequent long-term disease-free survival (DFS), whereas less-intensive therapy is less effective owing to subsequent BMT relapse. This suggests that occult marrow involvement is likely to be present at the time of testicular recurrence (Sanders—unpublished data, 1992). The current molecular methods for detecting minimal residual disease may be useful, although no data are available.

Several treatment methods have been reported for patients with recurrent Ph$^+$ chronic myelogenous leukemia (CML). Among patients whose Ph$^+$ chromosome has returned despite a morphologically normal marrow, discontinuation of immunosuppression (i.e., cyclosporine administration) has resulted in spontaneous disappearance of the Ph$^+$ chromosome in a substantial number of such patients.[12] When both the Ph$^+$ chromosome and abnormal marrow morphology occur, additional treatment with alpha interferon has been useful in controlling disease progression and rendering some patients Ph$^+$ negative. Infusion of donor lymphocytes has been successful in inducing an allogeneic "graft-versus-leukemia" effect with resultant disappearance of the Ph$^+$ chromosome and marrow evidence of CML.[33] This approach also induces a significant amount of acute GVHD, which requires treatment with immunosuppressive therapy. A final approach for CML patients in whom these measures fail is a second BMT. A recent report shows an actuarial DFS of 25% at 2 years after second BMT.[49]

Conventional chemotherapy has been reported to induce a complete remission for approximately 60% of patients who relapse more than 1 year after BMT, and for 20% of patients who relapse within the first year.[45] However, almost none of these remissions was prolonged, and most patients died of recurrent leukemia. It is unknown whether a significant number of patients with acute leukemia will benefit from infusions of donor lymphocytes to induce an allogeneic graft-versus-leukemia effect.[74] Response with clearance of leukemia cells has been observed for a few patients with acute myelogenous leukemia (AML). The efficacy of interleukin-2, which has demonstrated activity in AML, has not yet been sufficiently tested in post-BMT relapse patients to reach conclusions.[24] Another approach is performance of a second BMT from the same or another donor. The results from second BMTs for patients with acute leukemia demonstrate that recurrent leukemia continues to occur among 50% to 76% in one large series and from 54% to 95% in an analysis from the International Bone Marrow Transplant Registry.[46,49] Post-second-transplant DFS was significantly better for patients younger than 10 years of age than for patients 11 to 20 years of age and patients older than 20 years of age (57%, 7%, and 10% respectively; $P = 0.03$); patients who did not develop severe venocclusive disease (0.0001); and patients who did not develop severe GVHD (0.008).[49] These data demonstrate that a second transplant should be considered for young children, and that methods to decrease posttransplant toxicities and relapse are needed for older patients.

Suggested studies (see Table 15-3)

Test	Indication
Bone marrow examination	Abnormal blood counts
	Clinical suspicion
Cytogenetics	Ph$^+$ CML, pretransplant cytogenetic abnormalities, donor and recipient of opposite sexes

Suggested treatment (see Table 15-4)

Relapse type	Treatment
Isolated testicular	Orchectomy, RT, CT
Ph$^+$ CML	
Isolated Ph$^+$ CML recurrence	Discontinue immunosuppression
Overt marrow involvement	Interferon $\pm$ hydroxyurea
	Infusion donor lymphocytes
	Second transplant
Acute leukemia	
Overt marrow involvement	Conventional CT
	Second transplant

Summary

BMT has become a life-saving procedure for an increasing number of patients during the last two decades. As an ever larger number of patients are surviving long term, late effects related to the transplant preparative regimen, to the transplant procedure, and to the original disease are emerging. In addition to defining these problems, strategies to both decrease their likelihood and treat them are emerging. An awareness of potential sequelae is necessary to permit appropriate counseling of the patient before the BMT, and also to anticipate and recognize the late effects when they become apparent. The evaluation and treatment suggestions are just one way of approaching and treating the problem. As more experience is gained in this developing field, changes in the incidence of, approaches to, and treatment of many of the individual problems are expected.

REFERENCES

1. Anasetti C et al: Effect of HLA compatibility on engraftment of bone marrow transplants in patients with leukemia or lymphoma, *N Engl J Med* 320:197-204, 1989.
2. Atkinson K et al: Obstructive airways disease. A rare but serious manifestation of chronic graft-versus-host disease after allogeneic bone marrow transplantation in humans, *Transplant Proc* 16:1030-1033, 1984.
3. Atkinson K et al: T-cell subpopulations identified by monoclonal antibodies after human marrow transplantation. I. Helper-inducer and cytotoxic-suppressor subsets, *Blood* 59:1292-1298, 1982.

4. Beatty PG et al: Marrow transplantation from related donors other than HLA-identical siblings, *N Engl J Med* 313:765-771, 1985.
5. Beatty PG et al: Marrow transplantation from HLA-matched unrelated donors for treatment of hematologic malignancies, *Transplantation* 51:443-447, 1991.
6. Belohorsky B et al: Comments on the development of amenorrhea caused by Myleran in cases of chronic myelosis, *Neoplasma* 4:397-402, 1960.
7. Berry DH et al: Growth in children with acute lymphocytic leukemia: a pediatric oncology group study, *Med Pediatr Oncol* 11:39-45, 1983.
8. Bourguignon J-P: Linear growth as a function of age at onset of puberty and sex steroid dosage: therapeutic implications, *Endocrinol Rev* 9:467-488, 1988.
9. Bradstock KF et al: Fatal obstructive airways disease after bone marrow transplantation, *Transplant Proc* 16:1034-1036, 1984.
10. Chan CK et al: Small-airways disease in recipients of allogeneic bone marrow transplants. An analysis of 11 cases and a review of the literature, *Medicine* 66:327-340, 1987.
11. Clark JG et al: The clinical presentation and course of obstructive lung disease after allogeneic marrow transplantation, *Ann Intern Med* 111:368-376, 1989.
12. Clift RA et al: Allogeneic marrow transplantation in patients with chronic myeloid leukemia in the chronic phase. A randomized trial of two irradiation regimens, *Blood* 77:1660-1665, 1991.
13. Crawford SW, Clark SG: Bronchiolitis associated with bone marrow transplant, *Clin Chest Med* (in press).
14. De Sanctis V et al: Gonadal function after allogeneic bone marrow transplantation for thalassaemia, *Arch Dis Child* 66:517-520, 1991.
15. Deeg HJ et al: Cataracts after total body irradiation and marrow transplantation: a sparing effect of dose fractionation, *Int J Radiat Oncol Biol Phys* 10:957-964, 1984.
16. Deeg HJ et al: Increased incidence of malignant tumors in dogs after total body irradiation and marrow transplantation, *Int J Radiat Oncol Biol Phys* 9:1505-1511, 1983.
17. Dumont FJ et al: The immunosuppressive macrolides FK-506 and rapamycin act as reciprocal antagonists in murine T cells, *J Immunol* 144:1418-1424, 1990.
18. Endo M et al: Possible association of human growth hormone treatment with an occurrence of acute myeloblastic leukaemia with an inversion of chromosome 3 in a child with pituitary dwarfism, *Med Pediatr Oncol* 16:45-47, 1988.
19. Eppinger T et al: 8-methoxypsoralen and ultraviolet A therapy for cutaneous manifestations of graft-versus-host disease, *Transplantation* 50:807-811, 1990.
20. Etteldorf JN et al: Gonadal function, testicular histology, and meiosis following cyclophosphamide therapy in patients with nephrotic syndrome, *J Pediatr* 88:206-212, 1976.
21. Fairley KF, Barrie JU, Johnson W: Sterility and testicular atrophy related to cyclophosphamide therapy, *Lancet* i:568-569, 1972.
22. Fisher DA et al: Leukaemia in patients treated with growth hormone, *Lancet* i:1159-1160, 1988.
23. Fleming ID et al: Thyroid dysfunction and neoplasia in children receiving neck irradiation for cancer, *Cancer* 55:1190-1194, 1985.
24. Foa R et al: Treatment of acute myeloid leukaemia patients with recombinant interleukin 2: a pilot study, *Br J Haematol* 77:491-496, 1992.

25. Gleichmann E, Gleichmann H, Schwartz RS: Immunologic induction of malignant lymphoma. Identification of donor and host tumors in the graft-versus-host model, *J Natl Cancer Inst* 54:107-116, 1975.

26. Hancock SL, Cox RS, McDougall R: Thyroid diseases after treatment of Hodgkin's disease, *N Engl J Med* 325:599-606, 1991.

27. Jack MJ, Hicks JD: Ocular complications in high-dose chemoradiotherapy and marrow transplantation, *Ann Ophthalmol* 13(6):709-711, 1981.

28. Johnson FL et al: Chronic obstructive airways disease after bone marrow transplantation, *J Pediatr* 105:370-376, 1984.

29. Joss E et al: Final height of patients with pituitary growth failure and changes in growth variables after long-term hormonal therapy, *Pediatr Res* 17:676-679, 1983.

30. Katsanis E et al: Thyroid dysfunction following bone marrow transplantation: long-term follow-up of 80 pediatric patients, *Bone Marrow Transplant* 5:335-340, 1990.

31. Kernan NA et al: Analysis of 462 transplantations from unrelated donors facilitated by The National Marrow Donor Program, *N Engl J Med* 328:593-602, 1993.

32. Kirk JA et al: Growth failure and growth-hormone deficiency after treatment for acute lymphoblastic leukaemia, *Lancet* i:190-193, 1987.

33. Kolb HJ et al: Donor leukocyte transfusions for treatment of recurrent chronic myelogenous leukemia in marrow transplant patients, *Blood* 76:2462-2465, 1990.

34. Kurzrock R et al: Obstructive lung disease after allogeneic marrow transplantation, *Transplantation* 37:156-160, 1984.

35. Link H et al: Obstructive ventilation disorder as a severe complication of chronic graft-versus-host disease after bone marrow transplantation, *Exp Hematol* 10:92-93, 1982.

36. Loughran TP et al: Value of day 100 screening studies for predicting the development of chronic graft-versus-host disease after allogeneic bone marrow transplantation, *Blood* 76:228-234, 1990.

37. Lowrey GJ: *Growth and development of children,* ed 8, Chicago, 1986, Mosby–Year Book.

38. Lum LG et al: Transfer of specific immunity in marrow recipients given HLA-mismatched, T cell–depleted, or HLA-identical marrow grafts, *Bone Marrow Transplant* 3:399-406, 1988.

39. Lum LG et al: T and B cell deficiencies in patients with chronic graft-versus-host disease after HLA-identical marrow transplantation, *Transplant Proc* 13:1231-1232, 1981.

40. Manenti F et al: Growth and endocrine function after bone marrow transplantation for thalassemia. In Buckner CD, Gale RP, Lucarelli G, editors: *Advances and controversies in thalassemia therapy: bone marrow transplantation and other approaches,* New York, 1989, Alan R Liss.

41. Martin PJ et al: Graft failure in patients receiving T cell–depleted HLA-identical allogeneic marrow transplants, *Bone Marrow Transplant* 3:445-456, 1988.

42. McGuire T et al: Neuropsychological function in children given total body irradiation for marrow transplantation, *Pediatr Res* 31:143A, 1992 (abstract).

43. Meyers JD, Flournoy N, Thomas ED: Nonbacterial pneumonia after allogeneic marrow transplantation: a review of ten years' experience, *Rev Infect Dis* 4:1119-1132, 1982.

44. Morris RE et al: Mycophenolic acid morpholinoethylester (RS-61443) is a new immunosuppressant that prevents and halts heart allograft rejection by selective inhibition of T and B cell purine synthesis, *Transplant Proc* 1990 (in press).

45. Mortimer J et al: Relapse of acute leukemia after marrow transplantation: natural history and results of subsequent therapy, *J Clin Oncol* 7:50-57, 1989.

46. Mrsic M et al: Second HLA-identical sibling transplants for leukemia recurrence, *Bone Marrow Transplant* 9:269-275, 1992.

47. Mulhern RK et al: Memory function in disease-free survivors of childhood acute lymphocyte leukemia given CNS prophylaxis with or without 1,800 cGy cranial irradiation, *J Clin Oncol* 6:315-320, 1988.

48. Paz HL et al: Bronchiolitis obliterans after autologous bone marrow transplantation, *Chest* 101:775-778, 1992.

49. Radich JP et al: Second allogeneic marrow transplantation for patients with recurrent leukemia after initial transplant with total-body irradiation-containing regimens, *J Clin Oncol* 11:304-313, 1993.

50. Ray H, Mattison E: How radiation and chemotherapy affect gonadal function, *Contemp Obstet Gynecol* 109:106-115, 1985.

51. Robinson LL et al: Height of children successfully treated for acute lymphoblastic leukemia: a report from the late effects study committee of Children's Cancer Study Group, *Med Pediatr Oncol* 13:14-21, 1985.

52. Roca J et al: Fatal airway disease in an adult with chronic graft-versus-host disease, *Thorax* 37:77-78, 1982.

53. Sale GE et al: Oral and ophthalmic pathology of graft versus host disease in man: predictive value of the lip biopsy, *Hum Pathol* 12:1022-1030, 1981.

54. Sanders JE: Endocrine problems in children after bone marrow transplant for hematologic malignancies, *Bone Marrow Transplant* 8:2-4, 1991.

55. Sanders JE, Seattle Marrow Transplant Team: The impact of marrow transplant preparative regimens on subsequent growth and development, *Semin Hematol* 28:244-249, 1991.

56. Sanders JE et al: Ovarian function following marrow transplantation for aplastic anemia or leukemia, *J Clin Oncol* 6:813-818, 1988.

57. Sanders JE et al: Growth and development in children after bone marrow transplantation, *Horm Res* 30:92-97, 1988.

58. Sanders JE et al: Growth and development following marrow transplantation for leukemia, *Blood* 68:1129-1135, 1986.

59. Sasaki U, Hara M, Watanabe S: Occurrence of acute lymphoblastic leukemia in a boy treated with growth hormone for growth retardation after irradiation to the brain tumor, *J Clin Oncol* 18:81-84, 1988.

60. Schubert MA et al: Gynecological abnormalities following allogeneic bone marrow transplantation, *Bone Marrow Transplant* 5:425-430, 1990.

61. Schubert MM et al: Oral manifestations of chronic graft-v-host disease, *Arch Intern Med* 144:1591-1595, 1984.

62. Shalet SM: Irradiation-induced growth failure, *Clin Endocrinol Metab* 15:591-606, 1986.

63. Shalet SM et al: Testicular function following irradiation of the human prepubertal testes, *Clin Endocrinol* 9:483-490, 1978.

64. Shalet SM, Clayton PE, Price DA: Growth and pituitary function in children treated for brain tumours or acute lymphoblastic leukaemia, *Horm Res* 30:53-61, 1988.

65. Shulman HM et al: Chronic graft-versus-host syndrome in man. A long-term clinico-pathologic study of 20 Seattle patients, *Am J Med* 69:204-217, 1980.

66. Sklar CA, Kim TH, Ramsay NKC: Thyroid dysfunction among long-term survivors of bone marrow transplantation, *Am J Med* 73:688-694, 1982.
67. Starceski PJ et al: Comparable effects of 1800- and 2400-rad (18- and 24-Gy) cranial irradiation on height and weight in children treated for acute lymphocytic leukemia, *Am J Dis Child* 141:550-552, 1987.
68. Storb R et al: Marrow transplantation for severe aplastic anemia and thalassemia major, *Semin Hematol* 28:235-239, 1991.
69. Sullivan KM et al: Chronic graft-versus-host disease and other late complications of bone marrow transplantation, *Semin Hematol* 28:250-259, 1991.
70. Sullivan KM et al: Immunomodulatory and antimicrobial efficacy of intravenous immunoglobulin in bone marrow transplantation, *N Engl J Med* 323:705-712, 1990.
71. Sullivan KM et al: Chronic graft-versus-host disease in 52 patients: adverse natural course and successful treatment with combination immunosuppression, *Blood* 57:267-276, 1981.
72. Sullivan KM et al: Alternating-day cyclosporine and prednisone for treatment of high-risk chronic graft-v-host disease, *Blood* 72:555-561, 1988.
73. Sullivan KM et al: Prednisone and azathioprine compared with prednisone and placebo for treatment of chronic graft-v-host disease: prognostic influence of prolonged thrombocytopenia after allogeneic marrow transplantation, *Blood* 72:546-554, 1988.
74. Szer J et al: Donor leucocyte infusions after chemotherapy for patients relapsing with acute leukemia following allogeneic BMT, *Bone Marrow Transplant* 11:109-111, 1993.
75. Taylor PM, Rose ML, Yacoub MH: Expression of MHC antigens in normal human lungs and transplanted lungs with obliterative bronchiolitis, *Transplantation* 48:506-510, 1989.
76. Thomas ED et al: Bone-marrow transplantation, *N Engl J Med* 92:832-843, 895-902, 1975.
77. Thompson CB et al: The risks of central nervous system relapse and leukoencephalopathy in patients receiving marrow transplants for acute leukemia, *Blood* 67:195-199, 1986.
78. Vogelsang GB et al: Thalidomide for the treatment of chronic graft versus host disease, *N Engl J Med* 326:1055-1058, 1992.
79. Wade JC, Meyers JD: Neurologic symptoms associated with parenteral acyclovir treatment after marrow transplantation, *Ann Intern Med* 98:921-925, 1983.
80. Warne GL et al: Cyclophosphamide-induced ovarian failure, *N Engl J Med* 289:1159-1162, 1973.
81. Wingard JR: Advances in the management of infectious complications after bone marrow transplantation, *Bone Marrow Transplant* 6:371-383, 1990.
82. Wingard JR et al: Growth in children after bone marrow transplantation: busulfan plus cyclophosphamide versus cyclophosphamide plus total body irradiation, *Blood* 79:1068-1073, 1992.
83. Witherspoon RP et al: Secondary cancers after bone marrow transplantation, *N Engl J Med* 322:853, 1990.
84. Witherspoon RP et al: In vitro regulation of immunoglobulin synthesis after human marrow transplantation. II. Deficient T and non-T lymphocyte function within 3-4 months of allogeneic, syngeneic, or autologous marrow grafting for hematologic malignancy, *Blood* 59:844-850, 1982.
85. Witherspoon RP et al: Recovery of in vivo cellular immunity after human marrow grafting: influence of time postgrafting and acute graft-versus-host disease, *Transplantation* 37:145-150, 1984.

86. Witherspoon RP et al: Cumulative incidence of secondary solid malignant tumors in aplastic anemia patients given marrow grafts after conditioning with chemotherapy alone, *Blood* 79:289-292, 1992 (letter).

87. Yee GC et al: Minimal risk of chronic renal dysfunction in marrow transplant recipients treated with cyclosporine for 6 months, *Bone Marrow Transplant* 4:691-694, 1989.

16

Follow-up Care of Patients at Risk for the Development of Second Malignant Neoplasms

Anna T. Meadows
Judith G. Fenton

Cure following childhood cancer is now possible in 60% to 70% of patients because of the effectiveness of chemotherapeutic agents, often combined with radiation therapy (RT) and surgery. Differences in the mechanisms of action of these therapeutic modalities produce variations in the long-term effects that childhood cancer survivors experience. The development of a second malignant neoplasm (SMN) may be the most serious of these delayed consequences for a survivor.

Overall, for children who have experienced a primary malignancy, the incidence of new neoplasms ranges between 8% and 12% at 20 years.[4,6,21] This risk is 10 to 15 times greater than that of age-matched controls.

However, not all individuals are at equal risk for the development of SMNs (Fig. 16-1). Retinoblastoma carries the highest risk, but this is true only for children with the genetic form of the disease who have an inherent risk even excluding treatment variables.[5,12] The majority of genetic cases are recognized by their bilaterality. Patients with Hodgkin's disease treated with nitrogen mustard, vincristine, prednisone, and procarbazine (MOPP) also have a high risk for the development of radiation-associated sarcomas and leukemia, the former having a longer latent period and not yet showing a plateau, whereas the risk for leukemia plateaus at 10 years.[13] The Late Effects Study Group (LESG) has reported that primary neoplasms with the greatest SMN risk included retinoblastoma, Hodgkin's disease, and Ewing's sarcoma, although few were noted following acute lymphoblastic leukemia (ALL).[12] However, the data for that report were collected prior to the widespread cure of children with ALL.

There is a need for caregivers and counselors to know the frequency of SMN for a variety of diagnoses and treatment modalities. Nevertheless, the evaluation of each long-term survivor should include consideration that a new tumor might develop. Individuals at greatest risk need special surveillance and sensitive counseling to facilitate early diagnosis without needlessly increasing anxiety while providing appropriate reassurance.

Because improved survival has only been realized over the past 15 years, the lifetime cancer risk for many groups of survivors is not yet known. The average

PRIMARY DIAGNOSIS (N = 387)

RB
- Bone 47%
- STS 21.8%
- Leukemia/Lymphoma 4.6%
- Brain 10.9%
- Other 15.6%

Wilms'
- Bone 14.5%
- STS 12.7%
- Leukemia/Lymphoma 20%
- Brain 7.2%
- Thyroid 10.9%
- Other 16.3%

Bone
- Bone 46.8%
- STS 21.8%
- Leukemia/Lymphoma 15.6%
- Brain 3.1%
- Breast 12.5%

STS
- Bone 36.9%
- STS 15.2%
- Leukemia/Lymphoma 13%
- Brain 17.3%
- Thyroid 4.3%
- Breast 2.1%
- Other 10.8%

Leukemia
- Bone 17%
- STS 22.8%
- Leukemia/Lymphoma 14.2%
- Brain 5.7%
- Thyroid 20%
- Breast 2.8%
- Other 17%

Brain
- Bone 8.7%
- STS 13%
- Leukemia/Lymphoma 17.3%
- Brain 21.7%
- Thyroid 6.5%
- Other 32.6%

NBL
- Bone 5.7%
- STS 9.6%
- Leukemia/Lymphoma 23%
- Brain 30.7%
- Thyroid 11.5%
- Other 19.2%

HD
- Bone 12.2%
- STS 7.0%
- Leukemia/Lymphoma 40.3%
- Brain 3.5%
- Thyroid 15.7%
- Breast 3.5%
- Other 17.5%

0% 5% 10% 15% 20% 25% 30% 35% 40% 45% 50%

% OF SMNs

child at first diagnosis is only 6 years old and has not yet reached the fourth or subsequent decades of life when cancer incidence begins to rise in the general population. However, much is already known and can be used to guide practitioners caring for individuals at risk for the development of SMNs (Table 16-1).

A subset of SMN in previously treated patients is often curable and produces only moderate sequelae; these include neoplasms of the skin and thyroid gland. Even central nervous system (CNS) meningiomas can be cured in the majority of cases. Other SMNs are considerably more serious, requiring more intensive therapy, and often prove fatal. They include bone and soft tissue sarcomas, non-Hodgkin's lymphomas, and acute myeloid leukemia (AML).

Those SMNs that are related to treatment allow for the study of mutagenic and carcinogenic actions of drugs. The great benefit to survival witnessed since the advent of widespread use of polychemotherapy clearly outweighs the risks it imposes. Other SMNs develop in patients who are susceptible or genetically predisposed (e.g., retinoblastoma patients), and in these cases genetic factors can be studied. Increasing our knowledge of the genetics of cancer adds new information that may someday prove extremely effective in detecting those patients at greatest risk. Nevertheless, early diagnosis is now possible in many instances because of current knowledge, and for some patients this may prove advantageous to long-term survival.

RADIATION

Radiation is a potential mutagenic agent for children who receive this mode of treatment. This was noted many years ago when thyroid carcinoma was observed to occur following irradiation to the thymus gland in infancy.[7] Radiation may also impose an additional risk for certain children with the genetic forms of embryonal tumors, although this has not been confirmed.

Mutation produced by radiation primarily affects dividing cells and leads to clones of once-hit cells. Radiation can also provide a second event in those with a preexisting abnormality (or "hit"). Children whose tissues are actively proliferating are more likely to develop expanded (mutated) clones that are susceptible to additional events on the pathway to cancer. The bones and soft tissues of growing children are, therefore, particularly prone to the development of SMNs with the latent period relatively short in tumor-prone states.

Epithelial neoplasms such as those of the lung and gastrointestinal tract may take many years to develop because of the limited number of stem cells available for mutation. The majority of epithelial cells exposed to radiation are end-stage cells without the ability to divide. Stem cells, capable of division in visceral organs, usually divide to produce only one undifferentiated stem cell and one mature end-stage cell. Other factors such as chronic inflammation or certain dietary constituents are required to expand this type of stem cell population. SMNs from these cell types (e.g., of the lungs, gastrointestinal tract, and genitourinary tract) generally occur at longer latent periods.

Table 16-1
Second Malignant Neoplasms

SMN	Predisposing Factor	Other	Signs and Symptoms	Recommended Follow-up
Bone or soft tissue sarcoma	RT	Doses > 3000 cGy; adolescents	Pain or mass in irradiated area	Radiograph, other imaging baseline every 5 years or if symptoms arise
	Retinoblastoma	Familial and bilateral cases		
	Li-Fraumeni syndrome	Family history may be revealing; constitutional p53 mutation(?)		
	Neurofibromatosis (NF)	Diagnosis based on clinical findings; influence of RT not established		
Pineoblastoma	Retinoblastoma	Bilateral and familial cases	Change in sleep pattern	
Brain tumor	RT	Younger children at greater risk	Seizures, headaches, altered mental status	Neuroimaging baseline then prn symptoms
	NF			
	Nevoid basal cell carcinoma syndrome	Ionizing RT increases risk and shortens latent period		
Thyroid	RT	Younger children at greater risk	Enlarged thyroid, nodules	Ultrasound, baseline, then prn symptoms ^{131}I-scan

Breast	RT	Preadolescent females; interaction with family history (?)	Breast mass	Mammography at age 25 every 2 years to age 40 then every year biopsy prn mass
Skin	RT	Ionizing RT increases risk and shortens latent period	} New lesion or change in skin color or texture	} Biopsy
	Nevoid basal cell carcinoma syndrome			
	Xeroderma pigmentosum	Risk associated with ultraviolet light		
Leukemia	Alkylating agents	Dose response; melphalan > nitrogen mustard > cyclophosphamide; associated with chromosome 5 and 7 abnormalities	} Pallor, bruising, fatigue, petechiae	} Complete blood count annually. Bone marrow evaluation for symptoms
	Epipodophyllotoxins	Associated with 11q23 abnormality; schedule or dose dependent (?)		
	NF	Juvenile chronic myelogenous leukemia (JCML) most common; xanthomas; may develop monosomy 7		

Important factors for the evaluation of risk of radiation-associated SMN in a long-term survivor include the dose of radiation, number of fractions, age at exposure, source of energy, other therapies used in conjunction with radiation, and underlying genetic predisposition.

Studies have demonstrated an increasing risk of cancer with increasing doses of radiation. For patients with bone and soft tissue sarcomas treated with doses greater than 30 Gy, the risk of secondary bone sarcomas is more than 100 times expected.[19] An exception to this dose relationship appears to be leukemia as an SMN; in the LESG studies no increase in leukemia was noted following doses greater than 10 Gy.[22] However, lower doses of radiation have been associated with an increased risk of leukemia in survivors of the atomic bomb.

Risk according to radiation schedule has not yet been quantified; however, it seems that increased numbers of fractions may produce more mutation because active cells are hit more often. For a given dose of radiation, megavoltage is believed to be less oncogenic than orthovoltage because the bone absorbs a higher dose with the latter; however, substantiation for this is difficult to find.

Younger age at exposure to a given dose of radiation has been shown to increase susceptibility to SMN. Children under 6 years who received cranial irradiation for leukemia were more likely to develop brain tumors[14]; children under 5 years who received irradiation that included the neck were more likely to develop thyroid cancer.[20]

In the case of breast cancer as SMN, children who receive chest irradiation during the second decade of life when mammary tissue is proliferating may be more likely to develop breast cancer than those who receive chest irradiation for neuroblastoma, Wilms' tumor, and other primary tumors early in childhood.[12]

Alkylating agents and anthracyclines have been implicated in increasing the risk of radiation-associated bone sarcomas[4,19] and decreasing the interval between treatment and SMN, respectively.[15]

CHEMOTHERAPY

Antimetabolites such as mercaptopurine, methotrexate, and thioguanine are not known to be directly carcinogenic, although some may behave as cocarcinogens. Vinca alkaloids, steroids, and antibiotics such as dactinomycin and doxorubicin have also not been implicated in increasing the risk of SMN except as noted above in association with RT. Alkylating agents, however, are well-known leukemogens. Nitrogen mustard, procarbazine, nitrosoureas (carmustine) and, to a lesser degree, cyclophosphamide are associated with the development of leukemias.[3] The latent period for the development of these secondary leukemias is relatively short, ranging from 3 to 10 years. A dose-response relationship has been established for alkylating agents and secondary leukemias, which are usually myeloid. Non-Hodgkin's lymphomas also occur.

The epipodophyllotoxins, etoposide and teniposide, have been in use for the treatment of childhood cancer for about 10 years. They are now emerging as the newest leukemogenic class of agents, increasing the risk of secondary myeloid leukemia.[16,17] The schedule of administration appears to be a significant factor in the risk. Intermittent administration (less than every 2 weeks) of these agents in children with ALL was associated with low frequencies of myeloid leukemia. On the other hand, twice weekly and weekly schedules led to a higher risk of secondary AML.[17] The forms of AML seen after alkylating agents and epipodophyllotoxins differ. The AML seen after alkylating-agent therapy often shows chromosome 5 and 7 deletions, but a monocytic form occurs following the epipodophyllotoxins, often with an 11q23 abnormality.

Although surveillance of children who have received potentially leukemogenic therapy seems prudent, at the present time it is doubtful that earlier detection can lead to an improved outcome. Although excessive concern on the part of the physician may have a negative psychologic effect, an abnormal blood count in an individual treated with these agents should arouse the suspicion of caregivers and further evaluation should be initiated.

PREDISPOSITION

Most of what is known about the genetic risk for SMN comes from our knowledge of retinoblastoma. Patients with bilateral disease, a positive family history of retinoblastoma or chromosome 13q14 deletion have the highest rate of SMNs.[4,5,12] These subsets include approximately 25%, 10%, and 5% of the retinoblastoma cases, respectively.[2,8] Patients with a negative family history, unilateral disease, and no visible 13q14 abnormality can develop SMN as a consequence of a new germline mutation but give no history or signs so that realistic counseling is also necessary for such individuals. The majority of soft tissue SMNs in retinoblastoma patients occur in the field of irradiation, although bone tumors also develop outside the field of irradiation. These bone SMNs are either osteosarcomas or chondrosarcomas, although malignant fibrous histiocytomas of bone are also seen.[4,5,12]

The retinoblastoma gene also predisposes to pineoblastoma, so called trilateral retinoblastoma. Although not a true SMN, since the pineal gland is composed of the same photoreceptor cells as the retina, pineoblastomas occur in a subset of genetic (primarily familial) cases, usually before 5 years of age.[1]

Although not yet determined, it is possible that children with the genetic forms of Wilms' tumor, neuroblastoma, and other embryonal tumors will also prove to be at greater risk than nongenetic cases for the development of SMNs. It seems prudent to follow more carefully survivors of bilateral or multifocal Wilms' tumor and neuroblastoma, as well as those survivors with any congenital anomaly.

Other genetic conditions appear to predispose children to multiple neoplasms. Neurofibromatosis (NF1) is one such condition with a known increased cancer risk.[18] This condition is dominantly inherited and predisposes to neurofibrosarcomas, CNS tumors, and JCML. The gene for this condition has recently been cloned and is located on chromosome 17q. The diagnosis of NF1, however, continues to be based on clinical findings and often requires a complete examination of the patient. The influence of radiation in increasing or decreasing the risk of SMN in NF1 patients has not yet been determined.

The Li-Fraumeni syndrome, also a dominantly inherited condition, has received much attention recently because of the association between this syndrome and a germline mutation in the p53 gene in several affected families.[11] The clinical picture is one of breast cancer, bone and soft tissue sarcomas, brain tumors, and leukemias occurring in several generations of family members. A negative family history does not rule out this syndrome, however, since individuals can acquire the gene as a new germline mutation. Consequently, when an individual develops two or more of the tumors found in the syndrome, it should be suspected.[10] There is presently no consensus regarding the real risk of cancer in individuals who carry a mutation of the p53 gene, and therefore no recommendations for screening or counseling can be made.[9] On the other hand, individuals in families in which the abnormal gene has been identified appreciate careful follow-up.

Other rare diseases with increased risk of multiple neoplasms include xeroderma pigmentosum and the nevoid basal cell carcinoma syndrome.[12] The latter condition predisposes to medulloblastoma, basal cell carcinoma, and ovarian fibromata, with ionizing radiation increasing the risk and shortening the latent period. In the former disorder, the risk for basal and squamous cell carcinoma, fibrosarcoma, and melanoma are increased, and these tumors are associated with exposure to ultraviolet light.

SUMMARY

For survivors of childhood cancer, the possibility of developing another cancer later in life may evoke an image somewhat different from others in the general population. As they themselves have been cured and have conquered an earlier illness, survivors may view the possibility as less threatening than it might be to those who see cancer as an inevitable struggle with pain and death. Some survivors are imbued with a sense of immortality as they have already overcome a serious illness earlier in their lives. There are those, however, who carry with them the fears and the uncertainties faced earlier, and they continue to do so throughout their lives. For many, it is not possible to separate the fear of a new cancer from the fear of a recurrence of the earlier illness, and these concerns blend together in their minds.

It is evident that several factors may contribute to a childhood cancer survivor's risk for the development of an SMN. Practitioners need to be aware of the known risk factors and of their patients' treatment so that more directed follow-up may lead to earlier diagnosis and intervention for a potentially curable neoplasm. The education of survivors should include information concerning the possibility that a new malignant neoplasm will arise. This education does not take place at a single visit but rather requires considerable reinforcement and reiteration over several years of follow-up clinic encounters. In addition to providing some balanced view of their future risk of new cancer, these long-term follow-up visits need to provide guidance for the patient with regard to his or her own role in early detection and prevention. A thorough annual physical examination with detailed history taking are integral components of follow-up care. The purpose of this is to establish the background with which to compare any changes that may occur in the future. In addition, careful history taking can help the practitioner elicit subtle signs and symptoms that will lead to appropriate studies and thereby define a potential problem in a timely manner. No one can imagine that a single annual visit will serve to uncover or detect a new malignant disease in a patient who has not experienced any symptoms or signs suggestive of illness. We view these annual visits as health assessment periods, wherein the status of the patient at a given point in time is recorded carefully and any late effects are specifically discussed. This provides a baseline for both the physician and the survivor, so that, should problems develop in the interval between visits, both will be aware of any changes that require further evaluation.

There are ways and means of reducing one's lifetime cancer risk, even in a generally susceptible population. Counseling survivors of childhood cancer should include the promotion of healthful life-styles such as not smoking, eating a well-balanced diet, and avoiding other risk-taking behaviors. This requires emphasis during annual visits, not merely because certain behaviors may actually decrease the survivor's subsequent risk of cancer, but because they are also positive means of investing the survivor with a measure of control and encouraging the development of a positive view of the future.

Many survivors have heard that, because of their prior disease or their treatment, they are at very much increased risk of developing new cancers. Although this may be true in the aggregate, and is certainly so for subsets of patients, there are many children who have been cured and whose risk for SMN is no greater than that in the general population. Patients themselves as they reach young adulthood should be cognizant of their medical history, particularly related to their own cancer and its treatment. They best can alert practitioners who care for them to their special needs.

REFERENCES

1. Bader JL et al: Bilateral retinoblastoma with ectopic intracranial retinoblastoma: trilateral retinoblastoma, *Cancer Genet Cytogenet* 5:203-213, 1982.
2. Bunin GR et al: Frequency of 13q abnormalities among 203 patients with retinoblastoma, *J Natl Cancer Inst* 81:370-374, 1989.
3. Curtis RE et al: Risk of leukemia after chemotherapy and radiation for breast cancer, *N Engl J Med* 326:1745-1751, 1992.
4. Draper GJ, Sanders BM, Kingston JE: Second primary neoplasms in patients with retinoblastoma, *Br J Cancer* 53:661-671, 1986.
5. Eng C et al: Mortality from second tumors among long-term survivors of retinoblastoma, *Cancer Res* (in press).
6. Hawkins MM, Draper GJ, Kingston JE: Incidence of second primary tumors among childhood cancer survivors, *Br J Cancer* 56:339-347, 1987.
7. Hildreth NG, Shore RE, Dvoretsky PM: The risk of breast cancer after irradiation of the thymus in infancy, *N Engl J Med* 321:1281-1284, 1989.
8. Knudson AG: Mutation and cancer: statistical study of retinoblastoma, *Proc Natl Acad Sci USA* 68:820-823, 1971.

9. Li FP, Fraumeni JF: Predictive testing for inherited mutations in cancer-susceptibility genes, *J Clin Oncol* 10:1203-1204, 1992 (editorial).

10. Malkin D et al: Germline mutations of the p53 tumor-suppressor gene in children and young adults with second malignant neoplasms, *N Engl J Med* 326:1309-1315, 1992.

11. Malkin D et al: Germ line p53 mutations in a familial syndrome of breast cancer, sarcomas, and other neoplasms, *Science* 250:1333-1338, 1990.

12. Meadows AT, Baum E, Fossati-Bellani F et al: Second malignant neoplasms in children: an update from the Late Effects Study Group, *J Clin Oncol* 3:532-538, 1985.

13. Meadows AT et al: Second malignant neoplasms following childhood Hodgkin's disease: treatment and splenectomy as risk factors, *Med Pediatr Oncol* 17:477-484, 1989.

14. Neglia JP et al: Second neoplasms after acute lymphoblastic leukemia in childhood, *N Engl J Med* 325:1330-1336, 1991.

15. Newton WA et al: Bone sarcomas as second malignant neoplasms following childhood cancer, *Cancer* 67:193-201, 1991.

16. Pui CH et al: Myeloid noeplasia in children treated for solid tumors, *Lancet* 336:417-421, 1990.

17. Pui CH et al: Acute myeloid leukemia in children treated with epipodophyllotoxins for acute lymphoblastic leukemia, *N Engl J Med* 325:1682-1687, 1991.

18. Schneider M et al: Childhood neurofibromatosis: risk factors for malignant disease, *Cancer Genet Cytogenet* 21:347-354, 1986.

19. Tucker MA et al: Bone sarcomas linked to radiotherapy and chemotherapy in children, *N Engl J Med* 317:588-593, 1987.

20. Tucker MA et al: Therapeutic radiation at a young age is linked to secondary thyroid cancer, *Cancer Res* 51:2885-2888, 1991.

21. Tucker MA et al: *Cancer risk following treatment of childhood cancer.* In Fraumeni JF, Boice JD, editors: *Radiation carcinogenesis: epidemiology and biological significance,* New York, 1984, Raven Press.

22. Tucker MA et al: Leukemia after therapy with alkylating agents for childhood cancer, *J Natl Cancer Inst* 78:459-464, 1987.

17

Issues in Survivorship

Kathleen S. Ruccione

Childhood cancer survivors and their parents often express concerns about the ability to marry and have healthy children; psychologic normalcy; schooling; relationships with family and friends; employment discrimination; the possibility of obtaining insurance; and access to future good medical care.[3,20] These concerns are the subject of this chapter.

PSYCHOSOCIAL CONCERNS

Normalization

The overriding psychosocial issue faced by childhood cancer survivors and their families is normalization.[19] Normalization implies incorporation of cancer as part of one's life history. It includes an ability to decide when disclosure of a cancer history to new acquaintances (e.g., in dating relationships) is appropriate and comfortable. A number of studies have shown that normalization may be aided by the ability to find meaning in the illness and survival.[5,8] The search for meaning, sparked at the time of diagnosis, may persist well into the decades of survival. However, as individuals live with the uncertainty and compromise imposed by the cancer, the question "Why me?" may be difficult to bring to resolution.

Living with Uncertainty

Living with uncertainty and living with compromise are two issues conceptualized by Fitzhugh Mullen, a physician and cancer survivor.[15] Some survivors of childhood cancer may respond to uncertainty with a heightened sense of vulnerability. The lingering fear of recurrence—the sense of living "with one foot on a banana peel"—may be expressed through hypervigilance and fear that any sign of illness signifies the return of the cancer. In the pediatric setting, overprotectiveness is a common response of parents to their perceptions of a child's vulnerability.[6] Some people manage uncertainty through denial, increased risk-taking behavior, or an inability to plan for the future.

Living with uncertainty can be a transforming experience. Survivors and their families have reported that their experience with life-threatening illness led them to reorder their priorities in life, redefine their goals, and reconsider their values. Several studies have reported that positive things can be gained from the experience, as Susan Nessim has observed: "a whittling away of the inessential in life, heightened appreciation of family and friends, new insights into the depth of our spiritual strength, physical resiliency, and courage."[16] Positive aspects of survival have been noted in several studies, as has support for the notion that most survivors are resilient and generally well adjusted.[7,8,17]

Living with Compromise

Learning how to live with compromise is a particular challenge because of the myth that following diagnosis and treatment of cancer, survivors can pick up where they left off.[4] This myth fails to acknowledge or legitimize the necessary losses imposed by biologic cure and the developmental disruptions cancer causes in young people. Living with compromise can have repercussions in self-concept, self-esteem, body image, and other aspects of personal life. Relationships with family, friends, and significant others often must be renegotiated. Old friends may disappear, but new friendships may grow. Some of the negative aspects of recovery noted in several studies include health concerns and concerns about late effects,[8,11,17] the need for continued adaptation to permanent disabilities after the cancer is cured,[12] feelings of being different,[14] and parents' marital or family adjustment problems (including marital stress in parents).[7]

Although it might be predicted that survivors with marked or residual physical disability would have a more difficult adjustment, results of studies in this area are inconclusive. Marriage and family decisions, one indicator of adult adjustment, have been studied, but findings are conflicting, perhaps because of differences in conduct of the studies. In the largest study reported, Byrne and colleagues interviewed 2506 cancer survivors and 3266 matched sibling controls and found that survivors were slightly less likely to marry than controls, with survivors of brain tumors least likely to marry.[2]

Overcoming Stigma

The stigma of cancer still exists and is a major hurdle for many survivors because, according to van Eys, as long as survivors are viewed as "strangers in a strange land," as persons rescued from the dead, they may be received with open arms but by virtue of their special status excluded from society.[18] Stigmatization places blame with the victim; it is a way of regarding people as different and a justification for treating them differently. Stigma is one of the reasons that some people feel the term survivor should be discarded, and in some centers the term graduate is being used instead.

For children who survive cancer, the biggest social hurdles to overcome are initially in school, and later, in the workplace. Public education, lobbying, and legal action are required to overcome general misconceptions and to deal with specific instances of discrimination. The public perception of the cancer survivor must become consistent with the improved treatment and outcome, with acceptance of the philosophy underlying the Cancer Survivors' Bill of Rights of the American Cancer Society (1988). Its four major precepts are that (1) survivors have the right to assurance of lifelong medical care; (2) in their personal lives, survivors, like other Americans, have the right to the pursuit of happiness; (3) in the workplace, survivors have the right to equal job opportunities; and (4) since health insurance coverage is an overriding survivorship concern, every effort should be made to assure all survivors adequate health insurance, whether public or private.

THE "PARTNERSHIP OF EMPOWERMENT"

Improving psychosocial aspects of survival after childhood cancer challenges health care providers to work with patients and families, as well as peer-support organizations, in what Monaco calls a "partnership of empowerment"[13] affecting several key areas of practice.

Preparation for Survival Begins Early

The issues in survivorship do not wait for an arbitrary 5-year mark. Patients and families must be assessed from the day of diagnosis onward. Assessment takes into account the general risk factors for personal and emotional problems, including temporal clustering of stressful medical and life events (the "pile up" of stresses); a cluster of poverty, ethnicity, and single-adult family structure; poor prior coping resources; preexisting emotional problems or family discord; extent of disease, treatment modality, and degree of physical distress or residual disability; and a lack of social support.[1,10] Thorough assessment demands an up-to-date knowledge base about potential long-term complications, as well as clinical expertise in detecting abnormalities. Physicians and nurses caring for children with cancer need to be well grounded in growth and development to promote normalization.[9]

Psychologic Cure: Education, Counseling, and Advocacy

From the beginning, patient and family education, counseling, and advocacy can make a difference in the quality and nature of long-term survival. For example, school reentry soon after diagnosis facilitates reintegration into normal life activities. Survivors who are informed about the possible biologic late effects may not experience or may be better prepared for the anger felt by many of the childhood cancer "pioneers," whose late effects were not foreseen. Families who understand that fears of recurrence and feelings of loss and grief are normal and are part of the recovery process will be better prepared for the future.

Learning trajectories, topics, resources. From diagnosis onward, anticipatory guidance about the disease, treatment, and likely aftereffects must be given. This information should be clarified, reinforced, and reinterpreted over time. Risk information changes, as does survivors' readiness to listen and make use of the information. Children, in particular, need to be taught and retaught in ways appropriate to their changing cognitive abilities. The box on p. 333 highlights topics that need to be included in patient and family education. Examples of print resources for survivors are given in Table 17-1. There is a continuing need for well-designed and well-evaluated educational materials for use in pediatric and low-literacy populations.

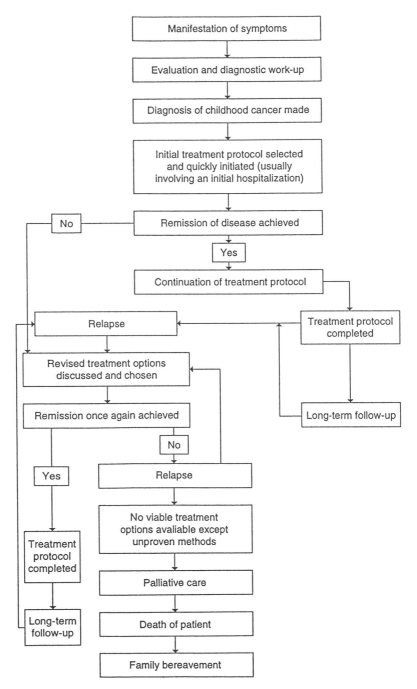

Fig. 17-1. Schema of potential medical milestones and psychosocial crises associated with childhood cancer.

Suggested Curriculum for Patient and Family Education

Pertinent summary of health history, including:
  Name of disease
  Date of diagnosis
  Date(s) and place of treatment
  Responsible physician/nurse
  Chemotherapeutic and/or biologic agents received
  Primary site, organs removed at surgery if any
  Amount of radiation therapy, areas treated if any
  Type of BMT, if any
  Any major treatment complications
Anticipated potential complications, and recommended medical follow-up
General health recommendations, according to American Cancer Society guidelines
Names, addresses of organizations providing information, support to survivors
How to notify treatment center of change of address and/or results of tests performed
  outside original treatment center

Reprinted from Ruccione K: Survivorship needs and issues after treatment for childhood cancer. *Proceedings of the sixth national conference on cancer nursing,* Atlanta, 1992, American Cancer Society.
BMT = Bone marrow transplant.

Table 17-1
Selected Recent Print Materials about Cancer Survivorship

Title and Author	Source
After the Storm (Dasenbrock AI, Flynn BE, Kitson JK)	The Derald Ruttenberg Cancer Center Box 1129 1 Gustave Levy Place New York, NY 10029
An Almanac of Practical Resources for Cancer Survivors (Mullan F, Hoffman B, editors.)	Consumer Reports Books 9180 LeSaint Drive Fairfield, OH 45014-5452
Cancer Survivorship: An Annotated Bibliography	National Cancer Institute NIH Publication No. 91-3173 1-800-4-CANCER
Cancervive: The Challenge of Life after Cancer (Nessim S, Ellis J)	Houghton Mifflin Company 2 Park Street Boston, MA 02108
Facing Forward: A Guide for Cancer Survivors	National Cancer Institute NIH Publication No. 90-2424 1-800-4-CANCER
Life in the Shadow: Living with Cancer (Soiffer B)	Chronicle Books 275 5th Street San Francisco, CA 94103

Continued.

Table 17-1
Selected Recent Print Materials about Cancer Survivorship—cont'd

Title and Author	Source
The Networker (newsletter)	National Coalition for Cancer Survivorship (NCCS) 1010 Wayne Ave., Fifth Floor Silver Spring, MD 20910 1-301-230-0831
Surviving (newsletter focusing on survivors of Hodgkin's disease)	Stanford University Medical Center Department of Radiology Division of Radiation Therapy, Room H013 300 Pasteur Drive Stanford, CA 94305
Taking Care of Yourself for Life: Your Personal Long-Term Follow-Up Guide and Treatment Record (Ruccione K, Hobbie W)	Kathie Ruccione, RN, MPH Children's Hospital of Los Angeles Division of Pediatric Hematology/Oncology Mail Stop 54, 4650 Sunset Boulevard Los Angeles, CA 90027
Taking Charge of Your Health: A Guide to Cancer Prevention for Men (Women) Who Had Cancer in Childhood. Part 1. (Meadows AT, Gallagher J, Jarrett P, Blumberg B)	Childrens Hospital of Philadelphia 34th and Civic Center Boulevard Philadelphia, PA 19104
Taking Charge of Your Health: A Guide to Medical Follow-Up for Adults Who Had Cancer in Childhood (Meadows AT, Gallagher J, Jarrett P, Blumberg B)	Childrens Hospital of Philadelphia 34th and Civic Center Boulevard Philadelphia, PA 19104
Taking Control: 10 Steps to a Healthier Life and Reduced Cancer Risk	American Cancer Society Publication No. 2019.05 1599 Clifton Road, NE Atlanta, GA 30329 1-404-320-3333
Tips on Health Insurance for Long-Term Survivors (Candlelighters Childhood Cancer Foundation Youth Newsletter vol. XIV, no. 1, Spring 1992)	Candlelighters Childhood Cancer Foundation 7910 Woodmont Ave., Suite 460 Bethesda, MD 20814 1-800-366-2223

Adapted from Ruccione K: Survivorship needs and issues after treatment for childhood cancer. *Proceedings of the sixth national conference on cancer nursing*, Atlanta, 1992, American Cancer Society.

Exit interviews. Many families experience very high anxiety during the period surrounding the completion of treatment, typically about 2 years after diagnosis. It is not unusual for families to relate that they were no more prepared for treatment to be finished than they were for the diagnosis in the first place. For this reason, some treatment teams offer patients and families exit interviews to address the issues and concerns that arise at this phase of survival.

Health passports. The value of ongoing health observation and maintenance must be conveyed. Annual checkups including an interval history and physical examination are essential. Additional specific follow-up guidelines should be individually tailored, based on the disease and treatment. Some treatment centers provide a "health passport" that summarizes the individual's disease and treatment history and includes recommendations for follow-up. Health passports may help survivors to be knowledgeable ambassadors to the world of adult health care. A vital part of the health teaching for survivors is health promotion and risk reduction to help minimize the chances of the preventable late effects and malignancy in the future.

Staying in touch. We need to make sure survivors understand why it is important for them to stay in touch with their original cancer treatment center or, if they have moved, a center involved in the same treatment regimens (with transfer of the detailed records). Most centers are—or will be—participating in long-range follow-up to learn more about disease and treatment sequelae. This new information can then be passed on to the survivors in a timely manner. In addition, cancer survivors continue to teach physicians and nurses about the long-term effects of therapy through their own observations and insights.

Counseling. Another part of appropriate rehabilitation is counseling. For most survivors, early referrals should be made to peer-support groups located in treatment centers or in the surrounding community. Such groups or one-on-one links between newer patients and long-term survivors can provide the buffering effect of social support with others who have gone through similar experiences. Peer support and networking are available in many areas of the country through the Candlelighters Childhood Cancer Foundation; under its auspices, there are parent peer-support groups, adolescent peer groups, and a network of adult survivors of childhood cancer.[13]

Ideally, a comprehensive rehabilitation program also refers individuals with high levels of psychologic distress to a therapist who is comfortable working with childhood cancer survivors and their families and who is familiar with the medical situations they face. Some treatment centers provide social skills training programs for children and adolescents to enable them to be assertive and overcome awkwardness resulting from their cancer experience, as well as school reentry and advocacy programs. These services may help prevent or mitigate long-term psychosocial complications.

As long-term follow-up clinics are established, an important function is to identify a cadre of knowledgeable counselors willing to be part of a referral network. "Drop-in" support groups for survivors and their significant others, available in some treatment centers, enable survivors to share and learn from mutual feelings and experiences. In addition to survivor support groups, support groups that focus on separate but related issues such as genetic conditions or infertility can be helpful.

Advocacy. Advocacy means that survivors and their families need to know that they have the potential for effective social change. Valuable resources for information and support, and to change public opinion, include the treatment center and such organizations as the Candlelighters Childhood Cancer Foundation, the National Coalition for Cancer Survivorship, the American Cancer Society, and the National Cancer Institute. In sheer numbers, cancer survivors have the potential to be a strong and effective political voice. Events such as National Cancer Survivors Day in June help make that voice heard.

Advocacy also means finding ways, in an era of cost containment, that treatment centers can provide coordinated care for survivors. Many treatment centers tell survivors they want to follow them for life, but few have organized surveillance programs for survivors. Among the logistic hurdles to overcome in providing services are the necessity for additional staffing and space. The role of the primary attending physician must be determined. Other challenges include adult survivors. The needs of adult survivors may include expanded ambulatory service hours, a different setting than one in which children are undergoing active treatment, and a referral network of adult medical practitioners. Exemplar programs do exist, however, and they can provide models and consultation to help health care providers, working with survivors, families, peer organizations, and with clinical administrators, meet the challenge of life-long monitoring given the constraints of limited resources.

Many Unanswered—and Researchable—Questions About Survivorship Remain

As treatment protocols evolve and more individuals survive more aggressive therapies, the constellation of potential biologic long-term effects may change, and this may affect survivors' psychosocial responses. Prospective longitudinal collaborative studies are needed; previous research has been limited by a lack of sensitive instruments and appropriate control groups. Nurses can make a unique contribution to research in this area because of their role as case managers who provide continuity of care over long periods, allowing for the establishment of trust and communication. Patients must be assured that the health care providers understand the cost of biologic cure and that it is acceptable and desirable to discuss all long-term concerns, including those of a psychosocial nature. Patients should not be viewed as ungrateful if they complain about the effects of curative therapies.

These psychosocial issues and suggestions for care are based on the notion, stated by Monaco, that "Life is a hollow gift unless cancer survivors emerge from treatment as competent and worthy individuals, able to obtain insurance, equipped to earn a living, and prepared to participate in a medical surveillance program to 'keep' the life they have won."[13]

REFERENCES

1. Barbarin OA: Psychosocial risks and invulnerability: a review of the theoretical and empirical bases of preventive family-focused services for survivors of childhood cancer, *J Psychosocial Oncol* 5:25-41, 1987.

2. Byrne J et al: Effects of treatment on fertility in long-term survivors of childhood or adolescent cancer, *N Engl J Med* 317:1315-1321, 1987.

3. Chesler M, Lozowski S: Problems and needs of children off treatment: Candlelighters research and proposed programs, *Candlelighters Childhood Cancer Foundation Quarterly Newsletter* 12:1-3, 1988.

4. Christ GH: Social consequences of the cancer experience, *Am J Pediatr Hemat Oncol* 9:84-88, 1987.

5. Comaroff J, Maguire P: Ambiguity and the search for meaning: childhood leukaemia in the modern clinical context, *Soc Sci Med* 15B:115-123, 1981.

6. Green M, Solnit A: Reactions to the threatened loss of a child: a vulnerable child syndrome, *Pediatrics* 34:58-66, 1964.

7. Greenberg HS, Kazak AE, Meadows AT: Psychological functioning in cancer survivors, *J Pediatr* 114:488-493, 1989.

8. Greenberg HS, Meadows AT: Psychosocial impact of cancer survival on school-age children and their parents, *J Psychosocial Oncol* 9:43-56, 1992.

9. Hobbie WL: The role of the pediatric oncology nurse specialist in a follow-up clinic for long term survivors of childhood cancer, *J Assoc Pediatr Oncol Nurs* 3:9-12, 1986.

10. Hymovich DP, Roehnert JE: Psychosocial consequences of childhood cancer, *Semin Oncol Nurs* 5:56-62, 1989.

11. Koocher GP, O'Malley JE: *The Damocles syndrome: psychological consequences of surviving childhood cancer,* New York, 1981, McGraw-Hill.

12. Maher E: Anomic aspects of recovery from cancer, *Social Science & Medicine* 16:907-912, 1982.

13. Monaco GP: The partnership of empowerment: caregivers and survivors, *J Psychosocial Oncol* 10:121-133, 1992.

14. Moore IM, Glazer ME, Ablin AR: The late psychosocial consequences of childhood cancer, *J Pediatr Nurs* 3:150-158, 1987.

15. Mullen F: Re-entry: the educational needs of the cancer survivor, *Health Educ Quarterly (supplement)* 10:88-94, 1984.

16. Nessim S, Ellis J: *Cancervive: the challenge of life after cancer,* Boston, 1991, Houghton Mifflin.

17. Schmale A et al: Well-being of cancer survivors, *Psychosomatic Medicine* 45:163-169, 1983.

18. van Eys J: Living beyond cure: transcending survival, *Am J Pediatr Hemat/Oncol* 9:114-118, 1987.

19. van Eys J: The truly cured child? *Pediatrician* 18:90-95, 1991.

20. Wallace MH, Reiter PB, Pendergrass TW: Parents of long-term survivors of childhood cancer: a preliminary survey to characterize concerns and needs, *Oncol Nurs Forum* 14:39-43, 1987.

18

Legal Issues

Barbara Hoffman

A growing number of children in the United States are being diagnosed with and successfully treated for cancer. Approximately 80% of all children diagnosed with cancer in 1990 will become long-term survivors.[1] By the year 2000, 180,000 to 220,000 childhood survivors will reside in the United States.[1] Unlike adult survivors, whose average age of diagnosis is near the retirement ages of 60 to 65, most childhood survivors offer decades of productive employment after cancer.[1]

Although past studies suggest that 25% of all cancer survivors face employment discrimination,[2] current studies and recent changes in federal law suggest that long-term survivors of childhood cancer will experience less discrimination than adult survivors. As we learn more about the working needs and abilities of the increasing numbers of childhood survivors, we can better prepare survivors and their caregivers to address the long-term economic consequences of treatment.

This chapter reviews current studies of employment problems reported by cancer survivors, describes why survivors encounter discrimination not faced by workers with other medical histories, lists legal resources available for those whose rights have been violated, and provides suggestions for reducing such discrimination. This chapter also discusses survivors' rights to health insurance and education.

THE SCOPE OF CANCER-BASED EMPLOYMENT DISCRIMINATION

Cancer Survivors in the Workplace

Two of the earliest studies of workers with a cancer history were conducted by Metropolitan Life Insurance and the Bell Telephone Companies. Between 1959 and 1972, the work performance of Metropolitan Life Insurance employees who had been treated for cancer differed little from that of colleagues of similar age with similar assignments.[16] Turnover, absence, and work performance rates of cancer patients were so satisfactory that the hiring of individuals with a cancer history could be recommended as sound industrial practice. At the time of this study, cancer survival rates were significantly lower than they are today. Of the 1351 Bell Telephone employees with a cancer history, 77% returned to work after their diagnosis and treatment.[13] Several studies have confirmed this rate of continued or reemployment.[3] Mor noted that 78% of white-collar and 63% of blue-collar workers remain in their jobs 12 months after diagnosis.[12]

Cerenex Pharmaceuticals conducted a study of cancer survivors, employees, and supervisors (unpublished, 1992). Of 503 cancer survivors, 60% reported that cancer did not affect their performance and an additional 21% reported that cancer had "very little" effect on their performance. Two thirds of the 201 supervisors surveyed, however, were very or somewhat concerned that an employee with cancer might not perform his or her job adequately. Twenty percent of the survivors reported discrimination, including changed job responsibilities, forced early retirement, denial of expected promotion, and termination after revealing their cancer histories to employers.

The Types of Employment Problems Encountered by Cancer Survivors

Young adult survivors entering the job market for the first time are a rapidly growing population. In 1990, 1 of every 1000 20 year olds was estimated to have been a childhood cancer survivor.[15] Although childhood survivors may not enter the job market for years or decades after their diagnosis, the history of cancer has the potential to affect employability at all career stages. Some disparate treatments, such as blanket hiring bans against all individuals with a cancer history, are irrational and blatantly discriminatory. Other employment decisions, especially actions by legally sophisticated employers, are far more subtle. As many as 20% to 45% of childhood survivors have encountered cancer-related barriers to employment.[4,10] Because childhood survivors must first enter the workplace, they are more concerned with how to obtain a job than with how to keep a job. Young survivors who are either employed or active in the labor market are more concerned than are older survivors about revealing their cancer history when searching for a job.[6]

The employment problems of cancer survivors take many forms. In a study of 403 survivors of Hodgkin's disease, Fobair reported a variety of job problems, including denial of a job offer (12%); denial of insurance (11%); denial of other benefits (6%); termination of employment following therapy (6%); conflict with supervisors or co-workers (12%); and rejection by the military (8%).[5] Eight of 40 (20%) survivors of childhood or adolescent Hodgkin's disease surveyed by Wasserman reported job discrimination.[15] Koocher and O'Malley found that 15 of 60 survivors of childhood cancer reported employment discrimination: 10 persons were refused a job at least once; 3 were denied benefits; 3 experienced illness-related conflict with supervisor; 4 reported job task problems; and 11 were rejected by the military.[10] Cancer may have a greater impact on blue-collar workers than on white-collar workers. Of white-collar respondents interviewed by Feldman, 54% described work problems that they attributed to the diagnosis of cancer, compared with 84% of the blue-collar respondents.[4]

Teta compared childhood cancer survivors with their siblings.[14] Of male survivors, 80% experienced rejection from the military, compared with 18% of their siblings. Thirty-two percent were rejected from nonmilitary job opportunities, compared with 19% of their siblings. Female survivors also faced disproportionate rejection from the military (75%, compared with 13% for their siblings), but the rejection rate from nonmilitary employment was the same for survivors as for their siblings (19%).

A recent survey by Hays suggests that long-term survivors of childhood cancer have few economic consequences of their cancer histories.[7] Hays surveyed 219 childhood survivors and matched controls who were treated between 1945 and 1975 and were at least 30 years old at the time of the survey. He found that childhood survivors, with the exception of survivors of central nervous system tumors, experienced relatively the same employment history as the controls. The controls, however, reported somewhat more annual income than did the survivors. Hays's results suggest that as the length of time between diagnosis and initial employment increases, the incidence of discrimination may decrease.

Only those survivors who sought entry into the military faced increased rates of discrimination (15.2% of survivors at one institute and 20.7% at another, versus 7.7% and 1.8% respectively of the controls). Although the Department of Defense presumes cancer survivors to be unfit for military service, it considers waivers on a case-by-case basis for childhood cancer survivors who have been out of treatment and cancer free for 5 years (2 years for Wilms' tumor and germ cell tumors of the testes).

WHY CANCER SURVIVORS FACE EMPLOYMENT DISCRIMINATION

The work experiences of cancer survivors suggest that the reasons for disparate treatment are rooted in myths about cancer, three of which have an impact on survivors' employment opportunities.

One myth is that cancer is a death sentence. Mellette found that in informal word association tests one of the most common thoughts associated with the word "cancer" is the word "death."[11] The impact of the death sentence myth is that employers are hesitant to invest in an individual whose death they believe is imminent; insurance companies increase rates or refuse to insure at all, banks deny loans, and society disallows long-term planning on the assumption of a short-term life.

The second myth is that cancer is contagious. For example, one man in Wasserman's study reported that he "was transferred from his job in a hotel kitchen for fear that he might 'contaminate' the food."[15] The impact of the contagion myth is that fellow workers physically and emotionally isolate those with cancer and employers succumb to co-workers' demands to fire or transfer cancer survivors.

The third myth is that cancer survivors are an unproductive drain on the economy. For example, a senior executive in a large corporation who had demonstrated to his employer that he could perform his job while undergoing radiation therapy for Hodgkin's disease was nonetheless forced to resign because his superior feared he would no longer be a productive executive.[8] The impact of

How to avoid employment discrimination

Do not volunteer cancer history.
Do not lie about medical history.
Keep focus on current health and ability.
Be prepared with letter from physician.
Seek employment with large employers.
Do not ask about health benefits prior to job offer.

Steps to take if confronted with discrimination

Consider resolving problem informally.
Suggest accommodations.
Seek support from health care providers, co-workers, legal resources, and other
    survivors.
Keep written records of actions.
Be aware of filing deadlines.
Carefully evaluate goals.

the unproductive worker myth is that the employed are fired, demoted, and denied benefits; the unemployed are faced with remaining so or considering lying about their medical history to obtain a new job; and the underemployed are drained of their self-esteem. The fact is that cancer survivors have relatively the same productivity rates as other workers.[3]

HOW TO COMBAT CANCER-BASED DISCRIMINATION

When Cancer-Based Discrimination is Illegal

Under federal law, and many state laws, an employer cannot treat a survivor differently from other workers in job-related activities because of a history of cancer as long as the survivor is qualified for the job. Individuals are protected by these laws only if 1) they can do the major duties of the job in question; *and* 2) their employer treated them differently from other workers in job-related activities because of cancer history.

The Americans with Disabilities Act (ADA) and the Federal Rehabilitation Act prohibit some types of job discrimination by employers, employment agencies, and labor unions against people who have or have had cancer (see box on the next page). On July 26, 1992, the employment provisions of the ADA took effect to cover all employers with 25 or more employees. Employers with 15 or more employees will be covered beginning July 26, 1994.

The ADA was modeled on the Federal Rehabilitation Act of 1973, which covers employers of any size who receive money, equipment, or contracts from the federal government. These employers include schools, hospitals, defense contractors, and state and local governments. The military does not have to obey either federal law, although civilian employees of the Department of Defense are protected.

Americans with Disabilities Act of 1990

What the ADA prohibits

Discrimination based on actual disability, perceived disability, and history of a disability

Which employers are covered by the ADA

Employers with 25+ workers (July 1992 to July 1994)
Employers with 15+ workers (after July 1994)

What the ADA requires

Employer must provide reasonable accommodations.
Employer may ask only job-related medical questions.
Employer may not discriminate because of family illness.
Employer is *not* required to provide health insurance.

How the ADA is enforced

Enforced by the Equal Employment Opportunity Commission (EEOC)
Local EEOC office: 1-800-669-4000
Enforcement information: 1-800-669-EEOC

Additionally, every state has a law that regulates, to some extent, disability-based employment discrimination. Some laws clearly prohibit cancer-based discrimination, although others have never been applied to cancer-based discrimination. State laws also vary as to which employers—public or private, large or small—must obey the law.

The ADA, the Federal Rehabilitation Act, and many state laws prohibit a prospective employer from asking applicants if they have ever had cancer. Under federal law and most state laws, an employer has the right to know only if the applicant is able to do the job at the time of application. A prospective employer may not ask applicants about health history, unless it could affect the applicant's current ability to perform that job. An employer may ask detailed questions about health status only after offering a job.

Federal law and most state laws require an employer to provide reasonable accommodations. An accommodation is a change, such as in work hours or duties, to help employees do their jobs during or after cancer treatment. For example, if the survivor needs to take time off for treatment, the employer may accommodate the survivor by allowing flexible work hours until the survivor completes treatment.

An employer does not have to make changes that would be an undue hardship on the business or other workers. For example, if the employer is a small business that is unable to obtain an insurance policy that will cover the survivor, the employer may not have to provide the survivor the same health benefits provided to other workers. As another example, if the survivor has to miss a substantial amount of work time and the work cannot be performed by a temporary employee, the employer may be able to hire a replacement. What constitutes a reasonable accommodation or an undue hardship depends on the individual circumstances of each case.

Federal law and most state laws protect cancer survivors who do consider themselves "handicapped" if they are treated differently because of their cancer history. The ADA, the Federal Rehabilitation Act, and most state laws prohibit job discrimination against persons who have a handicap, have a history of a handicap, or are regarded by others as having a handicap. Some state laws do not protect most cancer survivors, however, because they protect only people with serious physical handicaps.

A handicap or disability is a major health problem that affects one's ability to do everyday activities, such as drive a car or go to work. Survivors may be covered by these laws if their cancer currently affects their ability to do everyday activities (for example, walking up stairs); if at one time their cancer affected their ability to do everyday activities, but no longer does (for example, during treatment, the survivor could not walk up stairs, but can now); or if their employer believes that their cancer affects their ability to work, even if they believe it does not.

This is only a partial list of possible job-related activities that are illegal if they result from discrimination. Federal law and most state laws prohibit discrimination that results in not hiring an applicant for a job or training program; firing a worker; providing unequal pay, working conditions, and benefits such as pension, vacation time, and health insurance; punishing an employee for filing a discrimination complaint; or screening out disabled employees.

Under some circumstances, an employer may refuse to offer cancer survivors health insurance. At the time of this writing, employers are not required to provide health insurance, but when they choose to provide health insurance, they must do so fairly. For example, if an employer provides health insurance to all employees with jobs similar to a survivor's but does not provide health insurance to the survivor, then the employer's refusal may be considered discrimination under federal and state laws, unless it would cause an undue hardship on the employer. The Americans With Disabilities Act allows insurers to offer coverage based on risk assessment and actuarial data as long as the plan is "bona fide" and "not inconsistent with state law," and restrictions are not used as a "subterfuge" to evade the purposes of the ADA. If the survivor has health insurance through a group plan at work, a federal law—the Employee Retirement Income Security Act (ERISA)—prohibits the employer from firing the survivor to prevent the collection of health benefits.

One unique benefit of the ADA is that it prohibits discrimination based on relationship or association with a "disabled" person. Employers may not assume that an employee's job performance would be affected by the need to care for a family member who has cancer. State laws do not provide this type of protection.

In August 1993, the Family and Medical Leave Act (FMLA) became federal law. The FMLA mandates job security to workers in large companies who must take a leave of absence to care for a seriously ill child, spouse, parent, or self (see box on p. 347). The law requires employers with at least 50 employees to allow 12 weeks of unpaid leave during any 12-month period to care for a seriously ill dependent. Most important to cancer survivors, the FMLA requires employers to continue to provide benefits, including health insurance, during the leave period. Although the law does not guarantee an employee his or her exact job upon return, it does require employers to restore the employee to the same or equivalent position at the end of the leave period. The employee must make reasonable efforts to schedule foreseeable medical care so as not to disrupt the workplace. The FMLA may be enforced by private lawsuit.

HEALTH INSURANCE AND THE LAW

Barriers to Health Insurance

The more years that have elapsed since treatment, the better the chances that childhood cancer survivors can obtain health insurance on the same terms as other Americans (which may be equitable, but not adequate to meet medical needs). Hays found that 81% to 91.9% of long-term childhood survivors were covered as adults by health insurance policies without cancer-related restrictions (compared with 82.3% to 94.6% of the controls).[7] Among survivors, 6.9% to 14.3% described difficulties experienced by their parents in obtaining affordable health insurance for the entire family group during or after the survivor's illness (compared with 5.1% to 9.7% of the controls).[7]

Other surveys of childhood survivors, however, have reported more problems in securing health insurance. Holmes reported that 24% had difficulty in securing insurance.[7] Teta found that 14% of male childhood cancer survivors and 9% of female survivors were rejected for health insurance (as compared with 1% and 0% among the controls).[14] Although no law guarantees that all cancer survivors can buy adequate, affordable health and life insurance, some laws can help survivors secure and maintain health insurance. Survivors who do not have health insurance through a group policy (usually through work) are the most vulnerable. Insurance companies look for ways to save money by rejecting new applications, canceling policies, reducing benefits, increasing premiums, requiring long waiting periods before preexisting conditions are covered by the insurance, and excluding coverage for certain preexisting conditions.

Cancer survivors who have health insurance may find some of their claims rejected because the insurance policy does not cover "experimental treatment." What oncologists consider current standard aggressive cancer treatment is often considered experimental by insurance companies.

The Legal Right to Health Insurance

Currently, no law guarantees a legal right to adequate health insurance. Whether termination from a plan, denial of benefits under a plan, or refusal to issue

Resources

Federal agencies

Department of Education
Clearinghouse on Disability Information
Program Information and Coordination Staff
Room 3132 Switzer Bldg.
Washington, DC 20202
1-202-732-1723 or 1-732-1241
> Provides general information and referral services about disability programs and issues.

Equal Employment Opportunity Commission (EEOC)
Office of Communications and Legislative Affairs
1801 L Street NW
Washington, DC 20507
1-800-669-4000 (to obtain location of regional EEOC)
1-800-669-EEOC (to obtain information on enforcement of ADA)
> Enforces employment provisions of the Americans with Disabilities Act.

Job Accommodation Network
West Virginia University
809 Allen Hall
P.O. Box 6122
Morgantown, WV 26506
1-800-526-7234 or 1-800-ADA-WORK
> Provides information about jobs with accommodations for persons with disabilities.

United States Department of Justice
Coordination and Review Section
Civil Rights Division
P.O. Box 66118
Washington, DC 20530
1-202-724-2235
1-202-724-7678 (for the hearing impaired)
> Provides information about federal agencies that enforce the Rehabilitation Act of 1973.

United States Department of Labor
Pension and Welfare Benefits Administration, Room 5658
200 Constitution Avenue, NW
Washington, DC 20210
> Enforces COBRA.

National nonprofit organizations that provide information about the legal rights of cancer survivors

Candlelighters Childhood Cancer Foundation
7910 Woodmont Ave., Suite 460
Bethesda, MD 20814
1-800-366-2223

Operates a hotline that provides information and services to childhood cancer survivors and their advocates, including assistance with pursuing health insurance claims, employment discrimination problems, waivers into military service, and access to equal education. Candlelighters offers a variety of current publications, including *Insurance—Your Options and Your Child's.*

National Coalition for Cancer Survivorship
1010 Wayne Road, Fifth Floor
Silver Spring, MD 20910
1-301-650-8868

Provides information about legal rights and advocacy services for cancer survivors of all ages. Publications include *"Working It Out: Your Employment Rights as a Cancer Survivor," "Health Insurance and Cancer: What You Need to Know,"* and *"Charting the Journey: An Almanac of Practical Resources for Cancer Survivors."*

Family and Medical Leave Act of 1993

Applies to employers with 50 or more employees
Provides 12 weeks of unpaid leave during any 12-month period to care for seriously ill self, spouse, child, or parent
Requires employer to continue to provide benefits—including health insurance— during the leave period
Requires employer to restore employee to the same or equivalent position at the end of the leave period
Requires employee to make reasonable efforts to schedule foreseeable medical care so as not to disrupt the workplace
Enforced by private lawsuit

---

insurance violates a law is determined by two factors: the terms of the policy and the applicable law (federal law and state law).

Contractual rights. An insurance policy is a contract between the insured and the insurer. If a policyholder pays the premiums but the insurance company refuses to pay benefits (or perform another duty, such as renew the policy) in accordance with the terms of the policy, the policyholder may be able to sue the company for breach of contract.

Federal law. Although no federal law guarantees a right to adequate health insurance, cancer survivors can benefit from one federal law that allows employees

Different federal and state agencies regulate different types of insurers. In most states, insurance departments regulate private companies, including nonprofit insurers like Blue Cross and Blue Shield. Health maintenance organizations are regulated by state and federal law; however, state insurance departments can usually provide all necessary information. Self-insured plans—those financed by private employers or unions—are regulated by the Office of Pension and Welfare Benefits of the United States Department of Labor. Medicaid (MediCal in California) is regulated by state departments of social services. Medicare, Supplemental Security Income, and Social Security Benefits are regulated by the United States Social Security Administration. Veterans' Benefits and CHAMPUS are regulated by the Department of Veterans' Affairs.

to keep the health insurance they obtain at work, even after they are no longer employed.

The Comprehensive Omnibus Budget Reconciliation Act (COBRA) requires employers to offer group medical coverage to employees and their dependents who otherwise would have lost their group coverage because of individual circumstances. Public and private employers with more than 20 employees are required to make continued insurance coverage available to employees who quit, are terminated, or work reduced hours. Employers must extend coverage to surviving, divorced, or separated spouses and to dependent children.

By allowing employees to purchase group insurance coverage for a limited time, COBRA provides valuable time to shop for long-term coverage (18 months for employees; 36 months for dependents). Although employees must now pay for the continued coverage, the employee's rate may not exceed by more than 2 percent the rate set for former co-workers. The insurer must offer coverage regardless of any conditions, such as cancer.

COBRA is enforced by the Pension and Welfare Benefits Administration of the United States Department of Labor. The first step to resolving a COBRA complaint is to try to work out a settlement with the employer. If no adequate solution can be reached, employees may file a complaint with the Department of Labor (see box on p. 346).

State laws. Every state has an insurance commission or department that enforces state regulation of insurance companies. In most states, the commission determines what types of policies must be offered and when rates may be raised. States regulate insurance sold by insurance companies; they do not regulate self-insured policies (policies that companies fund and administer for their own employees). State regulations cover all aspects of health insurance, including rates, policy conditions, termination or reinstatement of coverage, and the scope of coverage and benefits. For example, New York, Michigan, California, Massachusetts, and Illinois are the first states to require insurers to reimburse for prescribed use of off-label cancer drugs that are recognized in the three major compendia or in peer-reviewed literature. Questions about an insurance company's possible violation of a state law should be addressed to the state insurance department.

One half of the states have laws that establish high-risk pools for those who are unable to obtain health insurance because of their medical histories. Risk pools usually provide a package of benefits with a choice of deductibles. Although the premiums are higher than those for individual insurance, most states impose a cap on the amount that can be charged. For individuals with a preexisting condition, most states have a waiting period after the policy is issued and before it will pay benefits. A waiting period of 6 months for preexisting conditions such as cancer is common. Contact your state insurance department for information about local high-risk pools.

RIGHT TO EDUCATION

Some childhood cancer survivors encounter educational barriers because of their cancer histories. Three federal laws provide survivors with equal access to education.

The Individuals with Disabilities Education Act (PL 94-142 and PL 99-457 amendments) requires states to provide children with disabilities a "free and appropriate education" between the ages of 3 and 21. The law includes students with cancer whose medical problems adversely affect their educational performance. For example, children who have had cranial radiation may experience learning disabilities and require special educational services. The school district must design an individual education plan that the family may challenge in court to ensure that the child receives an appropriate education.

Adult survivors of childhood cancer are protected from discrimination by public and private institutions. The Federal Rehabilitation Act prohibits schools that receive federal funding from discriminating against qualified students because of their cancer histories. The ADA, as well as many state antidiscrimination laws, prohibits private schools from such discrimination. For example, a Hodgkin's disease survivor who completed medical school successfully sued a psychiatric institute under New York law for denying her admission to its residency program solely because of her adolescent cancer history.[8]

A GUIDE FOR SURVIVORS

How to Avoid Becoming a Victim of Discrimination

Lawsuits are neither the only nor the best way to fight employment discrimination against cancer survivors. State and federal antidiscrimination laws help cancer survivors in two ways: they discourage discrimination, and they offer remedies when discrimination does occur. These laws, however, should be used as a *last resort* because they can be costly and time consuming and may not result in a fair solution. The first step is to try to avoid discrimination. If that fails, the next step is to attempt a reasonable settlement with the employer. If informal efforts fail, however, a lawsuit may be the most effective next step.

When seeking employment, survivors can take several steps to lessen the chance they will face cancer-based discrimination:

■ Do not volunteer the information that you have or have had cancer unless it directly affects your qualifications for the job. An employer has the right—under accepted business practices, federal law, and laws in most states—to know only if you can perform the major duties of the job.

■ Do not lie on a job or insurance application. If you are hired and your employer later learns that you lied, you may be fired for your dishonesty. Insurance companies may refuse to pay benefits or cancel your coverage.

■ If a job questionnaire asks, "Have you ever had cancer?" or "Have you had surgery in the past 5 years, and if so, for what?" answer truthfully, and then explain your current health and prognosis. Write in the margins if there are no blank lines.

Some suggestions are:

"I have not had cancer for xx years and have a normal life expectancy."

"I am presently fit to perform the duties of the job for which I am applying."

"I currently have no medical condition that would interfere with my ability to perform the duties of the job for which I am applying."

Instead of using the word "cancer," you may consider using the name of the specific type of cancer you have or had (such as "neuroblastoma" or "nephroblastoma") in the hope that the employer will not associate the term with cancer.

■ Apply only for jobs that you are able to do. It is not illegal for an employer to reject you for a job if you are not qualified for it, regardless of your medical history.

■ If you have to explain an educational gap or a long period of unemployment during cancer treatment, if possible, explain it in a way that shows your illness is past and you are in good health and expected to remain healthy. One way to deemphasize a gap in your school or work history because of cancer treatment is to organize your resume by experience and skills instead of by date.

■ Offer your employer a letter from your doctor that explains your current health status, prognosis, and ability to work. Be prepared to educate the interviewer about your cancer and why cancer often does not result in death or disability.

■ Seek help from a job counselor with resume preparation and job interviewing skills. Practice answers to expected questions such as "Why did you miss a year of school?" or "Why did you leave your last job?" Answers to these questions must be honest, but should stress your current qualifications for the job and not past problems, if any, resulting from your cancer experience.

■ If you are interviewing for a job, do not ask about health insurance until after you have been given a job offer. Then ask to see the "benefits package." Prior to accepting the job, review the benefits to make sure they meet your needs.

■ If possible, look for jobs with large employers because they are less likely than small employers to discriminate.

■ Do not discriminate against yourself by assuming you are handicapped. Although cancer treatment leaves some survivors with real physical or mental disabilities, many survivors are capable of performing the same duties and activities as they did prior to diagnosis. With the help of your medical team, make an honest assessment of your abilities in regard to the mental and physical demands of the job.

Fighting Back Against Discrimination

Survivors who suspect that they are being treated differently at work because of their cancer history should consider an informal solution before leaping into a lawsuit. They must walk a careful line to stand up for their legal rights without casting themselves as troublemakers.

Survivors who face discrimination may consider the following suggestions:

■ Consider using your employer's policies and procedures for resolving employment issues informally. First, let your employer know that you are aware of your legal rights and would prefer to resolve the issues openly and honestly rather than file a lawsuit. Be careful of what you say during discussions, so that something you say will not be used to hurt your claim should your discussions fail to resolve the problem.

■ If you need some kind of accommodation to help you work, such as flexible working hours to accommodate doctors' appointments for follow-up or late-effects treatment, suggest several alternatives to your employer. If your employer offers you accommodations, do not turn them down lightly. Such an offer may work in the employer's favor if the case ends up before a judge. The Job Accommodation Network, a free service of the President's Committee on Employment of the Handicapped, helps employers fashion accommodations for disabled employees (call 1-800-ADA-WORK for more information).

■ Educate employers and co-workers who might believe that people cannot survive cancer and remain productive workers. For example, you could give your employer a letter from your doctor explaining the type of cancer you have or had and why you are able to work. More than 8,000,000 Americans are cancer survivors, so there is a good chance that some of your co-workers may have had cancer and are now valued employees.

■ Ask a member of your health care team to write or call your supervisor to offer to mediate the conflict and suggest ways for your supervisor to accommodate you.

■ Consider seeking support from your co-workers. They have an interest in protecting themselves from future discrimination.

Survivors who are considering a lawsuit should take several precautions to protect their rights:

■ *Keep carefully written records of all job actions, both good and bad.* Good actions, such as positive performance evaluations, may help in a lawsuit to show that you were qualified for the job. Bad actions, such as being moved from a job involving much interaction with the public to a job involving little interaction with the public after your cancer history is disclosed, may be used against your employer to show illegal acts. Keep complete notes of telephone calls and meetings (including dates, times, and attendees), letters, and the names and addresses of witnesses. Make written notes as events occur instead of trying to recall the events weeks or months later.

■ *Pause before you sue.* Carefully evaluate your goals. For example, do you want your job back, a change in working conditions, certain benefits, a written apology, or something else? Consider the positive and negative aspects of a lawsuit. Potential positive aspects include getting a job and monetary damages, protecting your rights, and tearing down barriers for other survivors. Potential negative aspects include long court battles with no guarantee of victory (some cases drag on for 5 years or more), legal fees and expenses, stress, a hostile relationship between you and the people you sue, and a reputation in your field as a troublemaker.

■ *Consider an informal settlement of your complaint.* Someone such as a union representative, human resources or personnel officer of your company, or social worker may be able to assist as a mediator. Your state or federal representative or local media may help persuade your employer to treat you fairly. Keep in mind that the first step most government agencies and companies take when they receive a complaint is to try to resolve the dispute without a costly trial.

■ *Be aware of filing deadlines so you do not lose your option to file a complaint under state or federal law.* You have 180 days from the date of the action against you to file a complaint with a federal agency. You have only 30 days if you work for the federal government. In most states, you have 180 days to file a complaint with the state agency. If you file a complaint and later change your mind, you can drop the lawsuit at any time.

If an informal solution does not work, a lawsuit may be the most appropriate next step for some survivors. To enforce rights established under the ADA, the survivor must file a complaint with the EEOC. The EEOC will attempt to settle the dispute. If no settlement is reached, the EEOC may appoint an investigator to evaluate the claim. If the EEOC determines that the survivor's rights may have been violated, the EEOC may sue on the survivor's behalf or may grant the survivor the right to file a lawsuit in federal court.

The complaint should be filed with the closest regional EEOC office. To obtain the location of your regional EEOC office, call the EEOC Public Information System in Washington, DC (1-800-669-4000). The EEOC also offers publications that explain the ADA and procedures for enforcing rights under the law (call 1-800-669-EEOC).

If the survivor proves that he or she was qualified for a job but treated differently because of a cancer history, he or she may be entitled to back pay, injunctive relief such as reinstatement, and attorney's fees. The ADA does not, however, permit an award for compensatory or punitive damages without intentional discrimination.

Under the Federal Rehabilitation Act, employees of recipients of federal financial assistance have up to 180 days from the action against them to file a complaint with the federal government. Employees of the federal government, however, have only 30 days.

Survivors must file a complaint with the federal agency that provided federal funds to their employer. Individuals who do not know the name of that agency or would like more information can contact the Justice Department at the following address:

Coordination and Review Section
Civil Rights Division
Department of Justice
P.O. Box 66118
Washington, DC 20530

Remedies under the Federal Rehabilitation Act include but are not limited to back pay, reinstatement, and attorney's fees but do not include punitive damages.

Most states have a state agency that enforces the law. Some states permit survivors to file a lawsuit in state court to enforce their rights. Under most state laws, employees have up to 180 days from the action against them to file a complaint with the state enforcement agency.

For more information about the laws in your state, contact your state division on civil rights or human rights commission or an attorney who is experienced in job discrimination cases. The EEOC Public Information System (1-800-669-4000) can help you locate the appropriate state enforcement agency. Also check your local telephone book under "state government."

In some situations, a single act may support a claim of discrimination under more than one law. For example, a cancer survivor who is denied a job by an employer in New York City may have a claim under the New York Human Rights Law (state), the New York City Law on Human Rights (city), and the ADA (federal).

Survivors who have a choice of remedies may file a complaint with each relevant enforcement agency. One agency may "stay" (not act on) the claim until another agency issues a decision. A survivor may always drop a complaint at any time once he or she determines which agency is most responsive. Factors to consider when one is choosing a resource include what types of remedies are available, how quickly the agency responds to complaints (ask a representative of the agency how long the process usually takes), and which office is most convenient.

Survivors do not need to have a lawyer represent them before an enforcement agency or court. However, someone who is represented by a lawyer experienced in job discrimination is more likely to meet with success. Survivors can find a lawyer by contacting:

■ *Your local bar association.* Most county and state bar associations have a lawyer referral service that can provide the names of lawyers in your area who have experience in job discrimination. Many can also refer you to a local public interest law center. Look in the telephone book under "State" and "County" listings, as well as under "Lawyer Referral Services," "Legal Services," "Attorneys," and "Lawyers."

■ *Local organizations that provide cancer survivors support and services.* Some local cancer organizations and hospitals keep a list of lawyers who represent cancer survivors in job discrimination cases.

■ *National cancer organizations.* The Candlelighters Childhood Cancer Foundation (1-800-366-2223), the National Coalition for Cancer Survivorship (1-301-650-8868) and some units of the American Cancer Society (1-800-ACS-2345) may be able to help you find a lawyer in some areas.

Survivors should be cautioned that, as with any other situation involving legal rights, even if their legal rights were violated, there is no *guarantee* that a public agency or court will provide a fair remedy.

How to challenge a denied claim. Cancer treatment often involves numerous bills from a variety of parties: hospital; physicians (surgeon, anesthesiologist, oncologist, radiologist, and so on); support services (nurse, social worker, nutritionist, therapist, and so on); radiology group; pharmacy (drugs and medical supplies); and consumer businesses (wigs, breast inserts, special clothing, and so on). Insurance companies will pay some of these parties directly, in part or in whole. The survivor must pay other bills and submit copies to the company for reimbursement.

Keeping track of dozens of expenses, often amounting to tens of thousands of dollars, can be confusing and exhausting. The key to collecting the maximum benefits covered by the insurance policy is to keep accurate records of all medical expenses:

1. Making photocopies of everything you send to your company, including letters, claim forms, and bills
2. Keeping all correspondence you receive from your insurance company
3. Submitting all bills, even if you are unsure whether a particular expense is covered by your policy (the worst that can happen is your expenses will not be reimbursed)
4. Keeping accurate records of your expenses, claim submissions, and payment vouchers

A policyholder has a right to appeal a claim denial by a public or private insurer. Because claims are frequently delayed or rejected in part or in full because of errors in filling out the claim forms, care should be taken to accurately provide all the information requested by the insurance company. The following steps could help survivors who are having trouble collecting on their claim:

1. Contact your insurance company in writing and insist on a written reply. Send copies of all documents and keep the originals for your files.
2. Keep a record of your contacts with the insurance company (copies of all letters you send and notes from every telephone call). Write down everything you do, the names of people you talk to, dates, and other facts.

3. Contact the state or federal agency that regulates your insurance provider if you do not receive a satisfactory and timely answer from your insurer. Most state insurance departments or commissions help consumers with complaints. Look under "State Government" in the telephone directory.
4. Contact cancer support organizations in your community. Some, such as the Candlelighters Childhood Cancer Foundation, offer ombudsman programs to help survivors and their families maximize insurance reimbursement.
5. If your claim is still not settled, consider filing a complaint in small claims court or hiring a lawyer to sue your insurance company.

CONCLUSION

Survivors of childhood cancer diagnosed in the 1990s can expect fewer economic barriers than those encountered by previous survivors. The majority of childhood cancer survivors today will enter schools and the job market with a decreasing chance of facing discrimination and an increasing array of legal rights and remedies. Future survivors' access to health insurance remains an unknown at the time of this writing, subject to the effect of expected national health insurance reform.

This chapter is adapted in part from Hoffman B: Cancer survivors at work: job problems and illegal discrimination, *Onc Nur For* 16:1, 1989. For more detailed information about employment and insurance rights of cancer survivors, see Hoffman B: *Taking care of business: employment, insurance and money matters.* In Mullan F, Hoffman B, editors: *Charting the journey: an almanac of practical resources for cancer survivors,* Mount Vernon, 1990, Consumer Reports Books.

REFERENCES

1. Bleyer WA: The impact of childhood cancer on the United States and the world, *Cancer J Clin* 40(6):355-367, 1990.
2. *Hearing on discrimination against cancer victims and the handicapped: hearing on HR 192 and HR 1546;* before the Subcommittee on Employment Opportunities of the House Commission on Education and Labor, 100th Congress. 1st Session 28:1987 (statement of Representative Mario Biaggi, 31-33, and statement of Barbara Hoffman, National Coalition for Cancer Survivorship 41-53).
3. Crothers HM: *Employment problems of cancer survivors: local problems and local solutions.* In American Cancer Society: *Proceedings of the workshop on employment, insurance and the patient with cancer,* New Orleans, 1986:51-57, The Society.
4. Feldman FL: *Work and cancer health histories,* San Francisco, 1982, American Cancer Society, California Division (5-year study of the work experiences of 344 white-collar workers, blue-collar workers, and youths with cancer histories between 1975 and 1980).
5. Fobair P et al: Psychosocial problems among survivors of Hodgkin's disease, *J Clin Oncol* 4(5):805-814, 1986.
6. Greenleigh Associates: *Report on the social, economic and psychological needs of cancer patients in California,* San Francisco, 1982, American Cancer Society California Division (also in *Proceedings of Western States Conference on Cancer Rehabilitation,* San Francisco, 1982).

7. Hays DM et al: Educational, occupational, and insurance status of childhood cancer survivors in their fourth and fifth decades of life, *J Clin Oncol* 10(9):1397-1406, 1992.

8. Hoffman B: Employment discrimination based on cancer history: the need for federal legislation, *59 Temple Law Quarterly 1,* 1986.

9. Hoffman B: *Taking care of business: employment, insurance and money matters.* In Mullan F, Hoffman B, editors: *Charting the journey: an almanac of practical resources for cancer survivors,* Mount Vernon, 1990, Consumer Reports Books.

10. Koocher GP, O'Malley JE: *The Damocles syndrome: psychosocial consequences of surviving childhood cancer,* New York, 1982, McGraw-Hill.

11. Mellette S: *The semantics of cancer and disability.* In *Proceedings of the workshop on employment, insurance and the patient with cancer,* New Orleans, 1986, American Cancer Society.

12. Mor V: *Work loss, insurance coverage, and financial burden among cancer patients.* In American Cancer Society: *Proceedings of the workshop on employment, insurance and the patient with cancer,* New Orleans, 1986, American Cancer Society.

13. Stone RW: Employing the recovered cancer patient, *Cancer* 36(1):285-286, 1975.

14. Teta MJ, Del Po MC, Kasl SV et al: Psychosocial consequences of childhood and adolescent cancer survival, *J Chronic Dis* 39(9):751-759, 1986.

15. Wasserman AL, Thompson ET, Wilmas JA et al: The psychosocial status of survivors of childhood/adolescent Hodgkin's disease, *Am J Dis Child* 141:626-631, 1987.

16. Wheatley GM, Cunnick WR, Wright BP et al: The employment of persons with a history of treatment for cancer, *Cancer* 33(2):441-445, 1974.

19

Methodologic and Statistical Issues in the Study of Late Effects of Childhood Cancer

Richard K. Severson
Leslie L. Robison

With the striking improvements in the treatment of pediatric cancers, it is now clear that the prognosis for most children with cancer is excellent. Based on data from the National Cancer Institute's Surveillance, Epidemiology and End Results (SEER) program, improvements in therapy have increased the probability of cure from less than 30% in 1960 to over 65% in 1986.[8] Furthermore, SEER data predict that 80% of children diagnosed with cancer in 1990 will survive into adulthood. Because of the young age of these patients and thus the potential added years of life, the long-term consequences of therapy have a greater impact on their lives, and on society at large, than the acute complications of therapy they may have already experienced. Childhood cancer survivors are second only to breast cancer survivors with respect to the number of years of potential life saved.[2]

Appropriately, increasing attention is being focused on the continued follow-up and evaluation of childhood cancer survivors. Often this follow-up is done with the aim of providing data regarding the late effects of therapy. This information can therefore be used in making treatment decisions for future cancer patients, as well as formulating recommendations for appropriate follow-up of survivors.

The objective of this chapter is to provide an overview of some of the methodologic and statistical issues that should be considered when interpreting or conducting research in childhood cancer–survivor populations. Particular emphasis is placed on those methodologic and analytic issues relevant to the conduct and reporting of late-effect studies. This chapter will first cover basic concepts, then more on to issues of study design and conduct, and finish with methodologic and statistical issues in data analysis.

BASIC CONCEPTS

Measures of disease or condition frequency are commonly used to evaluate the occurrence of specific outcomes in groups and to compare and evaluate differences between groups. A useful measure for describing the occurrence of a disease or condition in a defined population is a *proportion,* which is a type of ratio in which persons included in the numerator are also included in the denominator. For example, in the evaluation of second malignancies in a population of childhood acute lymphoid leukemia (ALL) patients,[7] 43 second malignancies were identified, of which 24 were neoplasms of the central nervous system (CNS). Therefore, the proportion of CNS second tumors is 56%. A *rate* is a proportion that incorporates a specific period of time in the denominator. Rates may be expressed in any form that is convenient, so that both the time frame (per year, month, day, and so on) and the population denominator (per 100, per 1000, per 10,000, and so on) may vary. For example, the incidence rate for ALL in children under 15 years of age is 3.2/100,000 or 0.0032% per year.

Within the context of late effects, *incidence* and *prevalence* are the two most commonly used types of rates. Prevalence refers to the proportion of individuals (cases) who have a specific condition (e.g., thyroid dysfunction, second cancer, and so on) at a certain point in time, much like a snapshot of a given situation. Therefore, the prevalence rate measures the number of existing cases of the condition in the population per unit time. The prevalence rate may be used to estimate the probability that an individual has a specific condition at the given point in time. Prevalence rates are commonly used to express the extent of a condition in a given population, and, as such, they are very useful for activities such as planning and health care delivery considerations.

An incidence rate, on the other hand, refers to the number of individuals in the population who develop a specific condition (i.e., new cases) per unit time. Therefore, the incidence rate would be used to estimate the probability that an individual will develop a specific late effect during a given time interval. Incidence rates are generally used to measure the risk of developing an outcome and are very useful (usually more so than prevalence) in studies of etiology. The *mortality rate* refers to the number of individuals in the population who die within the time interval of interest and is similar to an incidence rate, except that it measures mortality rather than morbidity.

Within epidemiologic research, rates are often expressed in a variety of forms. One of these is the *crude rate,* which is simply a summary rate of the total number of cases of disease in the total population over a given time. If one wants to compare two groups, however, crude rates may have limitations because of differences in various characteristics of the populations being compared. For example, consider two populations, both of which range from 0 to 30 years of age. Although each population consists of both younger and older individuals, the first population may contain primarily young people and the second population may contain primarily older individuals. The second population may have a higher rate of a specific outcome of interest (e.g., second cancer) than the first population, not because of any important differences in exposure to risk factors, but simply because of differences in the age composition of the two populations. One method for dealing with this is to use *specific rates,* which are specific to various demographic subsets of the population (such as age-, gender-, or race-specific rates). For example, the age-specific incidence rates of ALL in children are 5.5, 2.8, and 1.7

per 100,000 per year for children aged 0 to 4, 5 to 9, and 10 to 14 years, respectively.

Often, a summary rate, which is based on the total population, is needed. *Adjusted rates,* which are also known as *summary rates* or *standardized rates,* represent rates that eliminate the effect of variables (confounding variables) that may be associated with both the exposure as well as the outcome. These rates may be compared directly across populations that may differ with respect to those characteristics for which adjustment has been made. Two commonly used adjusted rates are the *standardized incidence ratio* and the *standardized mortality ratio.* These rates are used to determine if the observed number of cases of a disease or condition (incidence) or death (mortality) within a particular population are substantially different from the expected number, which is usually derived from age-, gender-, and calendar-specific rates from the general population. These general population rates are often based on national data. As an example, consider again the occurrence of second malignancies in the 9720 children with ALL.[7] Based on the length of time the patients have been followed from the diagnosis of ALL and applying the age-, gender-, and calendar-specific cancer rates for the U.S. population, it was calculated that 6.18 cases of cancer would have been expected to occur in this group if they experienced the same rate of cancer as the general population. Therefore, comparison of the 43 observed second neoplasms to the expected number of cancers provides a standardized incidence ratio of 6.9 (43/6.18).

STUDY DESIGNS

Discovering the determinants of a disease or condition in a population is usually a gradual process that requires different types of study designs, depending on the nature and the current state of understanding regarding the disease etiology. If little is known about the disease, a *descriptive study* may be undertaken. These studies provide basic information on the occurrence of disease in a defined population and may be used to generate hypotheses relating to etiology. *Analytic studies* are designed to test hypotheses. In a general sense, it is possible to take either an experimental or observational approach in analytic studies. The main advantage of *experimental studies* is that study subjects are randomized to various exposure and treatment categories. However, experimental designs are often not feasible for many research questions, including those relating to late effects.

For analytic studies, the *relative risk* is the standard measure used for assessing the extent of association between a putative risk factor and the subsequent occurrence of a disease or condition in a specific population. The relative risk is defined as the ratio of the rate of a disease or condition in the group exposed to the risk factor of interest divided by the rate in the unexposed group. Relative risks may be derived directly in a *cohort study,* in which study subjects are classified into groups based on levels of exposure and observed over time to identify whether or not the outcome of interest occurs. For example, in the cohort study of second malignancies in children with ALL,[7] the relative risk is the rate of second malignant neoplasms (SMNs) in the children with ALL (the exposed group) divided by the rate of SMNs in all children in the U.S. (the unexposed group), which works out to be 6.9. Thus far, cohort studies in childhood cancer survivors are reasonably uncommon. Those cohort studies conducted have generally focused on the occurrence of second cancer. Another approach to investigate childhood cancer survivors is that of a *case-control study*. In this study design, one identifies two groups of subjects: 1) cases, defined as survivors diagnosed with the outcome of interest; and 2) controls, defined as children in whom the outcome of interest has not occurred and who are identified from the same population from which the cases arose. Data on individual characteristics and previous exposure and events for these cases and controls are then collected and compared. In this type of study design, relative risk cannot be calculated directly since the proportion of incident cases among the exposed subjects in the study sample is generally not equal to the incidence rate in the exposed population. However, it is estimated by the *odds ratio,* which is usually a close approximation of the relative risk for rare diseases. If an event occurs with probability p, then the ratio of p/q (where $q = 1 - p$) is the odds. For example, if $p = 1/10$ represents the lifetime risk of a certain cancer in the population, then the odds of this cancer are $1/9$ (($1/10)/(9/10)$). The odds ratio is defined as the odds of disease in the exposed group relative to the odds of disease in the unexposed group.

The third type of epidemiologic study is the *cross-sectional study*. In this study design, a group of subjects is identified based on some a priori reason, and both exposure status and disease status are simultaneously determined for each study subject. The odds ratio can also be used within this study design as an estimate of the relative risk. Within the literature, the cross-sectional study design is one of the most commonly used approaches for investigating late effects in childhood cancer survivors. Most likely, the reason that the cross-sectional design is common relates to 1) the lack of access to well-defined cohorts; 2) the conduct of studies within populations being seen in a specific setting (e.g., late-effects clinics); and 3) the interest in addressing specific questions within a relatively short period of time. An investigation of growth in ALL patients is an excellent example of a cross-sectional study.[9] In this CCG study, heights of patients were obtained approximately 7 years following diagnosis; and this provided data describing the population at a single point in time.

Comparing each of the study designs, a cohort study has the advantage of being able to calculate the relative risk directly. On the other hand, cohort studies can be very time-consuming and costly to execute because of the large number of subjects often required and the potential need for the extended follow-up. For example, if investigators were interested in following childhood cancer survivors for the occurrence of a relatively uncommon outcome that might occur between 18 to 35 years of age in the subjects, then the study population would have to be large (because of the rarity of the outcome of interest) and it would have to be followed for several decades to record the occurrence of all the outcomes of interest. A case-control study is usually less expensive and quicker to complete, but the investigators have to guard against various biases that may affect the risk estimates. Cross-sectional studies, although frequently used in studies of long-term survivors, need to be carefully considered since the potential exists for variations in the length of follow-up from exposure (i.e., diagnosis and treatment of cancer) as well as other potential for biases.

After the hypothesis to be tested has been formulated, one of the most important aspects of study feasibility is consideration of sample size and study power. Frequently, sample size and power calculations play an integral part in choosing the correct study design. The research team first establishes two separate hypotheses: 1) the *research hypothesis,* which contains the researchers' opinions of the true state of nature, and 2) the *null hypothesis,* which, usually stated, is that there is no relationship between the exposure of interest and the disease of interest (i.e., the relative risk equals unity). Considering the null hypothesis, the objective is to accept it when it is true and reject it when it is false. In pursuing this goal, there are two potential errors that can occur. The first is rejection of the null hypothesis when it is true. This is known as type-I or α error. The second error is acceptance of the null hypothesis when it is false. This is known as type-II or β error. The *power* of a study is defined as $1 - \beta$. As a general rule, a study should be designed to have more than 80% power. The power of a study is determined by the number of subjects included in the study, the level of the relative risk or difference that the researchers are willing to designate as important, the proportion of exposed subjects in the population of interest, and an arbitrary level of α (usually set at 0.05). Based on these quantities, it is possible to determine that the power is sufficient given the number of subjects to be included in the study. If not, the power of the study can be increased by increasing the number of subjects included in the study.

STUDY CONDUCT

A considerable amount of effort should be devoted not only to the design of a study, but also to the procedures for collecting the data. Summarized in the box below are some of the steps required in the typical epidemiologic study to investigate

---

Components of Epidemiologic Research

Choosing the research question
Choosing the study design
Choosing the study population(s)
Human subjects (ethical) considerations
Choosing the variables of interest
Conducting the power analysis and sample-size calculations
Developing the analysis plan
Developing data collection materials
Training the study staff
Collecting the data
Editing and data entry
Analyzing data and interpreting results

potential etiologic relationships between exposure and a subsequent outcome of interest. Once the research question has been defined, the study design selected, the variables of interest identified, and the power or sample-size calculations computed, the next step is usually to enter the data collection phase of the project.

Before initiating a study, it is critical to have well-defined definitions for the outcome(s) of interest (i.e., disease or condition), exposure, and other potentially important variables. Obviously, there are a multitude of intricate details and complexities that can serve to complicate the data collection process in a study of childhood cancer survivors. Because of this, it is important to employ a uniform written protocol to guide all study activities. Not only does this protocol serve as a guide to procedures during the course of this study, but it also provides a clear record of how the investigation was conducted should questions arise long after the study has been completed.

Usually included in a study protocol are guidelines for selection of study subjects, how exposure is to be determined, how disease is defined, the logistic methods used to contact subjects, the format for data collection materials (such as questionnaires, clinical and biologic procedures, and data collection forms), and informed consent procedures. At the same time, other documentation might include procedure manuals with instructions and guidelines for study personnel who will be interacting with study participants and coding procedures that incorporate detailed instructions for recording of study data. An important component of the data collection phase is the design and implementation of quality control procedures.

DATA ANALYSIS

After the data have been collected, following strict adherence to the study protocol with continual application of quality control procedures, the investigators may then proceed with analysis of the study data. Specific methods for the analysis of a study will depend on the type of study conducted and the way the data were collected. In general, analytic methods may be divided into either classical or multivariate methods. *Classical methods,* which include such techniques as contingency table analyses, parametric and nonparametric tests, and life table analyses, allow for the assessment of the effect of only one variable at a time (generally the exposure of interest) on the development of the disease. The confounding effects of other variables can be controlled for by stratification, which is the division of the original data into multiple subgroups, resulting in one analysis unit for each level of the stratifying variable.

Variables that are identified by a discrete number of classes are termed categoric. Examples include gender (male or female), race (white, black, or other) and age (younger than 2, 2 to 4, or older than 4 years of age). Contingency table analyses are frequently applied to these variables. The statistical test often used is a chi-square test (for homogeneity of proportions with a continuity correction such as Yates's). There are limitations in the application of the chi-square test in situations where the number of study subjects or observations is small. A general definition for "small sample size" is if the calculated expected number of subjects in any cell within the contingency table is less than five. Under these circumstances, an exact test (e.g., Fisher's) should be used. Frequently, comparisons are made in a variable measured on a continuous scale (such as age and blood pressure). These potential differences may be analyzed using either *parametric* or *nonparametric methods.* Parametric methods, such as the t-test, rely on relatively complex assumptions about distributional forms of the variables. If these assumptions are true, then the parametric methods are a powerful and appropriate tool for analysis. On the other hand, these assumptions are often likely to be clearly false. If so, then nonparametric methods, such as the sign test and the rank sum test (e.g., Wilcoxon, Mann-Whitney) may be more appropriate. In addition to not relying on specific distributional assumptions, these methods have the advantage of involving simple and rapid computations.

Classical methods have several advantages, such as the fact that they are easier to understand intuitively than the more complicated multivariate methods. Moreover, they also are not dependent on the more restrictive assumptions inherent in multivariate methods. Finally, they are usually simple enough that they may be computed by hand if a computer is not available. Classical methods also have several disadvantages. They do not work very well when the investigators need to adjust for several confounding factors at the same time. They also may not work well when the confounding variable cannot be well represented by a single categoric variable. An example would be a continuous variable such as age, which has a nonlinear relationship of a specific form (such as quadratic). Finally, classical methods do not work well when the confounders interact to jointly affect the outcome.

Multivariate methods, which include such techniques as linear regression, logistic regression, and Cox (proportional hazards) regression, use a mathematic model to adjust for covariates rather than stratification as used in the classical methods. As such, the effects on the outcome of interest of several different variables may be assessed simultaneously. The disadvantage of multivariate methods is that their use is based on more restrictive assumptions than those for classical methods.

Multiple linear regression was developed to study covariation among measures taken on the same subjects. It is appropriate for fitting linear models to describe the relationship between predictor variables and an outcome variable that has many levels. Unfortunately, linear regression is not useful in studies in which there are only two possible outcomes, such as either having or not having the disease of interest. Logistic regression is the preferred multivariate method for studies such as these in which the outcome is a dichotomous variable.

In cohort studies, it is often the situation that investigators know whether or not each individual in their cohort has experienced the outcome of interest, as well as how much time has elapsed between the initial exposure (i.e., diagnosis and treatment) and the development of disease or date of last contact. These data are commonly recorded as the number of person-years of observation, which allows the application of both life table and Cox regression methods. Life table methods are generally used in the analysis of clinical trials. However, they may also be used as a means of analyzing cohort studies. In many situations, these methods are referred to as survival analyses; however, mortality need not be the only endpoint of interest. The life table approach produces a graph of the survival curves for each group defined by the level of exposure. These curves, frequently referred to as a Kaplan-Meier curve, are graphs of the cumulative probability of remaining free of the event of interest up to specific points in time for members of each group. In addition to the visual comparison of these curves, a life table analysis includes a statistical test of the null hypothesis. Although several statistical tests may be employed, the most widely known and used is the log-rank test.

The main disadvantage of life table methods is that they have a limited capacity to incorporate covariates. Cox regression is a multivariate alternative to life table methods. The Cox model assumes that across follow-up times, the hazard rate, which may be thought of as the immediate risk of developing disease, is a constant multiple of a baseline hazard rate at all points. Cox regression is used when the dependent variable is expressed as the time from study entry to the development of the disease. Therefore, it is quite different from logistic regression where the dependent variable is dichotomous. Cox regression has two main advantages over life table methods. First, it allows for a more complete control for confounding effects of covariates. Second, it has the capacity to handle variables measured on a continuous scale, allowing for more complete evaluation of important features of an exposure-disease relationship such as a dose-response effect.

No matter what method is used to evaluate the data, one important piece of information that results is the estimate of the relative risk, as previously defined. Although the relative risk by itself conveys important information about the potential relationship between exposure and disease, it is also important to test the statistical significance of the risk estimate. Two ways to do this are to compute a probability value (p value) and confidence limits. A p value is simply the probability that the actual relative risk in the study population is really unity (i.e., not increased or decreased). When testing statistical significance, it is important to note that one may use either *one-sided* or *two-sided tests*. In a two-sided test, the null hypothesis may be that there is no difference or risk (i.e., either increased or decreased). In a one-sided test the research team is usually more certain about the direction of the risk or difference between groups. Therefore, the research hypothesis might be that the relative risk is strictly greater in one group, and the null hypothesis would be that the risk is less than or equal to unity. Most statistical testing procedures, such as Pearson's chi-square and Yates's continuity-corrected chi-square tests, are two-sided tests. However, the research team should be careful since a few tests, such as Fisher's exact test, are naturally one-sided tests. Some, but not all, statistical analysis packages convert the p values computed from one-sided tests into two-sided p values and report those two-sided p values. Perhaps more informative is the computation of *confidence limits*, which are the bounds of a range in which the actual relative risk is most likely to be found. The confidence limits are usually expressed in terms of the 95% confidence limit. Interpretation of study results requires consideration of both the estimated relative risk as well as the statistical significance of the estimate.

SUMMARY

Based on the incidence of cancer in children and the current projected survival rate, it can be estimated that by the end of this decade, approximately 1 out of every 900 individuals between the ages of 15 and 45 in the United States will be a survivor of childhood cancer. As this population of cured patients continues to increase, the importance of studies relating to the late sequelae gain greater importance. This is particularly true given the introduction of more intensive multiagent therapy for the treatment of childhood cancers, which may place patients at greatest risk for adverse late effects.

To maximize the knowledge that will be gained from the active follow-up of survivors, it is critical that the evaluations be performed in a systematic method through standardization of issues such as definition of endpoints, frequency of follow-ups, and assessment tools for late effects. Research in the area of late effects must be conducted at a level comparable to any other form of scientific research with detail given to study design, conduct, and analysis. This chapter provides only a general discussion of some issues considered to be important. A more in-depth review is available in textbooks on epidemiologic and statistical methods.[1,3-6]

As the number of late-effects clinics increases, the opportunities also increase for actively pursuing research into late effects of therapy. Collaboration between a multidisciplinary group of investigators, applying appropriate methodologies, should be actively pursued.

REFERENCES

1. Bailar JC, Mosteller F, editors: *Medical uses of statistics,* Waltham, 1986, NEJM Books.
2. Bleyer WA: The impact of childhood cancer on the United States and the world, *CA Cancer J Clin* 40:355-367, 1990.
3. Hollander M, Wolfe DA: *Nonparametric statistical methods,* New York, 1973, John Wiley.
4. Kelsey JL, Thompson WD, Evans AS: *Methods in observational epidemiology,* New York, 1986, Oxford University Press.
5. Lee ET: *Statistical methods for survival data analysis,* Belmont, 1980, Lifetime Learning Publications.
6. Mausner JS, Kramer S: *Epidemiology, an introductory text,* Philadelphia, 1985, WB Saunders.
7. Neglia JP et al: Second neoplasms after acute lymphoblastic leukemia in childhood, *N Engl J Med* 325:1330-1336, 1991.
8. Ries LAG et al: *Cancer Statistics Review 1973-88,* National Cancer Institute, NIH Pub. No. 91-2789, 1991.
9. Robison LL, Nesbit ME, Sather HN et al: Height of children successfully treated for acute lymphoblastic leukemia: a report from the Late Effects Committee of the Childrens Cancer Study Group, *Am J Pediatr Hematol Oncol* 13:14-21, 1985.

20

The Establishment of the Follow-up Clinic

Cindy L. Schwartz
Wendy L. Hobbie
Louis S. Constine

By the late 1970s, it became clear that survival curves for many pediatric malignancies were forming plateaus: after an interval of time, deaths due to recurrent cancer were no longer occurring. The patients living on the plateau of the survival curve were facing the challenges of adulthood, often encumbered by the medical and social problems related to the disease or the treatment. Although patients received an appropriate "pat on the back" and were occasionally enrolled in a study of a specific late effect, it became apparent to medical practitioners in several institutions that the chronic effects of treatment were significant and often complex; a systematic approach to the care of these survivors was necessary. Comprehensive clinical programs were designed in which risk factors were evaluated systematically in all long-term survivors. One such clinical program was established at the University of Rochester in 1988. The recommendations that follow are derived from the experiences at the University of Rochester (and similar clinics) and, it is hoped, will serve as the groundwork for the establishment of other follow-up clinics.

Survivors often have multiple health care and psychosocial needs that ideally should be addressed by a multidisciplinary team. The nucleus of such a team generally includes a nursing coordinator, a pediatric oncologist, a radiation oncologist, and various psychosocial personnel including a psychologist, social workers, and a school liaison. In addition, physicians from related disciplines such as cardiology, pulmonary medicine, orthopedics, neurology, and endocrinology must be associated with the team to assist in the evaluation of identified problems, both individually and in cohort groups. These subspecialists should be chosen with consideration of their interest in providing comprehensive care to long-term survivors as well as to participating in research projects that may improve the quality of life for current and future long-term survivors.

OPERATION OF THE CLINIC

Prior to each clinic visit, the nurse coordinator reviews the treatment record to determine a preliminary list of high-risk organs. Well-thought-out protocols for screening organs at risk are essential. A decision is made as to which team members should see the survivor and family.

At the time of the visit, the nurse coordinator meets the family and introduces the concepts of follow-up care, systematic evaluation, and late effects of therapy. A history is taken and a physical examination performed by the nurse; results are reviewed with the pediatric and radiation oncologists. Questions and concerns are answered by both the nurse coordinator and the oncologist. At this time, other team members who may contribute to the care of the patient are called in. The family is then sent off for evaluative studies, returning for wrap-up discussion. Following the visit, there is a postclinic meeting in which individual patients are discussed. Research questions may be formulated when the effects of therapy on individuals are considered. A follow-up plan is determined for each patient and recorded in the patient's chart. Follow-up letters are sent to the local physician, as well as to other involved health care professionals.

The follow-up clinic should be separate from the general functioning of the pediatric oncology clinic. The survivors and their families then feel that they are the priority of the clinic personnel and more easily recognize the importance of follow-up care. Many families appreciate being spared the emotional trauma of watching other families go through an ordeal that they themselves have only recently completed.

Although many clinics differ in their determination of who is appropriately included, children diagnosed with cancer before age 18 are considered long-term survivors when they are disease-free for 5 years and off therapy for 2 years. Medical records must be available. Patients who transfer to such clinics from outside institutions must forward medical records prior to being seen.

The Role of the Pediatric and Radiation Oncologists

Cindy L. Schwartz
Louis S. Constine

The child who survives a malignancy is both a confirmation of the success of medicine and a painful reminder of the limitations of our abilities as physicians. Such patients demand that we look not only at the successes of our treatments, but also at the effects these treatments have on their lives. As pediatric oncologists, we must return to our initial goal as pediatricians: to aid children in their developmental processes so that they can become functioning, happy members of adult society.

As the medical leaders of the long-term team, the pediatric oncologists must continually consider the pathophysiologic effects of cytotoxic treatment on the developing human. Expertise in dissecting and integrating the effects of chemotherapy, radiation therapy, and surgery demands a thorough understanding of these modalities, which is optimally provided by the interaction of a team of specialists.

This knowledge must be used to anticipate problems that may surface in the near or distant future and to consider preventative methodologies. In addition, the pediatric oncologist must serve as a resource for other health care professionals involved in the care of the child including primary care physicians, other specialists, nurses, and members of the psychosocial team. The oncologist can balance the relative risks and help the patient assess the likelihood that a potential toxicity will become a reality. For example, the risk of infertility will vary from patient to patient depending on the age at treatment, the extent of treatment, and the exact type of treatment. Consideration of these factors may assist a patient with his or her spouse to determine when they might attempt to begin a family and in what manner they should proceed.

While carefully considering the individual circumstances of a patient and how the individual's life might best be improved, the oncologist must also look at the treatment cohorts for clues as to previously unrecognized toxicities and potential mechanisms for overcoming the late effects or for preventing them in future patients embarking on therapeutic regimens.

The oncologist should see each patient as he or she comes to the clinic to renew old ties that may remain strong and to assure the patient that the physician is considering and understands the effect that treatment has had on the patient's life. Although the cancer may have been cured for some time, the fear of its return has rarely abated. As the children mature, they will need increasingly sophisticated information so that they understand the processes that affected their bodies. New concerns may also arise that may or may not be attributable to the original disease. Physician input is often required to fully assess any potential connection.

In addition to the benefits derived by patients who see their physicians in the long-term clinic, involvement in the care of long-term survivors gives the oncologist an understanding of cancer treatment that cannot be realized simply by caring for a patient during the year or two of treatment. Much of what physicians do during the early period has implications that are not recognizable at that time but become apparent with growth and development. The treatment of cancer does not end after the drugs and radiation have been administered. The treatment is only fully efficacious when the child has lived a full and healthy life.

The Role of the Pediatric Nurse Practitioner

Wendy L. Hobbie
Patricia J. Hollen
Jean H. Fergusson

HISTORICAL DEVELOPMENT OF THE ROLE OF THE PEDIATRIC NURSE PRACTITIONER IN ONCOLOGY

The nursing community recognized the need for an innovative role like the pediatric nurse practitioner in oncology (PNP/O) 2 decades ago. In 1976, a

Pediatric Nurse Practitioner Program in Oncology was established at Children's Hospital of Philadelphia in the Division of Pediatric Oncology, aimed at preparing pediatric oncology nurses to function in an expanded role. The program was designed to produce practitioners who were well-versed in primary care and pediatric oncology and who could share the clinical practice with pediatric oncologists. The educational goal for nursing was to expand the autonomy of oncology nurses through a more independent role directed at improvement of patient care. Through advanced education and shared practice, the PNP/O would develop a clinical expertise that fostered and supported the role of leader and innovator in pediatric oncology nursing.

THE ROLE OF THE PEDIATRIC NURSE PRACTITIONER IN ONCOLOGY WORKING WITH LONG-TERM SURVIVORS OF CHILDHOOD CANCER*

The PNP/O role has evolved in a fashion consistent with the trends described for advanced practice nursing in general. The role was originally envisioned modestly as one that identifies the population of long-term survivors, informs them of available services, and helps meet their unique needs. The early concept of the role included three interdependent functions: (1) clinician/caregiver, (2) educator, and (3) researcher. The functions of specialty care provider (formerly clinician/caregiver) and clinical/community educator remain strong; the role of researcher has been expanded, and new role components, clinical/program manager and consultant, have been added (Fig. 20-1).

From a systems perspective, the primary focus and energy of the role flows from direct care of individual survivors and high-risk subgroups to indirect care of the clinic population of survivors as a collective and of the community-at-large.

Specialty Care Provider

The direct care function for the PNP/O continues to be based on sound knowledge of the potential long-term consequences of cancer therapy. Clinical expertise is essential in detecting abnormalities obtained from a comprehensive history and physical examination. Early identification of both actual and potential late effects is imperative to make early intervention possible. The PNP/O needs to offer clear and concise explanations of these late effects at appropriate educational levels to gain the confidence of the survivors and their families; these explanations must be carefully given to reduce uncertainty. Interventions must be tailored for each survivor's actual or potential sequela of treatment. In addition, the PNP/O must have a broad background in growth and development to frame the late effects and counsel effectively.

The specialty care provider monitors long-term care of this formerly acutely ill population. The demarcation between the primary care provider's role and that of

---

*This section is modified by permission from Hobbie WL, Hollen PJ: Pediatric nurse practitioners specializing with survivors of childhood cancer, *J Pediatr Health Care* 7:24, 1993.

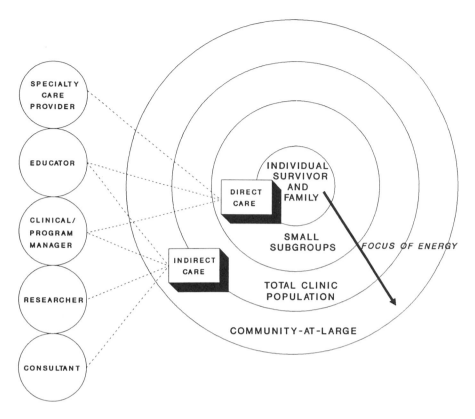

Fig. 20-1.   A systems model of the role of the pediatric nurse practitioner specializing in oncology (PNP/O) with the high-risk population of survivors of childhood cancer. (From Hobbie WL, Hollen PJ: *J Pediatr Health Care* 7:24, 1993)

the PNP/O in routine care is clear-cut. All routine care, including minor illness, is first filtered through the local primary care provider, a family's pediatrician or physician. However, if a family is concerned about an illness in relation to the past medical history of cancer, then even a minor illness should be evaluated by the PNP/O and other team members. The concerns of survivors, families, and health care providers today are the same as those identified by Hobbie in 1986[4]: (a) return of disease; (b) risk of second malignancies; (c) vital organ function; (d) linear growth and intellectual and psychosocial development; and (e) sexual maturation and fertility.

Restoration of normalcy to the family unit remains an important goal for the PNP/O. This entails assisting the survivors and their families as they deal with everyday consequences of cancer therapy. Putting past events in perspective is a difficult task with which most survivors need assistance. Success in this regard is essential if they are to accept their medical past and move forward in achieving future goals.

Parents are often thrown into a second crisis (the acute phase being the first) when they are informed of actual or potential late effects. Resolution of this second crisis is difficult but generally quicker as they journey toward acceptance and internalization of the cancer experience as chronic; knowing that the child has survived and that the family has withstood the earlier crisis accelerates this transition.[5] The PNP/O can facilitate this transition process by helping the family deal positively with actual late effects and by ensuring they are vigilant, but not overalarmed, about potential late effects.

Educator

The clinical/community educator aspect of this advanced practice role remains strong. Providing information to survivors and families continues to be a vital function of the PNP/O role. Certain concepts regarding survival need to be continually reinforced. Koocher and O'Malley[5] found that parents had lingering concerns of reoccurrence, second malignancies, and late effects, regardless of length of survival, a finding that continues to be supported through clinical experience. Factual information must be carefully woven with hope and support to reduce uncertainty as much as possible.

The PNP/O has an educational role within the community-at-large in addition to the function of patient and family educator. The stigma of cancer still remains, although major strides have been made in public awareness of cancer. A concerted effort is needed on the part of specialty care providers to promote accurate information and to provide innovative approaches to care in the community.

Teachers continue to be a significant group for whom the PNP/O needs to provide accurate information related to students' needs in the classroom. The attitudes of teachers and fellow students are critical in a survivor's concepts of normalcy. Moreover, some learning problems caused by central nervous system prophylactic therapy have been minimized by individualized instruction, tutoring, and parental support.[14]

Educating personnel in insurance companies to realistically evaluate actual and potential late effects continues to be a primary target of the PNP/O. The findings of Koocher and O'Malley's[8]—that survivors experienced discrimination while seeking health and life insurance, obtaining jobs, and entering the military service and other governmental positions—continue to be supported clinically.[8] The PNP/O needs to provide anticipatory guidance regarding this discrimination and either educate young adult survivors and their families on their legal rights or refer them to an attorney. Writing supportive letters and putting survivors in contact with available resources for information, such as the Childhood Candlelighters Foundation, American Cancer Society, Leukemia Society, National Cancer Institute, and the National Coalition of Cancer Survivors, is imperative.

The PNP/O in specialty practice plays a role in educating the professional community about survivorship in many ways. Corresponding with local physicians improves the continuity of care and ensures the consistency of information given to the family. Lecturing at professional meetings, interacting in cooperative study groups, and publishing important approaches to care continue to be effective ways to disseminate information about survivors.

Clinical/Program Manager of Nurse-Run Clinics

Follow-up clinics for long-term survivors have predominantly been nurse-run clinics to date. In one such clinic at Strong Children's Medical Center in Rochester, New York, the PNP/O is part of a multidisciplinary team that includes a pediatric oncologist, radiation oncologist, psychologist, social worker, school liaison, and identified specialty physicians (e.g., orthopedist). This team meets routinely to evaluate the physical, physiologic, and psychosocial effects of surviving cancer. However, the PNP/O compiles the pertinent information and begins to formulate a list of studies that will best evaluate an individual survivor at the time of the yearly visit. This information is compiled in a computerized data bank for easy retrieval in clinical and research use. During the weekly team meetings, the PNP/O generally acts as the leader/facilitator, presents each survivor's history, and validates the appropriate evaluations with the other team members. The PNP/O completes a patient history on the day of the visit as well as a thorough physical examination. The pediatric oncologist and radiation oncologist meet with the survivor and family and discuss any questions related to their areas of expertise or to evaluate areas of concern identified by the PNP/O. Following the visit, the PNP/O completes all follow-up tests, makes all referrals, and obtains all family feedback as case manager for each survivor and family. In essence, the PNP/O has overall responsibility for clinical effectiveness in collaboration with the oncology medical director.

Program case management can be conceptualized as providing care to groups and populations with similar needs. The PNP/O has the opportunity to synthesize the unmet needs of this population of survivors through a triangulation of methods.[2,7] Use of a triangulation of methods for a population of survivors could be (a) interviewing or surveying the survivors and their families in the clinic setting as consumers of services; (b) collating information from key informants (members of the multidisciplinary team or colleagues specializing in survivor care); and (c) integrating current literature related to actual and potential late effects. This use of multiple, complementary methods prevents bias in program development and production of unmarketable services.

Program case management, when it focuses on the special unmet needs of the survivor population, provides the basis for strategic program planning in collaboration with the program medical director and other team members. As program money becomes tighter, the PNP/O will need to base program development on a well-grounded needs-assessment and on proven marketing strategies to obtain needed funding.

Activities that promote a comprehensive program for survivors are necessary for effective program management by the PNP/O. Eliminating those aspects of the program that are obsolete and creating new ones based on documented needs keeps the program viable. Approaching local foundations or cancer organizations, if necessary, to obtain external funds to expand the program may be a future role for the PNP/O.

Ethically, the PNP/O creates a standard of care for the aggregate of survivors through the role of program case management, resulting in comprehensive and quality services for the clinic population. Using this standard within the role of clinical case manager, the advanced practitioner determines what services the survivor and family should receive in conjunction with the other team members.

Researcher

In the Hobbie description of the PNP/O role, the function of researcher was oriented toward data collection and management of clinical information for a given study with some involvement in research planning and data synthesis toward protocols for follow-up care.[4] This component of the PNP/O role has evolved to become more collaborative. Masters-prepared nurses have claimed a significant role as clinical experts with survivors and need to consider working with doctorate-prepared nurses or physicians on research projects. The desire, much less the expectation, to conduct clinical research as a principal investigator may not be realistic for clinicians providing holistic care to a high-risk population. However, the union between the specialty care provider and a doctorate-prepared nurse or physician provides an excellent way to conduct research as a coinvestigator or research associate.

Because the PNP/O is the case manager who knows the needs of the clinic population of survivors, the PNP/O is best able to assist in or determine research questions or hypotheses; monitor access to the survivors so that they are not deluged by researchers; coordinate the clinical studies conducted with this population at a given site to minimize time demands on both survivors and researchers; and ensure that protocols do not interfere with one another, thus protecting the researchers' outcomes. This comprehensive review of all studies for this aggregate is different from the intensive individual study review by a human subjects review board. The PNP/O needs to weigh the importance of a research study, family time expended, invasion of privacy or dignity, and interruption of staff time and its impact on clinic flow.

Consultant

The consultant function for the PNP/O has become more important over the last few years as more institutions recognize the importance of systematic evaluation in establishing clinics tailored to the specific needs of a population. In addition, community organizations often seek help in program planning for high-risk populations.

The PNP/O promotes better understanding of survivorship by participating in community organizations and by professional networking. As the PNP/O keeps current in this specialized field, accumulates clinical experience, and participates in research, the role of consultant becomes a reality on the local level, and gradually more distant sites and larger projects become possible.

DISCUSSION

The role of the PNP/O has been evolving since the late 1970s to meet the demands of an increasing cancer-surviving population with special needs related to actual and potential late effects. The aims of the PNP/O role are to decrease the full negative impact of long-lasting effects of therapy; to assist the survivor and family to cope effectively while monitoring and treating late effects; and to help the survivor and family gain perspective on the cancer experience so they can be vigilant toward potential late effects. Essentially, the central focus for the PNP/O is the survivor and family, which is extended to the clinic population and related groups. Any role on behalf of this clinical population should be assumed as necessary to provide comprehensive care.

The Role of the Psychologist and Social Worker

Paul Carpenter
Carla Levant

In the past 30 years scientific advancements in the identification of effective medical regimens for the treatment of childhood cancer have unveiled a myriad of long-term effects that can have significant impact on patients' physiologic, cognitive, emotional, and social maturation, development, and adaptation. To provide a mechanism for the comprehensive assessment and appropriate clinical management of these potential long-term treatment effects, a multidisciplinary, team-oriented model of patient care was adopted in pediatric oncology. This approach to patient care is a process that begins at the time a child is initially diagnosed. The surveillance and clinical management of a patient's disease status and treatment effects within the context of a clinic specifically designed for childhood survivors should be a natural extension of this process. To facilitate the visualization of the complexities involved in the long-term care of children with cancer, a schema of anticipated medical milestones and potential psychosocial crises that are often associated with childhood cancer is presented in Fig. 20-1.

Clinical/pediatric psychologists and social workers should be integral components of the multidisciplinary team in the long-term clinic and be involved in the day-to-day multidisciplinary evaluation and formulation of all patients' comprehensive health care planning. Although salary support for a social worker, whose professional role in patient care is a mandated requirement for hospital accreditation, is generally available, limited hospital budgets often cannot provide salary support for a clinical psychologist. Other potential sources of salary support for a clinical psychologist that can be pursued include insurance reimbursement for direct clinical services, psychologic and neuropsychologic testing, consultations, and individual, group, and family psychotherapy provided by a licensed clinical psychologist; monies from community-based childhood cancer support organizations, which are often eager to subsidize the expansion of hospital programs to help provide the best possible care for children with cancer; and grants or contributions from businesses or individuals in the community.

To be effective, the psychologist and social worker must have primary hospital appointments and clinical responsibilities within the hospital unit or division that provides treatment and clinical care for children with cancer. All psychosocial professionals should function within the context of a psychosocial team with an appointed Director of Psychosocial Services. In addition to participating in team meetings pertaining to patients seen in the long-term clinic, the psychosocial team should also have a separate weekly meeting to review and discuss team activities and to provide an opportunity for in-service training. As a group, the psychosocial team is responsible for the psychosocial evaluation of all long-term clinic patients; providing input into the formation of patient care plans; providing direct psychosocial interventions; giving patients and their families referrals to other professionals or organizations in the community; and interactions and collaborations with organizations in the community that provide supportive services and activities for children with cancer and their families. To minimize redundancy of professional activities among members of the psychosocial team and to maximize the team's efficiency and effectiveness, the psychologist and social worker should have designated roles and clinical responsibilities.

To coordinate and integrate the professional training, skills, and roles of the psychologist and social worker, a conceptual framework for guiding the psychosocial assessment, formulating a psychosocial plan, and recommending psychosocial interventions for children with cancer should be adopted. For example, a patient/ family systems, life-span developmental model provides such a framework for integrating information that can yield a comprehensive patient/family systems developmental profile. Guided by this assessment model, the interrelationship of four broad functional/developmental patient-focused domains (physiologic, cognitive/academic, emotional/behavioral, and social), which are evaluated within the context of a patient's family/community system, provide the structure in developing these profiles. Profiles that are developed and periodically updated when a patient is in active treatment provide an important source of information pertaining to the patient's and the family's baseline psychosocial development and functioning that help to identify potential psychosocial problems that may arise in the long-term clinic. Some of the more common, yet sometimes subtle, potential long-term treatment effects and psychosocial problems are neurocognitive/ academic (memory, attention/conceptualization, speed of mental/motor processing, learning disabilities, and so on); biophysiologic (sexuality, growth, amputation, physical appearance, and so on); social (peer acceptance, employment, insurability, and so on); and psychologic (self-competence, identity, uncertainty about the future, frustration in coping with diminished cognitive/academic abilities, and so on). In addition, there are also a host of psychosocial problems that may arise in the long-term clinic specific to the long-term effects of childhood cancer on the family and their intricate interpersonal relation (siblings' perception of emotional isolation owing to parental attention on child with cancer, overprotectiveness of the child with cancer by parent resulting in increased dependency, marital/family conflicts, and so on).

The psychosocial issues among the patients and their families seen in the long-term clinic are quite different from the issues associated with treatment. For example, a childhood cancer survivor and his or her family may need assistance in the restoration of normalcy within the family structure and in coping with changes resulting from the long-term effects of therapy.

The clinical/pediatric psychologist, with doctoral-level training in the scientist-practitioner model, plays an important role in contributing to and directing the comprehensive team's efforts in scientifically, educationally, and clinically addressing the psychosocial issues and problems of patients seen in the long-term clinic. The psychologist should have overall leadership and responsibility for the psychosocial team's activities. The clinical responsibilities of the psychologist are (1) to provide appropriate supervision and guidance for all members of the psychosocial team; (2) to assess the emotional, behavioral, social, and neuropsychologic development and functioning of patients seen in the long-term clinic with identified concerns or specified by a therapeutic protocol; (3) to consult with long-term patients and/or their families with respect to questions or concerns regarding their psychosocial development and functioning; (4) to provide individual, group, or family psychotherapy; (5) to provide consultation to medical personnel and recommend appropriate strategies for the clinical management of psychosocial issues and concerns that emerge in the long-term clinic; and (6) to provide consultation to hospital and community professionals, agencies, or organizations regarding the psychosocial issues of childhood cancer survivors.

The social worker is often the psychosocial team member who has the most direct clinical contact with patients, their families, and medical personnel in the long-term clinic. The social worker should be given the role of coordinating the psychosocial team's clinical activities. The social worker has primary responsibility for obtaining the necessary information for developing the psychosocial profiles for every patient seen in the long-term clinic. Based on this profile, the members of the psychosocial team can collaborate in formulating an appropriate psychosocial plan that may involve direct interventions provided by the social worker or psychologist or a referral to other community professionals, agencies, or support organizations. The social worker may also be needed for assistance in obtaining medical and life insurance. For example, graduation from college will result in the need for an independent (nonparental) insurance policy. Prior knowledge of this may prevent a lapse in coverage. In addition to insurance, patients may face problems with entering the military, receiving services for vocational rehabilitation, and obtaining employment. Knowledge of local resources and programs is essential. Insurance, for example, may not cover the expenses required for activities of daily living after amputation. A survivor in our clinic required special tools for cooking after forequarter amputation. By contacting a local organization that organizes numerous programs for children with cancer, assistance was found. This enabled the patient to achieve independence and to attenuate feelings of inadequacy and helplessness. The social worker is often called upon to write letters to insurance companies, places of employment, and school settings to assist survivors in achieving developmental goals and independent living. Patients may benefit from peer groups supervised by the psychosocial team that assist survivors in understanding the universality of survivorship issues. In addition to general assistance in coping, referral to the team psychologist (or to a psychiatrist) may be necessary, particularly if there is a need for lengthy and intense psychiatric therapy. Suicide ideation or inability to function (as a result of family issues or fear of disease return) may require such involvement.

An understanding of the late concerns of patients and families will enable social workers to help new patients and families understand what the future may hold. In some instances, simple intervention, such as helping families of newly diagnosed children recognize the importance of discipline and maintaining normalcy in the family structure, will prevent severe adjustments in later years.

The Role of the Educational Liaison

Deborah Karl

The role of the educational liaison in the long-term survivor clinic is to offer expertise in identifying and addressing the unique educational concerns of the childhood cancer survivor. Survivors' educational, occupational, and personal achievements assume great significance when an extended or normal life span is anticipated. The diverse developmental and educational issues presented by increasing numbers of childhood cancer survivors can pose multifaceted challenges for affected individuals of all ages, as well as for their families and schools. It is advantageous to include in the long-term survivor clinic team an educational specialist knowledgeable about the educationally related effects of childhood cancer treatment; comprehensive assessment of neurocognitive late effects of treatment; intervention appropriate for addressing specific needs; and means of accessing available support in the school systems and community agencies. Although many pediatric cancer centers offer school reintegration services for patients involved in treatment, few programs exist that address the long-term educational needs of survivors. The educational liaison is a relatively new role that has largely been assumed by health professionals in a position to note and advocate for patients' educational needs. With the inclusion of a professional educator in the systematic follow-up team, specialized assessment, information, referral, and advocacy services can be provided to assist the patient and family in addressing the potential impact of childhood cancer on long-term educational functioning.

Research studies and clinical experience with long-term survivors of childhood cancer demonstrate that there are academic and vocational concerns unique to various subsets of this population.[10,11] In particular, children who have received central nervous system (CNS) treatment often exhibit lifelong problems with learning and performing in school.[9,11,12,15] Other survivors may experience developmental or educational effects because of changes in sensory or perceptual abilities, limb loss, various physical residua, speech or motor impairment, and complications of disease and treatment, as well as issues relating to premorbid status. Although many studies have documented changes in neurocognitive measures of CNS-treated children, there is a paucity of research pertaining to broad, long-term educational and vocational outcomes.[3] There is need for well-designed investigation of a wide range of functional difficulties that may be experienced by this population during secondary and postsecondary study and in the occupational domain, regarding achievement, social adjustment, and independence. Concerns in these areas are often reported during visits to the long-term–survivor clinic. It is important to screen all long-term survivors for the presence of educational problems and to further study the potential impact of childhood cancer on school and work functioning. Hence, educational monitoring through the long-term clinic can be a vital part of the follow-up process.

EDUCATIONAL SURVEILLANCE METHOD

Within the long-term clinic, the educational liaison reviews and assesses factors associated with risk of educational difficulty (see box below). The results of vision and hearing screening are reviewed to determine the need for further evaluation of sensory or perceptual abilities, critical because such deficits can affect learning and school performance. An indepth patient/parent interview is conducted with specific questions regarding particular areas of school functioning, academic achievement, educational support services received, learning strengths and challenges, extracurricular activities, and socialization. Relevant information concerning educational functioning and related psychosocial domains are also acquired through the use of standardized behavior scales, such as the Achenbach Child Behavior Checklist,[1] completed by the parent; by adolescent self-report; and, with proper consent, by the school. Administration of a normed instrument, such as the Wide Range Achieve-

---

Cancer-Treated Children at Greatest Educational Risk Are Those with

- Disease, surgery, chemotherapy, or irradiation of the CNS
- Diagnosis of brain tumor or acute lymphoblastic leukemia
- Sensory deficit or neurologic impairment
- Cancer diagnosed before mastery of basic academic skills
- Prior history of developmental/educational delay
- Persistent, severely compromised stamina
- High rate of school absence
- Family history of school difficulty
- Significant economic deprivation or family dysfunction

CNS, Central nervous system.

ment Test—Revised, provides standardized screening of basic academic skills.[6] When educational screening indicates significant delays or concerns, the patient is referred for further psychoeducational, neuropsychologic or interdisciplinary developmental evaluation, whether as an adjunct service of the cancer center or by referral to other medical center, school, or community resources. The educational liaison must often assist the advocacy efforts of the student and family to ensure access to entitled educational services, detailed further in Chapter 18 (see sections on educational intervention and special educational needs).

The educational liaison also refers individuals who are beyond school-age for appropriate services and community resources. Individuals whose educational or occupational functioning has been significantly impaired by cancer and its treatment are entitled to the same services and civil rights protection as citizens with disabilities.

A newly identified educational disability that may have been acquired due to cancer treatment and has lifelong consequences can reactivate the sense of loss of a normal, healthy childhood. Because a grieving process often accompanies detection of a disability, a fundamental role of the educational liaison is to provide or locate emotional support for individuals and their families.

The role of the educational liaison within the long-term survivor clinic can be best served by a professional who has training in the field of educational psychology, with experience and credentials in special education or school psychology. Experience in interdisciplinary team functioning and effective collaborative-consultation skills are invaluable, along with an essential working knowledge of education law and mediation and advocacy skills.

A major role of the educational liaison is to educate parents and school personnel about the potential educational effects of CNS treatment for childhood cancer (see box below). Ideally, this will have occurred long before enrollment in the late-effects clinic, so that students will have received ongoing, thorough monitoring of educational development from the time of diagnosis.

Educational Effects of CNS Treatment for Childhood Cancer

CNS Treatment-Related Brain Injury Can Adversely Affect:
- Rate and quality of cognitive information-processing
- Regulation of attention and concentration
- Timely initiation of mental activity
- Memory and retrieval of information
- Graphomotor speed and performance
- Abstract, visuospatial abilities
- Planning and organizational skills
- Social development
- Measured IQ
- Stamina

Educational follow-up is an important component of regular long-term care. The educational liaison can facilitate detection of educational problems and related psychosocial issues and provide linkage with resources appropriate for addressing identified concerns. With specialized help, the functional sequelae of childhood cancer treatment can be better addressed and thereby enhance survivors' quality of life.

Computerization

Howard Panken

The medical team caring for long-term survivors of childhood cancer must have easy access to the previous treatment history of the individual as well as the outcomes for similarly treated cohorts. Sufficient concentration of specialized resources in one dedicated clinic allows for the capture and organization of medical data, through the use of a computer. A clinical data base allows easy access to a complex treatment record that may span years. In addition, it is an essential part of the process that allows for the formal scientific identification of late effects in the patient population.

PURPOSES

The development and maintenance of a clinical data base are significant undertakings that advance the goals of the clinic. Collection of medical information gleaned from the patient's clinical record, for entry into a data base, provides the opportunity for clinic medical staff to retrospectively review and evaluate portions of the history. A nurse, physician, or physician's assistant may perform the task of extracting relevant clinical information from the medical record.

The data base can then produce a clinical summary for an individual patient, useful for dissemination of information to current medical staff as well as for future health care providers. This report provides:

- A uniform summary of the patient's original disease
- The course of treatment
- Any side effects, including second malignancies found to date
- Psychosocial status of the patient
- Other significant information relating to an individual patient's care

The uniform format of the standard clinical summary prevents historically significant information from being overlooked even if treatment has occurred at a number of institutions or over a long period of time. In addition, the clinic can use its computerized data base to request current information from primary health care providers and to disseminate screening recommendations.

A properly maintained data base is a significant asset, enabling researchers to study specific patient cohorts. With a clinical data base, statistically valid analyses of the effects of therapy can replace anecdotal approaches to clinical medicine.

CONTENT

Fields that support the patient name, birth date, diagnosis, and date of diagnosis are necessary for the permanent patient record. Because it may be important to contact registered patients periodically for immediate administrative or medical needs, clinic contacts should be frequent enough to maintain a current address. Providing a field to store the referring pediatrician or current physician data will allow efficient distribution of progress notes or other correspondence. The format of our clinical data base mimics a classic history and physical, with a detailed description of the treatment and outcome (see Table 20-1 and Fig. 20-2).

Associations between treatments and late effects require that treatments are carefully described. Cumulative drug dosages must be determined from the medical history. A person familiar with the treatment given should methodically collect and calculate this data. This process may be tedious, but the accuracy of any derivative research will depend on it being correct.

RELATIONAL DATA BASES

Relational data bases are the most powerful commercially available data bases today. In this type of data base, multiple tables organize specified types of related

Table 20-1
The Clinical Summary

Patient information
Presenting symptoms
Past medical history
Family history
Physical examination
Initial workup
   Blood chemistry
   Radiologic testing
   Surgery
   Histology/morphology
   Staging
   Marker studies
   Chromosomes
Treatment
Radiation therapy
Relapse
Complications
Psychosocial
Long-term effects by organ system

information. To keep information from being duplicated, valid data items may be referenced to data items in other tables.

Many separate tables comprise the clinical data base. One such table might be the "Name and Address" table incorporating the patient demographic information (name, address, phone number, referring physician). Other tables could hold Chemotherapies, Radiation Therapy, Presenting Symptoms, and Surgical Procedures. The data manager can add a record of therapy, for example, to the Radiation Therapy table every time a patient receives a course of radiation therapy. The Radiation Therapy row (or record) will include a reference to the patient in the "Name and Address" table. In this manner, all of the information kept by the data base is part of a specific table. The relations of each individual item to information in other tables describe the patient's clinical record.

All data bases offer numeric, fixed-length alphanumeric, date, and logical data types. A programmer will create a data base schema to describe how to store information within the data base. The data base schema for each table will assign a data type to every column name. Quantitative fields are assigned to numeric fields. Alphanumeric fields are used when information is quantifiable or described succinctly, such as diagnosis, stage of disease, drugs, and drug dosages. Fields to be used to search for specific cohorts within the data base require entries that are extremely consistent; computer data bases are unforgiving on textual variations of entries. For example "Male," "MALE," "M," or "MAN," are not recognizable as equivalent terminology. The data base design should offer, as much as possible, suggestions as to valid entries for individual fields to promote consistency. A mechanism to ensure the uniform entry of alphanumeric data will protect the integrity of the data base. Studies will lose patients who do not match retrieval criteria precisely.

Descriptive information that otherwise defies computerization is entered into free-form memo fields. This type of field may be useful for presenting symptoms, past medical history, and physical examination findings.

APPLICATIONS

Applications may report relevant subsets of the clinical data base information in a variety of useful formats. Some of these reports are run frequently. To save time, computer files called scripts, containing frequently run commands, are set up in advance for routine data base applications.

Follow-Up Study and Outcome

The use of a clinical data base will greatly facilitate the clinical studies of the effects and outcome of cancer therapy. The retrieval of clinical information from the data base may yield survival rates, plotted against any number of significant criteria, including sex, stage, and treatment protocol.

The organization of a clinical data base allows the identification of patients as part of a cohort group. This selection process provides an unbiased method of performing demographic studies. The group under study may consist of people

Long-Term Follow-up Clinical Summary

Name: *Johanna Doe*   Sex: *F*   Race: *W*
DOB: *02/18/70*   Unit Num: *1234123*
Diagnosis: *Sarcoma-Ewings*
Date of DX: *02/01/83*
Pediatrician: *Dr. Smith*
Current MD: *Dr. Jones*

Presenting symptoms:

Hx: Minor trauma Oct 82, progressive severe thigh pain, swollen medial thigh

Past medical history: Family history: Cancer in 1st deg. rel: Yes
Cancer in 2nd deg. rel: No
Cervical carcinoma in situ in mother

Physical examination:

Tender, swollen medial thigh

Initial workup:

CBC: WBC 7700   Hg 13.0   HCT 38.0   PLT 229,000   ESR 14
      DIFF
Chem: Creat 0.6   Alk Phos 129   LDH 127   AST 13   Urate 3.3   Ca 10.6
CSF: ND
BM: Norm

Radiologic tests done:

2/1/83-X-ray: Left femoral lesion, CXR: normal
Bone scan CT, Arteriogram: large extra medullary mass

Surgery:

1. Biopsy   2/1/83: Bx of left femoral mass
2. Other   2/10/83: Thoracotomy: removal of metastatic lesion
3. Other   2/10/83: Broviac insertion
4. Biopsy   11/3/84 Necrotic bone tissue

Histology/morphology: Ewings sarcoma

Stage: Metastatic   IV
Metastatic Sites: Pulm
Marker Studies: ND
Chromosomes: Done?   ND

Treatment:

First Protocol: VCR, ADR, CPM, 5-FU, AMD

Fig. 20-2.   Format for a long-term follow-up clinical summary.

Long-Term Follow-up Clinical Summary—cont'd

Cumulative Drug Doses:

BSA: Initial 1.40   End of Tx 1.50

Drug	Dose	Number of Doses
Nitrogen mustard	0 mg/m²	Number of Doses: 0
Actinomycin	12.0 mg/m²	Number of Doses: 6
Daunomycin	0 mg/m²	Number of Doses: 0
Adriamycin	375 mg/m²	Number of Doses: 5
Other anthracycline	0 mg/m²	Number of Doses: 0
CCNU/BCNU	0 mg/m²	Number of Doses: 0
Cyclophosphamide	205 mg/m²	Number of Doses: 43
Vincristine	90 mg	Number of Doses: 52
Cisplatin	0 mg/m²	Number of Doses: 0
Bleomycin	0 IU/m²	Number of Doses: 0
Procarbazine	0 mg/m²	Number of Doses: 0
Ara-C	0 mg/m²	Number of Doses: 0
Ara-C	0 mg IT	Number of Doses: 0
Methotrexate	0 mg/m² IV/IM	Number of Doses: 0
Methotrexate	0 mg IT	Number of Doses: 0

Radiation therapy:

Site	Dose (rads)
1. Left femur	4500
2. Femur boost	5520
3. Lung whole	1500
4. Lung boost	3500

Complications:

Neurologic? N	GI Tract? N	Infectious (not F&N)? Y
Cardiac? N	Hepatic? N	Bone? Y
Pulmonary? N	Renal? N	Muscle? Y
Endocrine? N	Growth? N	2nd Malig? N
Dental? N	EENT? N	Skin? N

Hypoplasia and leg length descrepancy. Fitted with orthosis for leg since diagnosis for stability, scoliosis, intermittent edema of left leg.
7/19/84: Septic shock with pseudomonas.

Psychosocial:

Marital Status: S
Pregnancies: 0   Viable Offspring: 0
Occupation: Student   Employed? Y
Education: Highest Level: College-3   Special Education? N

Date off therapy: 08/19/86

Number of hospitalizations off therapy: 0
Problems off therapy: edema left ankle; hypoplasia left thigh; decreased ROM leg.

Last visit: 07/5/93
Consider leg-shortening procedure.

Fig. 20-2, cont'd.   For legend, see opposite page.

within a selected demographic group, with a specific disease, treated by a given protocol or with specific agents or cumulative doses of a pharmacologic agent under study. Follow-up studies of targeted cohort groups use the clinical data base to capture additional data. Issues under study may be addressed by adding a study sheet to the patient's medical record, including notes on laboratory tests that should be obtained at the next visit. These results are entered into the data base as they are obtained. When the results of a follow-up study are in the data base, the analyses of data are facilitated.

The management of clinical data outcome reporting is a natural consequence of holding a long-term survivor's clinic. When a well-maintained clinical data base exists, clinical research usually does not require significantly increased data management resources.

Callbacks

In addition to their routine visit, individuals within a cohort group may be called into clinic as appropriate for the objectives of a study. This application will use patient-selection criteria to generate a smaller table for a callback list. The administrative staff uses this list to call back selected patients by phone or by letter. It is a small extension of this process to export this list to a word processor for use in a form letter.

Referral Letters

The patient population receiving long-term follow-up care may be highly mobile. When a patient is changing his or her primary health care provider, is being referred to a specialist, or requires that information be provided to an outside agency, the system may print out a standard clinical summary in a highly readable format.

COMPUTING EQUIPMENT

Hospital-Based Mainframes

The power and availability of a hospital-based mainframe makes an excellent environment for a long-term survivor's clinical data base. The addition of the data base described earlier could be a natural extension to a system that already provides computerized medical records and lab tests. A clinic, with access to an information specialist who can set up electronic retrieval of the data previously mentioned, would have an ideal situation.

Clinic-Based Personal Computers

Many clinics do not have easy access to the data kept in a hospital-based mainframe. Medical records are rarely in electronic formats. When medical records are electronically stored, different departments may keep their data in uniquely accessed data systems. These situations can create an electronic "Tower of Babel," where the data are available but not comprehensible to other computer systems. For these situations, a personal computer is often more practical.

The current availability of fast and inexpensive personal computers allows for implementation of a modest clinical data base. An IBM-compatible PC with a 386 or 486 processor or equivalent Macintosh microcomputer would be adequate for most clinics. Personal computers may use a network to improve access to information in multiple locations. In many clinics, access through a single computer is adequate to accumulate information slowly over time. These factors, along with the ultimate size of the data base and the selection of PC data base software, will help determine the type of the machine(s) selected.

DATA BASE SELECTION

The selection of a data base for a mainframe is usually easy, because most mainframes already have a data base available for applications. Application developers are usually familiar with the data base and the development tools. If more than one data base is available on a mainframe, other applications in use should be examined to choose the data base most appropriate for the long-term clinic. Each candidate should be evaluated on ease of use, data integrity, and facility of modifying the system at a later time.

When there is no mainframe with a relational data base available, the Data Manager should select a relational data base after considering a number of significant issues, including the following.

Availability. The system needs to be available to the clinic staff. A single computer running the application needs to be accessible to the entire staff. In situations where a single personal computer is inadequate, further issues are raised. Will the system allow access over a network? Will the system protect the data base from multiple simultaneous updates? How will the system protect the privacy of the data base?

Development tools. The forms, screens, reports, and data base layouts should be customized to the requirements of the clinic. The availability of developmental tools and trained people to use these tools is an important consideration.

Cost. Each computer data base installed requires the purchase of a right-to-use license from the manufacturer. The development of a system that meets the specifications of an individual clinic will require adequate financial resources. The recurring costs of software and hardware maintenance should not be over-looked.

User interface. The data base system should have a consistent, easy-to-use interface. Once a data base expert has set up the system, personnel familiar with the data base should routinely enter information. Although some training in the use of computer-based information is always desirable, extensive training should not be a requirement.

Reports. The system should have the capability to report useful and accurate information when required for clinical use. Form letters, lists of patients identified under a particular study, and clinical progress notes are data base reports. The report system should be operable by personnel with minimal computer skills.

Full-featured relational data bases are available for all computers, mainframe or personal. Some popular relational data bases available include Ingress, Oracle, Sybase, and Informix.

Although the above data bases offer extensive networking support, one or more personal computers can adequately serve a clinic with a simpler configuration. The IBM-compatible PC offers many less-complicated data bases that can help develop a suitable clinical data base application. This widely available software often makes application development a simple process. Although these data bases might be more familiar to the clinic's data management staff, the selection criteria mentioned earlier are still appropriate. Some of the popular packages available for the PC are DBASE IV, Paradox, FoxPro, Access, and R:BASE.

Fourth Generation Languages (4GL)

Fourth Generation Languages are a powerful tool used to describe an application to a computer. This development tool acts as an automatic generator of information systems. The developer will describe the data. The 4GL will generate data base structures, entry screens, and reports. The system is then modified to meet clinical needs.

REFERENCES

1. Achenbach TM: *Manual for the child behavior checklist and revised child behavior profile,* Burlington, VT, 1988, University of Vermont.
2. Goeppinger J, Schuster GF: *Community as client: using the nursing process to promote health.* In Stanhope M, Lancaster J: *Community health nursing: process and practice for promoting health,* ed 3, St Louis, 1992, Mosby–Year Book.
3. Gotay CC: Quality of life among survivors of childhood cancer: a critical review and implications for intervention, *J Psychosoc Oncol* 5:5-23, 1987.
4. Hobbie WL: The role of the pediatric oncology nurse specialist in a follow-up clinic for long-term survivors of childhood cancer, *Assoc Pediatr Oncol Nurses* 3:9, 1986.
5. Hopson B, Adams J: *Towards an understanding of transition: defining some boundaries of transition dynamics.* In Adams J, Hayes J, Hopson B, editors: *Transition: understanding and managing personal change,* Montclair, NJ, 1976.
6. Jastak S, Wilkinson GS: *Manual for the Wide Range Achievement Test Revised Edition,* Wilmington, Del., 1984, Jastak Associates.
7. Kimchi J, Polivka B, Stevenson JS: Triangulation: operational definitions, *Nurs Res* 40:364, 1991.
8. Koocher GP, O'Malley JE: The damocles syndrome: psychosocial consequences of surviving childhood cancer, New York, 1981, McGraw-Hill.
9. Madan-Swain A, Brown R: Cognitive and psychosocial sequelae for children with acute lymphocytic leukemia and their families, *Clin Psychol Rev* 11:267-294, 1991.
10. Mulhern RK et al: Social competence and behavioral adjustment of children who are long-term survivors of cancer, *Pediatr* 83(1):18-25, 1989.
11. Mulhern RK et al: Neuropsychological status of children treated for brain tumors: a critical review and integrative analysis, *Med Pediatr Oncol* 20:181-191, 1992.

12. Packer RJ et al: A prospective study of cognitive function in children receiving whole-brain radiotherapy and chemotherapy: 2-year results, *J Neurosurg* 70:707-713, 1989.
13. Peckham VC: Educational deficits in survivors of childhood cancer, *Pediatrician* 18:25-31, 1991.
14. Peckham VC et al: Educational late effects in long-term survivors of childhood acute lymphocytic leukemia, *Pediatrics* 81:127, 1988.
15. Waber DP et al: Neuropsychological diagnostic profiles of children who received CNS treatment for acute lymphoblastic leukemia: the systemic approach to assessment, *Dev Neuropsychol* 8(10):1-28, 1992.

Index